Reproductive Hormones

Edited by Courtney Marsh

Published in London, United Kingdom

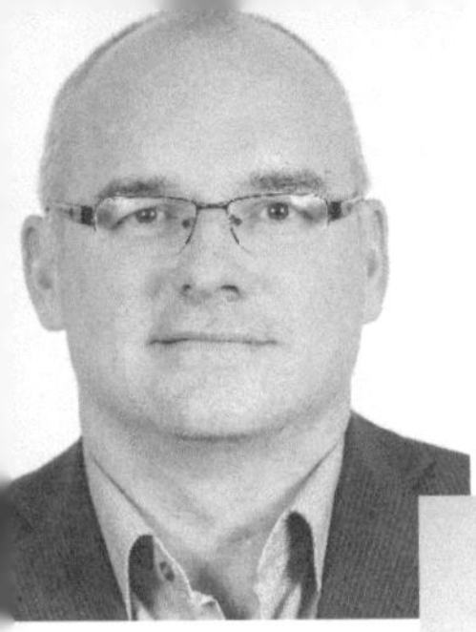
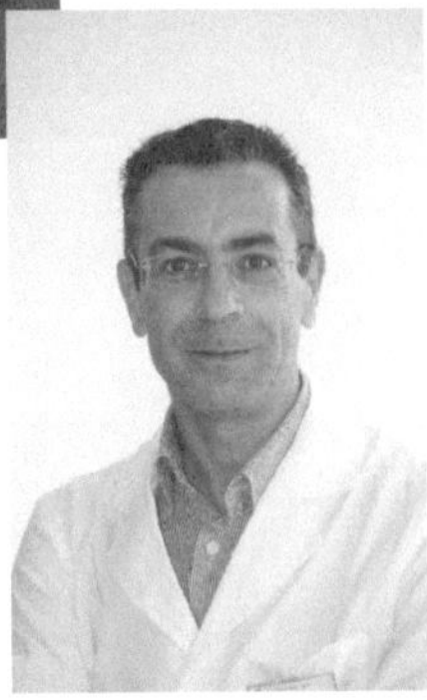
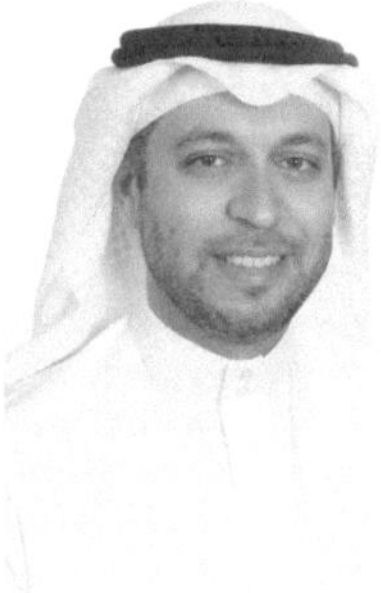
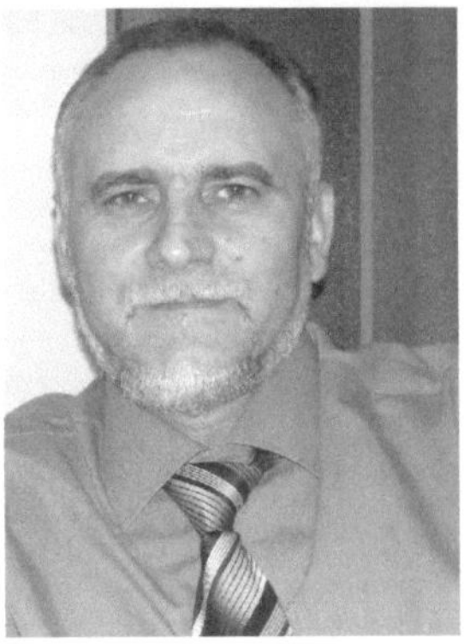
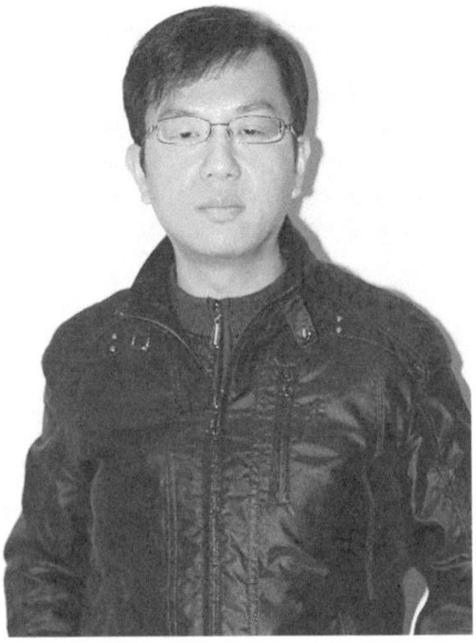
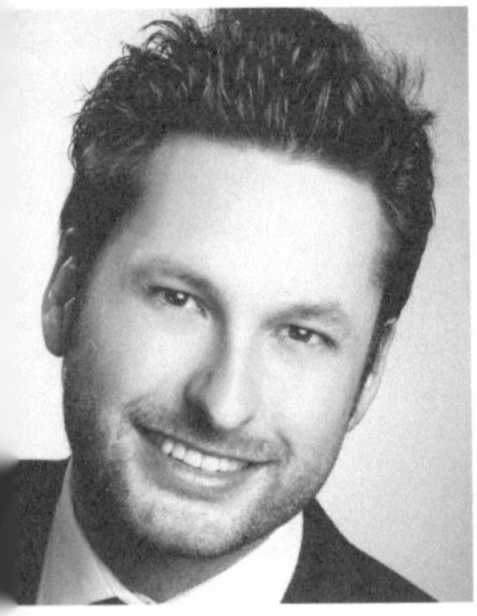
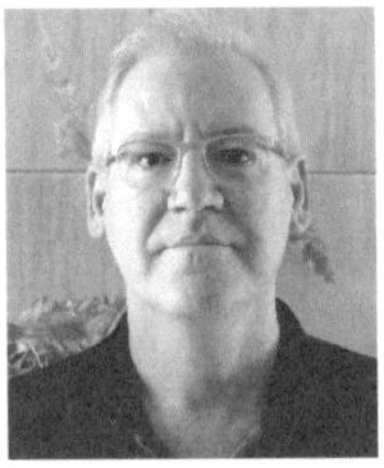

IntechOpen

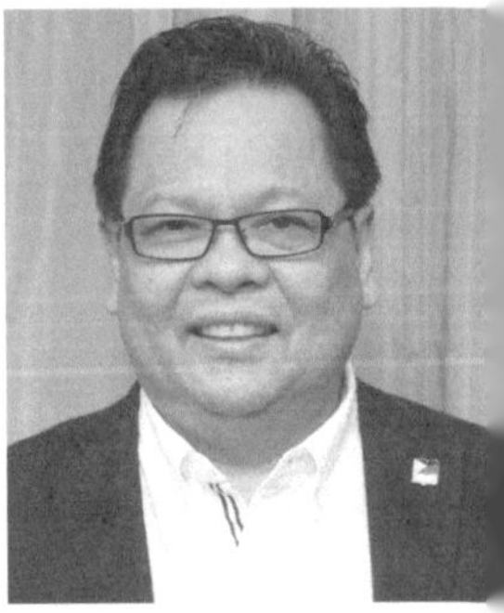
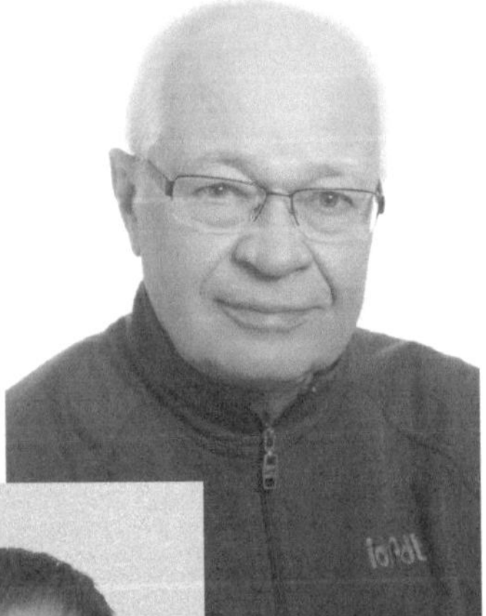
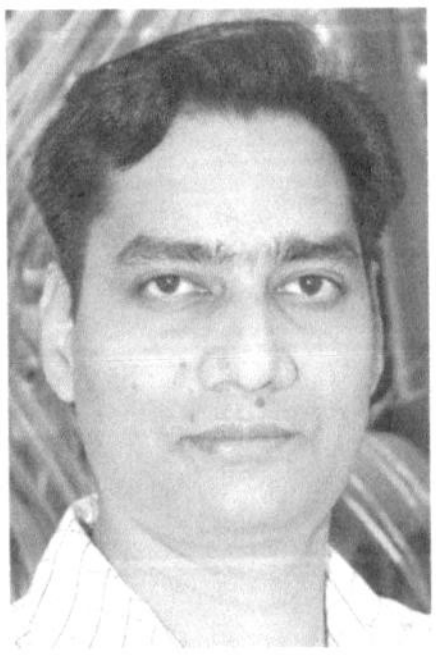
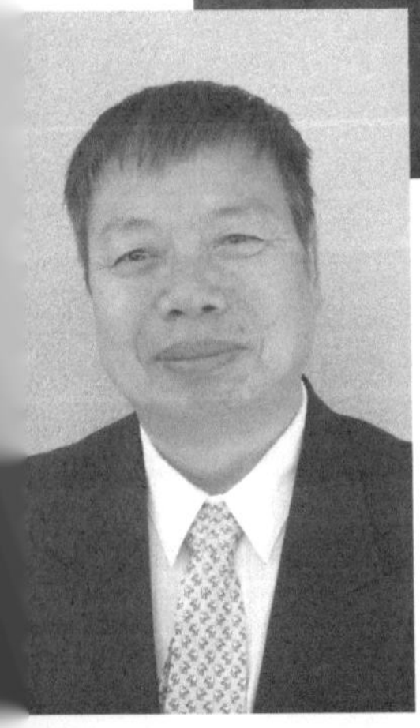
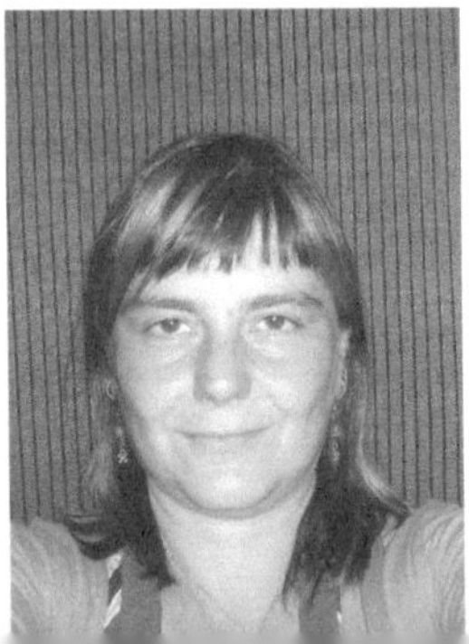
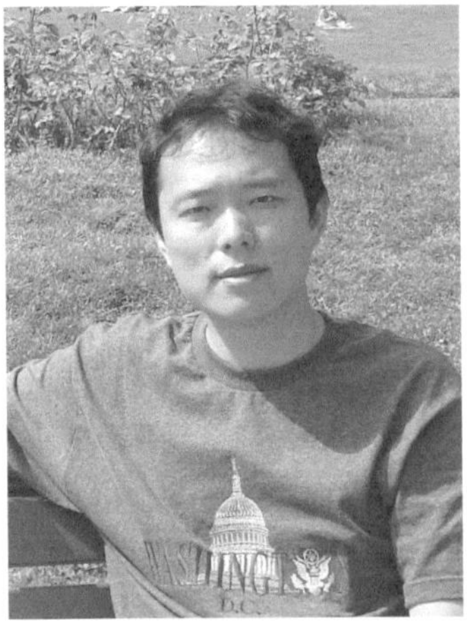

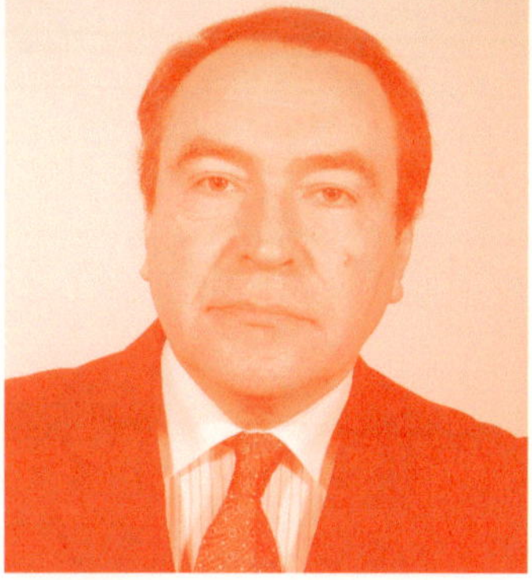

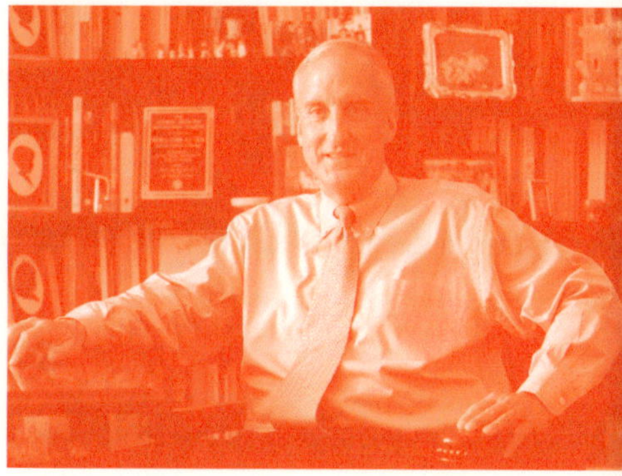

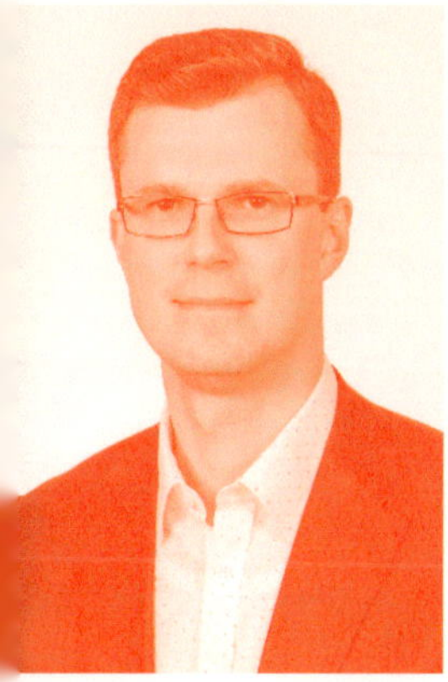

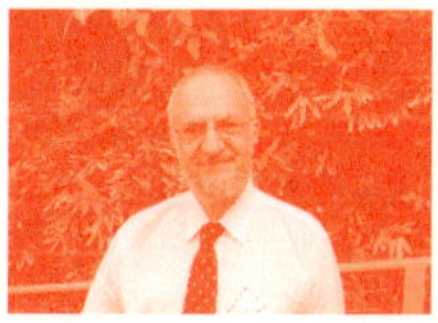

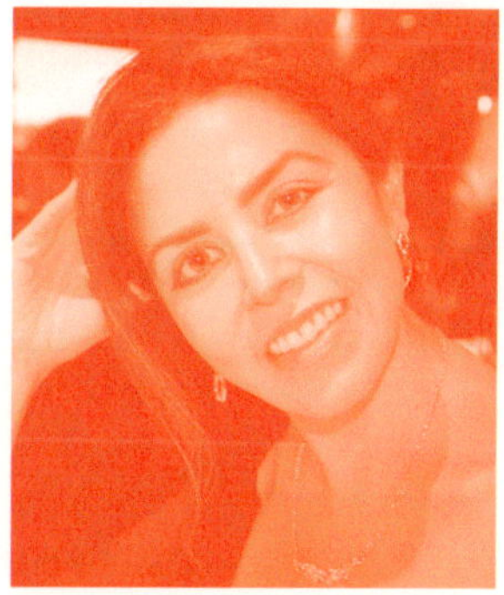

Supporting open minds since 2005

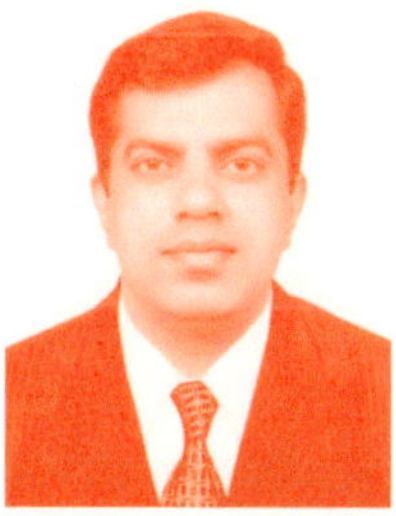

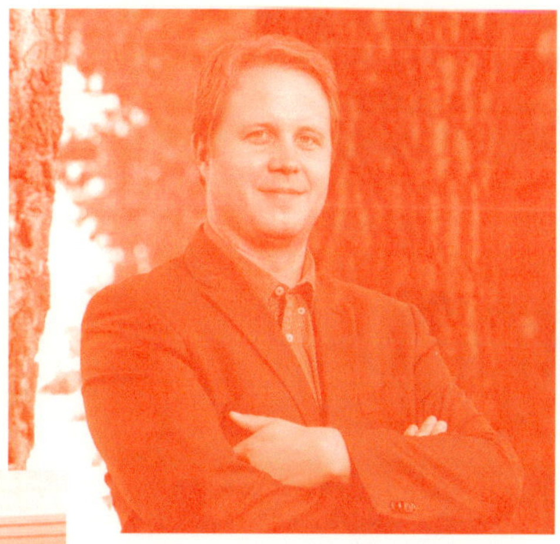

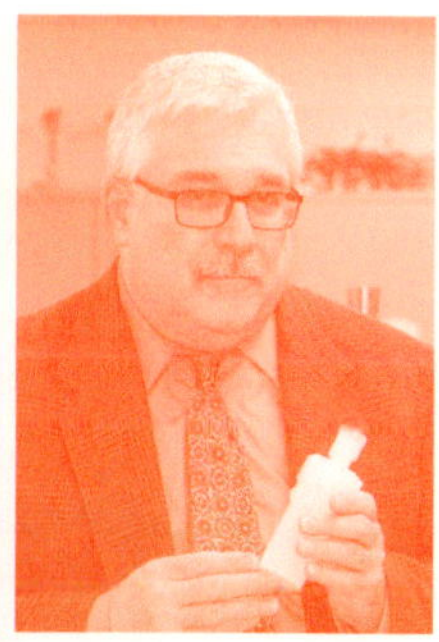

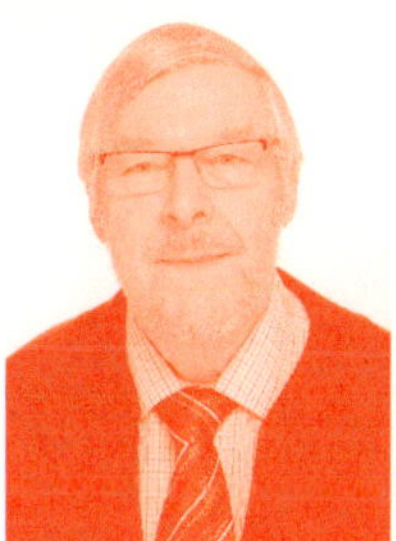

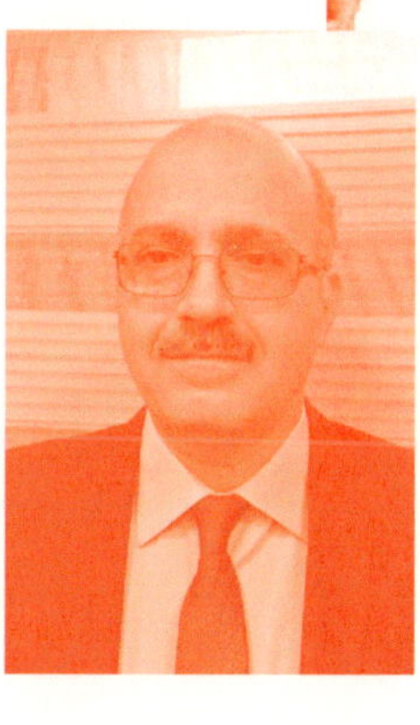

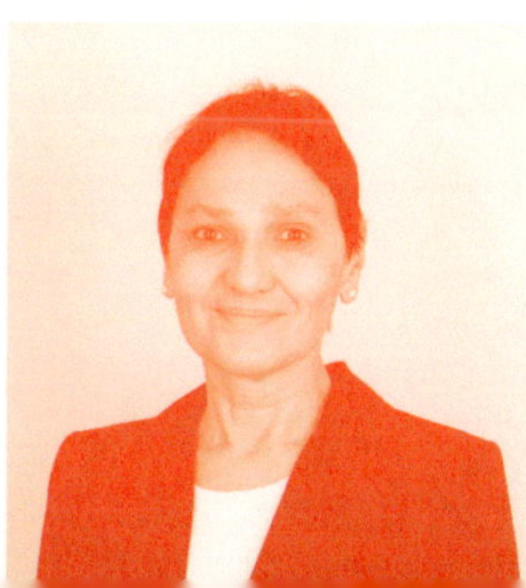

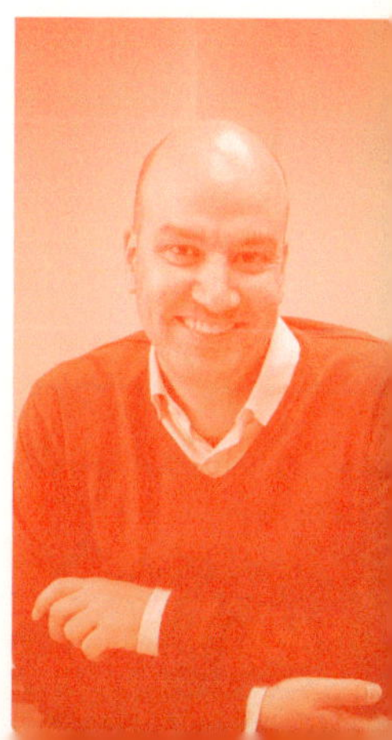

Reproductive Hormones
http://dx.doi.org/10.5772/intechopen.91499
Edited by Courtney Marsh

Contributors
Waleed Al-Khyatt, Syed Yusef Iftikhar, Luz Irene Pascual Mathey, Abdulsamed Kükürt, Mushap Kuru, Ömer Faruk Başer, Mahmut Karapehlivan, Gerrit J. Bouma, Agata M. Parsons, River Evans, Imaobong Etti, Chukwuemeka Nwafor, Grace Essien, Cheryl A. Frye, Jennifer K. Torgerson, Vincent F. Lembo, Kelly Drew, Kizito Omona, Gislaine Almeida-Pereira, Lucila L.K. Elias, José Antunes-Rodrigues, Licy L Yanes Cardozo, Alexandra M. Huffman, Jacob E. Pruett, Damian G. G. Romero, Nassrin Malik Aubead, Sara Luz Morales-Lázaro, Óscar Enciso-Pablo, Karina Angélica Méndez-Reséndiz, Tamara Rosenbaum

First published in London, United Kingdom, 2021 by IntechOpen
IntechOpen is the global imprint of INTECHOPEN LIMITED, registered in England and Wales, registration number: 11086078, 5 Princes Gate Court, London, SW7 2QJ, United Kingdom
Printed in Croatia

British Library Cataloguing-in-Publication Data
A catalogue record for this book is available from the British Library

Additional hard and PDF copies can be obtained from orders@intechopen.com

Reproductive Hormones
Edited by Courtney Marsh
p. cm.
Print ISBN 978-1-83962-229-8
Online ISBN 978-1-83962-230-4
eBook (PDF) ISBN 978-1-83962-287-8

Meet the editor

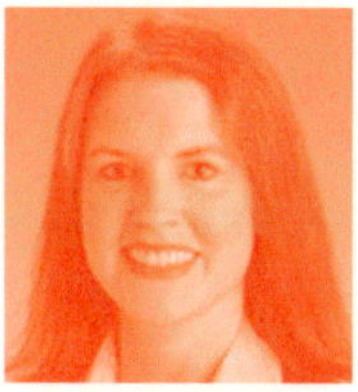

After graduating from the University of Kansas School of Medicine (KUMC), Dr. Marsh went on to complete her obstetrics and gynecology residency at Emory University, Atlanta, Georgia. For fellowship, Dr. Marsh trained in reproductive endocrinology and infertility at the University of Michigan. As a fellow, she researched hypothalamic feedback of estrogen as related to the pubertal onset and menstrual cyclicity. She also completed research using neuroimaging techniques to better understand polycystic ovary syndrome (PCOS). She has several publications in the scientific literature and is also a member of many medical associations. Dr. Marsh specializes in treating women with infertility and PCOS. She is proud to provide both medical and surgical options in treating infertility including assisted reproductive technology.

Contents

Preface

Reproductive hormones are important derivatives of the cholesterol pathway with widespread implications for the human body. The production of sex steroid hormones is an integral product of the hypothalamic-pituitary-gonadal axis with gonadotropin-releasing hormone (GnRH) released in a pulsatile fashion from the hypothalamus. At the pituitary gland, GnRH stimulates the release of follicle-stimulating hormone (FSH) and luteinizing hormone (LH). FSH and LH bind to receptors in target tissues to increase expression of the steroidogenic acute regulatory protein (StAR) to transfer cholesterol to the inner mitochondrial membrane; a rate-determining step in sex steroid production. In this book, we explore the interactions of estrogens, androgens, and progestins on their receptors and the downstream effects on multiple organ systems.

Courtney A. Marsh MD, MPH
Associate Professor,
University of Kansas School of Medicine,
Kansas City, KS, USA

Section 1

Sex Steroid Hormones

Chapter 1

Role of Sex Hormones in Human Body

Nassrin Malik Aubead

Abstract

Gonadal Steroids hormones play an important role in the reproductive and non-reproductive systems. Estrogen has important rule in cardiovascular system as it has vasodilator effect and reduces or prevents platelet activation. In addition, it improves the profile of circulating lipoproteins. All of which may explain why women at premenopausal age are less likely to have heart disease than menopause women or men. E2 play a grate effect on the skeletal system as it is one of the strongest regulators of osteoblast and osteoclast function, and it is responsible for the reduction of adipose tissue and regulation of the body weight, and also has dermatological effect,hence it stimulates the proliferation of keratinocytes and prevents their apoptosis, in addition to the progesterone which increases collagen synthesis. Estrogen is necessary for the functioning and integrity of the tissues of the urinary system specially of the lower urinary tract. Sex steroid are crucial for nervous system, as progesterone is important for production of neurosteroid, and estrogen is currently used in Parkinson's and Alzheimer's disease because of its effects on mental health. The androgens also have a crucial biological effects on neural, muscle, bone, adipose tissue,prostate, cardiovascular, haemopoietic, and the reproductive systems. The gonadal steroid hormones play an important role in immune system and regulating the immune response against different viral or bacterial infections.

Keywords: sex hormones, cardiovascular, brain, bone, urinary tract, immunity

1. Introduction

Gonadal Steroid hormones (GSH) play an important role in reproductive and non-reproductive systems. As this effect occurs early in the fetus' life, gonads are initially present at the fifth weeks and developed on the medial surface of mesonephric ridges.

Therefore, sexual development and discrimination are depending on the type of hormones and gonads that present. GSH play an important role in determining sexual function and behavior. Structures of the central nervous system, such as the hypothalamus, midbrain, amygdala, cortex and anterior pituitary gland, contain androgens and estrogen receptors. The GSH must bind to specific receptors to produce cellular response. While binding of receptor antagonists generally lead to inactivation of these receptors [1].

This chapter explain the effect of sex hormones on the human body and the differences in their action in both genders.

2. Physiological effects of sex hormones

Sex hormones are chemical structures derived from cholesterol, and they are a group of steroidal hormones act as chemical messengers in the body. The activity of steroid hormones is carried out by receptors on extracellular proteins belonging to the family of nuclear substances. Through genomic and non-genomic action, these receptors intervene transduction of signals in a manner of specific context [2].

2.1 Estrogen receptor

2.1.1 Genomic activity

Estrogen binds to SHBG in the blood and in the interstitial fluid, where it penetrates the cell membrane and enters the cell nucleus and binds to receptors. These 2 genes are encoded for 2 estrogen isoforms α and β.

The hormone- receptors structures forms dimer (usually ERα-ERα, ERβ- ERβ or ERα- ERβ) that bind to a specific nucleotide sequence, namely, Estrogen-response elements (EREs) in regions that control different genes regulation of transcription [3] (see **Figure 1**).

Estrogen acts through several nuclear receptors. Estrogen affects the endometrium, the vagina and the breast [4]. And it interact with Calcitonin, parathyroid hormone, vitamin D and interleukin. Estrogen stimulates the division and growth of the skin cells, connective tissue and mucosal membrane [5].

2.1.2 Non genomic activities

The rapid effects of estrogen, such as the removal of Ca^{2+} granular cells and uterine blood-flow are mediated by non-genomic actions [3].

Non-genomic activity occur without bind to cellular receptors of estrogen. The beneficial effects of estrogen on blood vessels are an important non-genomic effect [5]. It affects not only blood vessels in the reproductive system, but also the cerebral, coronary and carotid arteries.

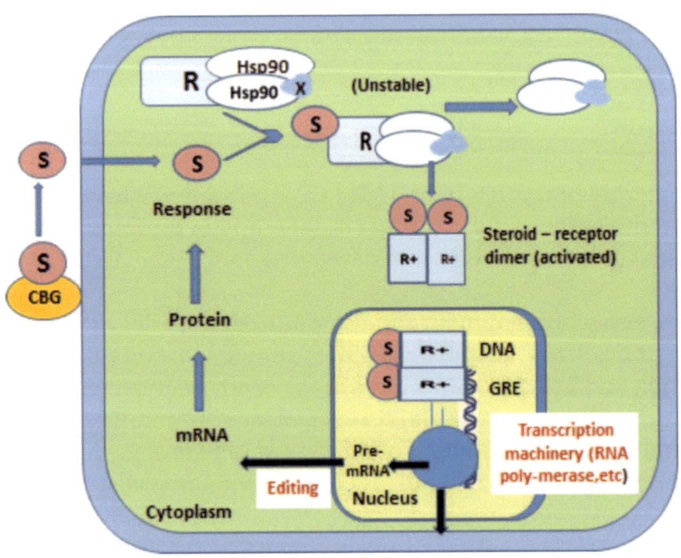

Figure 1.
Genomic action of steroid hormones (estrogen) in the cell.

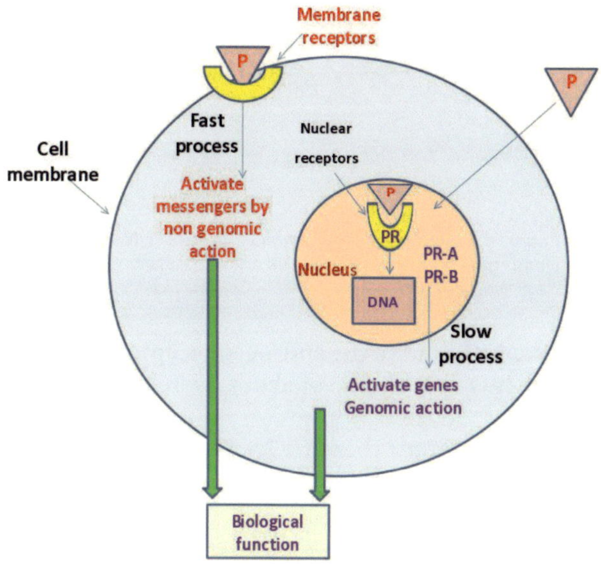

Figure 2.
Mode of progesterone action by genomic and non- genomic action.

Production of nitrous oxide, mediates vasodilation and endothelial protection. Estrogen also stimulates the production of prostacyclin vasodilating, prevents vasoconstriction and prevents platelet aggregation. Also Acetylcholine dilates blood vessels only in the presence of estrogen [6].

2.2 Progesterone receptors

Like estrogen, progesterone act through nuclear receptors, progesterone action is by 2 isoform of progesterone receptors (PR-A and PR-B). These 2 isoforms differ in fact that PR-B has an extra (164) amino acid at N-terminal region termed the B-upstream segment,and this is absent in PR-A.And any mutations of amino acids in B-upstream segment lead to loss of PRB specific gene regulation activity. Normally in human tissues, PR-A and PR-B are as a rule present at same levels but impairment of this ratio regulation lead to tissue abnormalities like that occur in breast cancers [7].

Like estrogen progesterone receptors has genomic and non -genomic activities as shown in **Figure 2**.

2.3 Androgen receptors

Androgen is one of steroid hormone nuclear receptor family. The location of androgen receptors is on the X chromosome. And these receptors composed of 3 functional domains: the ligand binding domain, the DNA binding domain, and N-terminal transcriptional regulation domain (**Figure 3**).

The DBD is the most highly protected part among the various types of the steroid hormone receptors in the nucleus,while the N-terminal domain in androgen receptor is the mostly changeable. And due to the highly protected quality of DNA binding domain among steroid hormone receptors (nuclear receptors), and having selective androgen response elements, this will result in particular activation of the androgen receptors.

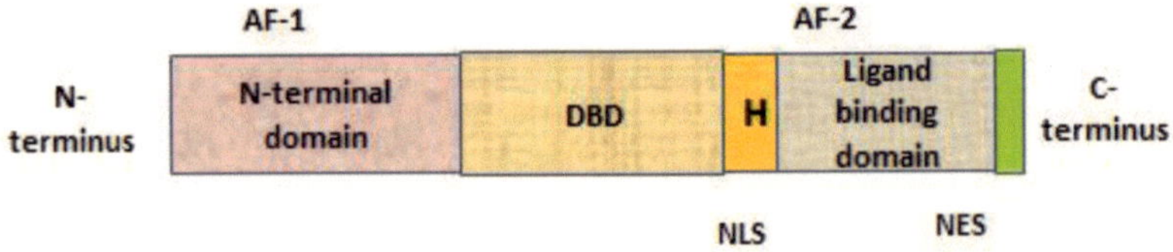

Figure 3.
Functional domains of the androgen receptor (AR): N-terminal domain, DNA binding domain (DBD), ligand binding domain. AF-1 – Transcriptional activating function 1. AF-2 – Transcriptional activating function 2. H – Hinge region. NLS –nuclear localization signal. NES – Nuclear export signal.

The dihydrotestosterone bind to the androgen receptors with a twofold and more affinity with less dissociation of about fivefold in comparison with testosterone.

Like estrogen and progesterone there are 2 ways of ligand-dependent androgen receptors action, DNA dependent (genomic) and DNA independent (non-genomic) binding (**Figure 4**).

The androgens have a crucial biological effects on, muscle, bone, adipose tissue,prostate, neural, cardiovascular, haemopoietic,immune, and the reproductive systems [8].

The biological effects of the AR mutation lead to insensitivity of receptors to androgens in men, resulting feminization of external genitalia of the male (XY female) [9].

Studies in animals with AR deficiency have shown that androgenic signaling is associated with a greater number of women with premature ovarian senility, associated with follicular atresia. Subsequent analysis of AR-free mice showed defects in lutenization of the ovarian follicle [10–12].

As a result of the development of the reproductive system, androgens (especially testosterone and 5α-dehydrotestosterone), induces and maintain secondary sexual characteristics, stimulate male reproductive activity and assist in the production of the sperms. The prostate epithelium is also sensitive for androgen, and androgen signaling is necessary to maintain cell homeostasis in the adult prostate. As the apoptosis in epithelial cells affects the prostate, can be altered by the supplementation of androgens [13].

A predictive model of AR in the prostate showed that strategic paracrine signals control the proliferation of epithelial cells [14].

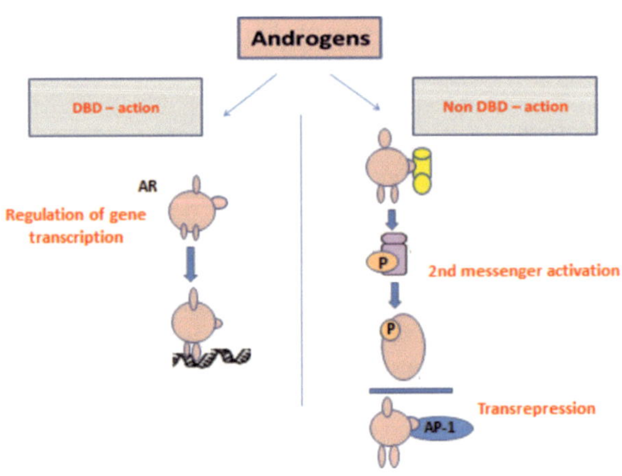

Figure 4.
Mechanisms of ligand-dependent androgen receptor (AR) action.

The effect of AR on the prostate pro-survival, plays a vital role in the pathogenesis of the prostatic cancers. It has been shown 75 years ago that prostate cancer regeneration occurs due to androgen deprivation after castration [15].

In many ways, this is due to the transport of androgens to the prostate, which are involved in metabolism, in the formation of the cell cycle and in the control of growth factors signaling [16].

In addition, the epithelial AR signal is correlated with an 'infection' in the prostate, which is independent of the parasitic AR signal in the stroma. AR increases VEGF-related angiogenesis and increases prostate growth, therefore, AR is an important treatment for prostate cancer. AR signaling has been shown to cause cancers in other organs, including breast, bladder, pancreas, ovary and endometrium [17, 18].

3. The biological effects of sex steroids

Although estradiol and progesterone levels vary during menstruation, estrogen and progesterone levels are always higher in women than in men [1] (**Table 1**).

Estradiol and progesterone have many effects depend on its relation to the venereal system. All steroid hormones have a great effect on the ovaries, fallopian tubes, uterus, external genitalia, hypothalamus and pituitary gland. Estrogen, progesterone and androgen, have significant effects on non-reproductive tissues [1].

3.1 Cardiovascular system

A significant lower risk of CVD has shown in premenopausal women than men and postmenopausal women. Estrogen support the vasodilation effect through relaxation of smooth muscle via increases the production of nitric oxide, which helps maintain low platelet activity, and the angiogenesis is stimulated by estrogen production.

Variation in the epidemiology, incidence and sequel of cardiovascular diseases in both sexes indicate changes in susceptibility to hereditary cardiovascular diseases that can result from several factors. In other cases, gender differences are important in expression of genes (especially X-chromosome genes), incidence of heart disease,as explained previously at the same age, cardiovascular disease is more common in men than in women [19].

Gonadal steroids	Normal range, conventional units
Estradiol	Women, basal 20–60 pg./mL Women, ovulatory surge >200 pg./mL Men <50 pg./mL
Progesterone	Women, luteal phase 2–20 ng/mL Women, follicular phase <2 ng/mL Men <2 ng/mL
Dihydrotestosterone	Women 0.05–0.3 ng/mL Men 0.25–0.75 ng/mL
Testosterone	Women <1 ng/mL Men 3–10 ng/mL

Table 1.
Normal ranges of sex steroid in male and female.

Therefore, it has been suggested that variation in sex steroid hormones have the key role on cardiovascular pathophysiology. Androgens and estrogens are mainly male and female sex hormones respectively, they are found in different levels and with different biological effects in the body in men and women.

Unlike androgens, which are dangerous due to the risk of heart disease and atherosclerosis, estrogens have a protective effect. In fact, a decrease in plasma Estrogen and elevated androgen is associated with an increase in cardiovascular disease in men and women during their menopause time (average age of menopause is between 51 and 52 years). This indicates an enhancing risk of getting cardiovascular disease in postmenopausal women and also in women who have developing hyperandrogenism [20, 21].

3.1.1 Characteristics of the action of sex hormones on the cardiovascular system, development of atherosclerosis and coagulation

Due to their metabolic and vasoactive properties, sex hormones directly or indirectly affect cardiac function through genomic and non-genomic mechanisms [22–24].

This effect is mainly depend on the receptors, such as estrogen/testosterone are found in different cardiac cells in humans and animals.

The contractions of the vascular walls was same in male rats (in normal and castrated), but it more evident in female with removed ovaries, indicating specific differences in vascular tone with estrogen in both sexes [25, 26].

3.1.1.1 Oestrogenic effects

Estrogen affects vascular function through genomic and non-genomic mechanisms [27–29].

In fact, administration of estrogen in vivo leads to vascular dilatation that occurs 5 to 20 minutes after ingestion and is not associated with any change in gene expression. The responses shown to be sex-related. In this regard, intracoronary, administration of estradiol increases coronary blood flow in women, but has not been demonstrated in male with coronary diseases [30].

Acute vasodilation effect of estrogen is endorsed by endothelial related and unrelated mechanism. The properties related to estrogen retention and transport of secondary ions (antagonist action of this hormone on ca^{2+}), while the endothelial related mechanism are highly dependent on the types of endothelial cells associated with the active estrogen receptor (EPs) by the activity of endothelial nitric oxide.

In addition, effect of 17β-estradiol on endothelial, NO synthesis and releases has been suggested to be happen through ER alpha activation [31, 32], while ER-β shows stronger role in the non-genomic effects of estrogen include changes in blood vessels. The expression of extracellular genes and proteins is initiated by two different nuclear ER (α and β) [27–29].

Both ERα and ER β have significant physiological effects on blood vessels. Animal studies have shown that ERα protects against vascular damage and atherosclerosis [33, 34].

ER- also controlled genes are involved in the regulation of blood volume and blood pressure [35, 36].

Since the expression of sex hormone receptors may vary with sex, and type of gonad, so the sex-related changes in vascular response may be related to specific receptor density in vascular tissue, why do women have more ER than in men [37] in addition, although this activity is low in postmenopausal women, ER intensity decreases dramatically in women with cardiovascular and cerebrovascular disease.

These data may indicate a decrease in the protective effect of estrogen in women who have deprive from it for a long time. In fact, estrogen's effects on endothelial function depend on duration from starting menopause rather than chronological age of the menopause [38, 39].

In general, estrogen dilates the systemic arteries [24, 27], improves the coronary artery and peripheral endothelial function, prevents coronary artery spasm and reduces endothelial secretion in women with coronary heart disease [27, 28, 40–42].

Estrogen also affects blood vessels in men. Previous studies have shown that defective mutations in estrogen synthesis or receptor expression are associated with vascular endothelial dysfunction and atherosclerosis [43, 44].

Male estrogen levels are depend on androgen production. Almost 80% of plasma 17-estradiol in men formed from testosterone aromatization and androstendione into estrogen. In addition, estradiol is produced directly in male blood vessels, where it stimulates ERs of endothelial smooth muscle cells. It has been noted that aromatase deficiency and endothelial dysfunction in men with atherosclerosis, low dose of estrogen improves endothelial function [45, 46].

Furthermore, endothelial dysfunction occurs in normal men who receive aromatase inhibitors [23, 47, 48].

Sex hormones can affect the level of vasomotor tones, altering different responses to vascular factors, such as norepinephrine, angiotensin II (AII) or aldosterone. In fact, norepinephrine less likely to cause constriction of blood vessels in women, than men.

Endogenous estrogen helps in control of blood pressure in premenopausal women due to its vasodilation effect. High blood pressure in women occurs after about ten years and is higher in older women than in men at the same age [49–51].

Human and animal studies have shown that atherosclerosis affected by gender. Many animal models with atherosclerosis cause early and more severe symptoms, regardless of male or female fat and hypertension.

Estrogen and androgen motivate metabolic, hemodynamic and humeral effect which affect in turn the CV profile. In addition, these hormones can directly affect the development of atheromas through various blood stimuli. In women, the loss of estrogen (menopause or after surgery) is associated with hardening of the arteries. When estrogen/hormone therapy is started immediately after menopause, the severity of atherosclerosis decreases [52, 53].

HRT starts in younger women (50–59 years) lead to a low rate of cardiovascular event and lower mortality within 10 years after menopause [54, 55].

For this reason, there is sometimes a balance between the positive and negative effects of exogenous estrogen on blood vessels. The use of hormone replacement therapy prevents hardening of the arteries. Before the appearance of atherosclerosis, only when hormones are started before the advancing atherosclerosis over time after menopause. The current concept is that there is a 'window of opportunity' in the peri-menopausal or early postmenopausal years through which the taking of hormonal replacement therapy might reduce the diseases and fatality from cardiovascular diseases by preventing the formation of atheroma [20, 24, 56, 57].

The significant effects of estrogen can only be achieved with oral medicines that are caused by first liver passages of hormones, that stimulate enzyme activity in the organs. In some patients, antithrombin III decreases, factor VII and X are dose dependent increase [58].

3.1.1.2 Mediated Effects of testosterone

The function of the endothelium derived NO in testosterone induced vasodilation is unclear in many studies. Inhibitors of NO synthesis and endothelium-denuded tissue are used in some studies and have suggested a partial contribution, while other studies did not link the role of NO to vasodilation induced by testosterone [59, 60, 61]. Testosterone-induced, an endothelium independent relaxation,not related to gender, and not mediated by hormonal receptor but appear to include the opening of K + channels and L-type calcium channel block [62, 63].

There is a difference in the amount of estrogen in the expression of androgen receptors in the blood stream, which indicates the density of different types of receptors in men, proposing sex linked response to androgen [23, 24, 59, 64].

Although the effects of testosterone in men are not fully understood, the effects of androgens in women are less clear, but appear to be related to estrogen levels. In woman changing her sex rule to male (transsexual) who receive long-lasting testosterone, same plasma concentration is obtained. The diameter of brachial arteries is larger with impaired nitrate induced vasodilation, Nonetheless, the shape and pattern are similar to that in female at the same age. In postmenopausal women treated with estrogen, blood testosterone is about five times increase in concentration than normal levels with improved vasodilation [65, 66]. Testosterone has an estrogen-like effect in women [67] and, in place of estrogen levels, the estradiol/testosterone ratio plays an important role in the androgenic effects of women with atherosclerosis.

Negative correlations have been found between levels of free testosterone and coronary heart disease in men undergoing coronary angiography [68, 69]. In addition, low androgen levels have been reported in men who have larger intima media thickness.

Potential androgenic effects in women are assessed based on observations from women with serious medical conditions, such as PCOS. Women with PCOS suffer from heart disease and atherosclerosis due to high testosterone levels, and elevated risk of having myocardial infarction (MI), a risk factor was used on (33) females have PCOS, and (132) with same age normal females. The risk factor sample was determined from independent risk factors for MI in a prospective population study of (1462) females done in Göteborg, Sweden, the factors were age, diagnosed hypertension, and diabetes mellitus, increased waist/hip circumference ratio (central obesity), serum level of triglyceride. A frequently elevated risk (relative risk of 7.4) of having MI was seen for females with poly cystic ovary syndrome in compression to the normal females with same age [70].

3.2 Lipid metabolism and sex hormones

Sex hormones can directly or indirectly affecting the lipid profile, lipoprotein, HDL, LDL, and triglycerides, the last two are important in development of CVD. This is mainly due to the impaired production of estrogen [71, 72]. Estrogen stimulates lower triglyceride levels, synthesis of HDL and apoliporotein A-I in the liver. It also improve reversion of transport of cholesterol. As a result, these hormones reduce total cholesterol levels and LDLc levels too, levels of triglycerides and it increases the levels of HDL. Testosterone can affect fat metabolism due to its specific androgenic effects and the role as aromatization substrate to Estradiol (E2).

Elevated plasma testosterone levels are believed to influence the profile of lipoproteins, and cardiovascular disease is more common in both sexes. Male data show that plasma testosterone levels correlate positively with HDL-c serum levels and negatively related to triglycerides, LDL, total cholesterol, fibrinogen and PAI-1 [59, 73–75].

Several studies show that the overall effect on fat metabolism is part of the unexplained effects on excess weight and insulin resistance but clinical studies have shown that testosterone treatment do not affect HDL cholesterol in older men. The positive effects of these properties have the necessary effect [76]. The effect of testosterone therapy on female lipid profile (mainly by lowering HDL cholesterol) depends on the level of estrogen and therefore estradiol/testosterone ratio. However, HDL-c deficiency is androgenic. The reduction in HDL-c should not be assumed as a direct pro-atherogenic risk factor because it can exhibit a reduction in sub fraction of HDL3 and therefore is not associated with a significant reduction in cholesterol transport [77].

3.3 Obesity

Gender differences in body fat distribution are related to sex hormones. Although androgens have been linked to the formation of abdominal fat,. Android's fat distribution is associated with androgen deficiency [78]. The distribution and amount of female fat is related to ovarian function. During menstruation, women gain weight, fat is distributed is gynoid, with peripheral obesity, while in menopause is in the middle (abdomen) [79–81].

In both genders, high abdominal circumference or waist/hip ratio are markers of android's fat distribution which are associated independently with insulin resistance, serum triglycerides, low-density lipoprotein cholesterol, hypertension and increase in sympathetic drive, in addition to participating in the negative metabolic changes mentioned above, also affect hormonal metabolism due to the lack of sex hormones [82, 83].

Male testosterone supplements are designed to reduce belly fat, stimulate lipolysis and thus reduce fat accumulation. Testosterone also has beneficial effects on metabolic parameters, such as glucose and lipid metabolism, therefore, hormone replacement therapy causes weight gain in women and prevents the spread of menopausal pattern body fat. The exact mechanism of this effect is not generally known [84–87].

3.4 The effect of sex hormones on bone regeneration and resorption

Deficiency of the hormone estrogen (E2) causes osteoporosis in postmenopausal women and helps to promote osteoporosis in older men. As E2 deficiency result in enhancement in the number of osteoclast cells (OC), and at the same time there is reduction in apoptosis of these cells and also increases their activity [88–90]. Sincethe formation of osteoblasts, including functional estrogen receptors (see **Figure** 5).

In 1988, the understanding of the molecular basis for estrogen activity has been rapid, but fragmented and incomplete. The importance of metabolism is centered on the specific role of cytokines: IL-1, IL6, TNF-A, granulocytes, macrophage stimulating factor (M-CSF) and prostaglandin E2 (PGE2) these substances Increase in OC volume and their activity in bone marrow [91].

An elegant study by Cenci et al [92], reported that production of TNF-α by T-cells increase bone resorption in overiectomized (OVX) mice.

The authors raised the hypothesis that in overiectomized animals bone loss can be inhibited by giving either E2, TNF-a binding protein, or by inhibiting the antibodies that is specific to the TNFa.

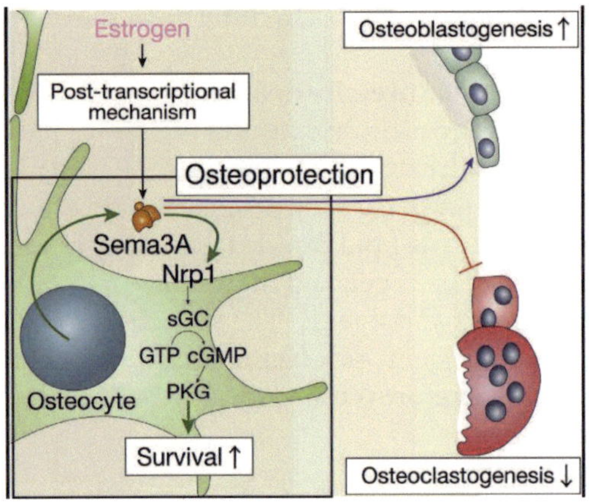

Figure 5.
Biological effect of estrogen on the bone.

T cell deficient OVX mice increase TNF-a production in T cells, which can increase the number of T cells instead of TNF. In this case, the tumor necrosis factor-α is not controlled by bone marrow monocytes. It increases the production of RANKL depending OC, augmenting M-CSF. TNF-a has a direct effect on OC precursors.

Estradiol B (E2) alters the bone protective effects of men and women, reducing the estrogen signal, especially in bone cells. ER A is needed to convert bone cells into bone marrow. However, the formation of osteocytes that require estrogen is difficult [93].

3.5 Sex hormones role in skin

Estrogen and progesterone, makes the skin healthy and soft and maintains the natural thickness of dermis and epidermis. Estrogen motivate, multiplies and prevent apoptotic keratinocytes. When estrogen increase collagen synthesis in the skin, progesterone inhibits matrix metalloproteases and together with estrogen decrease breaking down of collagen. Estrogen increases the production and accumulation of glycosaminoglucan in the dermis. Estrogen also promotes healing of wounds.

Several studies have shown that estrogen has an important protective function and is beneficial for skin physiology [94–96].

They have been shown to accelerate the healing of skin lesions [97]. Most women recover from inflammatory skin conditions, such as psoriasis, during pregnancy, also estrogen, shows some protective effect to photo aging of skin [98–105].

3.6 Effect of sex hormones on the uro-genital tract

The urogenital tract of females developed initially from the primitive urogenital sinuses at the 4th week of intrauterine life. The estrogen receptor is located in both systems, and their levels fluctuating in the circulation.

During the menstruation, the symptoms are vary, and mainly developed in pregnancy or after menopause, when there is genital atrophy, lower urinary tract and vaginal symptoms are frequently reported. Nonetheless, aging may affect these changes. Which result in difficulty to prove the causation [106].

3.6.1 Pathophysiology

Estrogen receptors are steadily presented in the squamous epithelia of vagina and urethra in addition to the bladder-trigone in areas with metaplasia [107, 108].

However, they are not found in the epithelium of the transitional dome of the bladder, which clearly reflects the germinating roots of this tissue. The pelvic floor is also under effect of estrogens [109, 110]. In woman lower urinary tract, Estrogen raise the activity of cell cycle [111], and there is increment in the number of superficial and intermediate cells, the changes are similar to vaginal changes in postmenopausal women [112–114].

During menstruating, changes in cytology of urinary tract are almost identical with that in vaginal cytology [115]. Changes also occur in sediment after estrogen therapy [116]. Frequent changes in urinary symptoms during menstruation can be detected by the urethral pressure profilometry (UPP) [117].

The functional, anatomical, and physiological length of the urethra increases with mid menstruation and earlier luteal phase, indicating changes in serum concentration of estrogen. Changes also occur during pregnancy [118, 119], which sanctifies a relative increase in urinary out-put and gravid uterus pressure.

A recent article by the University of London School of Medicine suggested possibility of influencing hormones on bladder that mediated by progesterone [120]. Progesterone receptors are expressed in the lower urinary tract and may be associated with estrogenic status in women. Androgen receptors are found in the bladder and urinary tract of women, but their function is currently unknown [108, 121].

3.6.1.1 Estrogen and urinary incontinence

In women, during menopause are usually complaining of frequent symptoms in the urinary system. The most common are frequent micturition, bed wetting, stress and urge incontinence, they may also experience urinary tract infection and vaginal symptoms, such as itching or dryness. The specific diagnosis of the underlying pathology is based on a comprehensive clinical study and the study of urodynamic. There are many causes for urinary incontinence; these include bladder dysfunction, instability with constipation, excessive urination, fistula (between vagina and the bladder, or between vagina and ureter or with urethra) or due to diverticulum or immobility.

The causes of transient enuresis in the elderly include urinary tract infections, estrogen deficiency, restricted mobility, medications, and depression. The two most common symptoms are stress and\ or urge incontinence.

Urinary tract and pelvic tissues are sensitive to estrogen, as it play an important role in the storage mechanism. For a woman to be on the continent, the pressure of the urethra must be greater than that of the bladder. The urethra consists of four functional layers sensitive to estrogen that are involved in maintaining positive pressure, by its effect on epithelium, blood vessels, muscles and connective tissues [122].

Extracellular changes in the urinary epithelial layer have been reported in response to estrogen. There is some evidence that estrogen affects the blood vessels in the system, and can treat urinary incontinence in women by hypersensitivity to the alpha-adrenergic receptors of the ureteral smooth muscles, stimulation of collagen production around the urinary tract, increased sensitivity of the bladder, increased pressure in the urethra [123, 124].

3.6.1.2 Estrogen to prevent and treatment of enuresis

Although less research is done, the role of estrogen in the treatment of enuresis is controversial. Some have shown reliable results, but this may be due to different estrogens, different doses, and instructions over the duration. This disease is more difficult to treat. There are now two methods of meta-analysis to clarify the situation. It was the first report by the Hormones and Urogenital Therapy (HUT) Committee.

The use of estrogen has been discussed to treat all causes of enuresis in postmenopausal women [125].

Of the 166 articles in English published between 1969 and 1992, only six were considered, but this was not the case. The results showed that real stress is a major psychological development for all patients with urinary incontinence. However, the analysis of the target parameters showed no change in urine volume. The maximum pressure to close the urethra increases, but only one test significantly affects the result. In the second meta-analysis [126], potentially controlled cases and 14 indirect studies related to estrogen therapy were considered. They also found that estrogen therapy does not relieve stress, but it can help with sudden and recurring symptoms. This method can be useful for women with low stress or who need surgery. Estrogen to prevent rapid urination, and has been used to treat menopause for many years, but several controlled studies have shown its benefits. A combination of estradiol (2 mg) and 1 mg estriol (Imagine Daily) reduced urinary retention in 7 of 11 women, compared with 1 in 10 in the placebo group [127, 128].

3.6.1.3 Estrogen for urinary tract infections

Changes in urine production in women after childbirth increase the risk of developing UTI in women, especially during intercourse. The pH of the vagina increases and the number of lactobacilli decreases, that is colonization induces Gram-negative bacteria that play a pathogenic role in urine. In response to these changes, estrogen can be used for treatment or prophylaxis, which can occur in adult women with recurrent steroid intake [129].

3.7 Effects of testosterone on erythropoietin (EPO) and on muscle

High levels of testosterone, important for hemoglobin and hematocrit and stimulate EPO and reduction of cellular exhaustion. Testosterone increases iron absorption by red blood cells, stimulates EPO and restores EPO-bound hemoglobin [130].

As a large amount of DNA accumulates in adult muscles after birth and is made up of dependent cells, satellite cells, which are an important area for controlling muscle growth, and protein regulation in muscle fibers. Testosterone is a blood transporter that binds directly to muscles and therefore increases protein [131].

3.8 Sex hormones and brain

Estrogen is involved in many processes throughout life. Minds of men and women. For example, neurological developmental and synaptic changes resulting in sexual behavioral differentiation [132, 133].

Progesterone is important for synthesis of neurosteroid, and estrogen regulates rapid and prolonged neuroplastic processes in the central nervous system, including synaptic-cyclical changes [134, 135].

Estrogen affects many neurological functions and behaviors, such as mood, cognitive function, blood pressure regulation, motor coordination, pain and sensitivity to opioids. Many of these characteristics have small gender differences that lead to uncertainties about hormones and genetic factors, including the mitochondrial genome [136].

Brain aging is often associated with many diseases of the nervous system resulting from disorders in the workplace. Recent evidence suggests that estrogen replacement therapy may reduce the risk of degenerative diseases such as Alzheimer's disease and cognitive decline in women [137–139].

Estrogen is the broadest group of drugs used to prevent Alzheimer's disease (AD). These steroids are powerful neurotransmitters in vitro and in vivo and have been shown to have similar effects in preventing attention deficit disorder. This includes suppression of the amyloid expression of the pro-amyloid protein (A), Epidemiological evidence supports the use of estrogen to lower the stress at the beginning of menopause and treatment of Alzheimer's disease [140].

Epidemiological studies have shown that women are 1.5 to 2 times Lower than men to develop Parkinson's disease (PD), indicating a protective effect of estrogen. Experimental data show that estradiol has a protective effect on neurons and dopaminergic proteins. Studies have shown that higher levels of estrogen are associated with fewer symptoms of Parkinson's disease and an increased risk of Parkinson's disease in postmenopausal women. These data indicate that estrogen may have a protective effect on dopaminergic neurons [141].

3.8.1 Neuromprotective effect of estrogen

Obviously, estrogen has other functions, such as stimulating nerve cells and protecting them from stimuli caused by other diseases, such as seizures, stroke and Alzheimer's [142, 143].

The exact role of cellular nuclear ERs detected on inhibitory effect between neurons is unclear, but one key is the function of E2 to enhance neuropeptide Y (NPY) expressing and releasing, because NPY has antiexcitatory actions [144, 145].

The second fact that E2 is neuroprotective its function is translocate ER-β to mitochondria, in addition its ability to sequestrate mitochondrial Ca^{2+} ion, including Bcl-2 translocation [146].

Studies on estrogen's ability to prevent stroke and fight Alzheimer's and Parkinson's disease have shown that the brain can produce estrogen and possibly cholesterol [147, 148]. Like E2, androgens have a protective effect on nerve cells, the pyramidal neurons are an important type of CA1 AR nucleus. In men, nuclear ARAS may play an important role in the development of spinal synapses, not in NMDA, but in cholinergic activity [149–151].

3.8.2 The behavioral effects of sex hormones

Genital steroids affect children's brains, especially the hypothalamus, and cause gender differences. The differences in behavior between men and women are related to the sexual ability of the three families of steroid hormones (estrogen, androgen and progesterone) in the nervous system. The classic family of receptors is associated with elements that act as transcription factors after the breakdown of layers, nuclear translation and hormonal effects of DNA [152]. Gender differences in the brain are usually anatomical, neurochemical or molecular.

The neurochemical change in sex occurs at the level of neurotransmitters, enzymes or local hormones. Molecular changes in sex, gene expression and epigenetic changes in phase signaling occur with any gender difference in the hypothalamus regulated by the regulatory effects of estradiol.

Estrogen has long been known to have a psychoactive effect. Therefore, it is believed that the inappropriate metabolism of estradiol may play a role in the development of mental illness. Differences in brain area, size, cell number or radiation intensity (for example, differences in cell size, neural complexity or morphology, dendritic cell length and number of contacts) [153].

3.9 The effect of sex hormones on the immune system

The role of estrogen in the negotiations between the internal system and the immune system was described about 15 years ago [154, 155].

Estrogen effects: macrophages, CD8 + lymphocytes and ERF3 B lymphocyte rings are also expressed in lymphoid tissue and can be membranes linked to the receptor. Estrogen and anti-estrogen binding sites (AEBS) are also found in lymphocytes [156, 157].

Regarding cytokines: TNF levels in endotoxin coatings increase significantly with estrogen, while levels of IL-6 (due to ethylene 17 in the blood) decrease [158, 159]. Active ER stimulates nuclear transcription factors and maintains NF-IL6, NF-ICB and C/EBPf3 [160, 161].

Physiological levels of estradiol in cultured human cells significantly increase the activity of the IL-1 receptor antagonist (mRNA) but it suppressed by higher estradiol concentrations [162]. Estradiol 17F3 produces IL-5 mRNA in vitro [163]. Estradiol and glucocorticoids activate secretory substances that prevent leukemia, sagging and overuse in humans [164].

And in uterus the uterine epithelial cells stimulate antigen secretion and preserve uterine E2 cells [165].

In adults, the activity of natural killer cells increases after in vitro treatment with 17G3-estradiol [166]. Estradiol increases the sensitivity of natural human prostate killer cells in classic ER [167, 168]. Cytotoxic activity of estrogen-dependent CD4 + cells [169].

The chemotactic activity of human polymorphonuclear leukocytes is greatly reduced due to the physiological concentration of estradiol (10-IOM) [170].

In short, antiestrogens act on specific estrogen receptors and lymphocytes when they affect the nervous and endocrine systems and on target cells, or tissues in the transplant system.

As the nervous system and the immune system produce a regulatory response, immune changes cause changes in the nerves and vice versa. This is a phrase was made possible by for example, the thymus is an organ that produces the steroid hormone. In addition, the immune system can convert steroid precursors into active hormones [171].

Steroid hormones are the ones that most control the immune system, as they can control signaling at the level of nuclear transcription factors [172]. However, it is not clear whether estrogen is necessary for the normal functioning of the immune system or if its effect on primary levels of estrogen in the regulation of the vaccine varies. We are not aware of the potential differences between the different steroids and estrogen receptors in the immune system. Estrogen regulates immune function differently in men and women [170–176].

Estrogen is important for building the body's immune system against viral infections. Stabilization of the cytokine storm has been shown to control and mediate immunological changes against the influenza virus and pneumonia. Due to the effects of estrogen, SARS-CoV-2 is lower in women than in men. Some believe that SARS-CoV-2 cause stress in the endoplasmic reticulum (ER), which inturn aggreviate the infection.

This problem can controlled by estrogen as it cause degradation of phosphatidylinositol 4,5-bisphosphate (PIP2) into diacylglycerol (DAG) and inositol triphosphate (IP3). IP3 in-fluxing Ca + 2 ions and helps activate UPR (unfolded protein responce). Data from 392 patients were analyzed and found that 26% of females and 74% of men were affected by SARS-CoV-2. It indicated that women are less affected due to the possible effect of E2 hormone in females [177].

4. Summary

Sex steroids roles have not limited to their reproductive function, but their roles are also shown to be extend to a lot off effects on other body systems including cardiovascular, neural, musculoskeletal, adipose tissue, dermatological, immune, and haemopoietic systems, The sex hormones include the androgens, estrogens, and progestogens, their effects are exert by either slow (genomic process) via nuclear receptors, or by rapid non-genomic process through membrane related receptors and signal cascades.

Androgens and oestrogens impact biology of the blood vessels, predominantly in a sex specific way. And this effect is a cardioprotective, while oestrogens having benefit effect in both males and females, but the effect of androgens different in the two genders. As the effect of testosterone in females rely on the estrogen levels and thereby on estradiol to testosterone ratio. Estrogens and androgens exert potent influences on the post-natal building of muscles and bones and important for their sexual dimorphism, these 2 hormones also vital for the homeostasis of both tissue in addition to the skin, adipose tissues, and regulation of body weight through adulthood, as well as integrity and function of female genitourinary system (specially the estrogen).

The nervous system is a target for effect of sex hormones. Estrogens, progestins, and androgens, all effect the function and physiology of the brain,these steroids are powerful neurotransmitters in vitro and in vivo and have been shown to have similar effects in preventing attention deficit disorder. Experimental data show that estradiol has a protective effect on neurons and dopaminergic proteins. Sex hormones also play a vital role as modulators of the immune system, as the sex steroids and immunity are closely connected, and their mutual regulation is involved in the maintenance of immune balance.

5. Conclusion

The sex steroid are considers balance of the functions and protection of the body systems, and can use for prevention and treatment of many systemic disorders, and the possibility of applying of their effects on the incidence of many organic and infectious diseases.

Author details

Nassrin Malik Aubead
Department of the Obstetrics and Gynaecology, Medical College of Hammurabi, University of Babylon, Hilla.Babylon, Iraq

*Address all correspondence to: nissrenmalik@uobabylon.edu.iq; maliknassrin@yahoo.com

References

[1] Bruce A. White, PhD. Introduction to the endocrine system, Endocrine and Reproductive Physiology, fourth edition, 2013,1,1-25e2.

[2] Shannon Whirledge, John A. Cidlowski. Steroid Hormone Action, Yen & Jaffe's Reproductive Endocrinology, 2019, eighth edition, chapter 5,115-131.

[3] George P. Chrousos, MD. The Gonadal Hormones & Inhibitors; Basic and clinical pharmacology, ed. 13,2015;40: 1024-64.

[4] Hohlweg W (1943) Ober das Sexualzentrum. Zbl Gynak 67:1357-1387.

[5] C. Lauritzen. M. Oettel and E. Schillinger History of Estrogen Research, Physiology and Mechanisms of Action of Estrogens and Antiestrogens, Experimental Pharmacology, 1999, Volume 135\I, 1, 1-14.

[6] Sarrel PM (1990) Ovarian hormones and the circulation. Maturitas 12:122:287-292.

[7] Britta M. Jacobsen and Kathryn B. Horwitz. Progesterone Receptors, their Isoforms and Progesterone Regulated Transcription.Mol Cell Endocrinol. 2012 June 24; 357(1-2): 18-29.

[8] Rachel A Davey and Mathis Grossmann. Androgen Receptor Structure, Function and Biology: From Bench to Bedside. Clin Biochem Rev 2016;37(1).

[9] Jaaskelainen J: Molecular biology of androgen insensitivity. Mol Cell Endocrinol, 2012,352(1-2):4-12.

[10] Shiina H, Matsumoto T, Sato T, et al: Premature ovarian failure in androgen receptor-deficient mice. Proc Natl Acad Sci USA, 2006.103(1):224-229.

[11] Hu YC, Wang PH, Yeh S, et al: Subfertility and defective folliculogenesis in female mice lacking androgen receptor. Proc Natl Acad Sci USA, 2004. 101(31):11209-11214.

[12] Panda B, Rao L, Tosh D, et al: Germline study of AR gene of Indianwomen with ovarian failure. Gynecol Endocrinol, 2011, 27(8):572-578.

[13] Sugimura Y, Cunha GR, Donjacour AA: Morphological and histological study of castration-induced degeneration and androgen-induced regeneration in the mouse prostate. Biol Reprod1986. 34(5):973-983

[14] Lai KP, Yamashita S, Vitkus S, et al: Suppressed prostate epithelial development with impaired branching morphogenesis in mice lacking stromal fibromuscular androgen receptor. Mol Endocrinol 26(1):52-66

[15] Huggins C, Hodges CV: Studies on prostatic cancer: I. The effect of castration, of estrogen and of androgen injection on serum phosphatases in metastatic carcinoma of the prostate. 1941. J Urol 2002.168(1):9-12

[16] Zhou Y, Bolton EC, Jones JO: Androgens and androgen receptor signaling in prostate tumorigenesis. J Mol Endocrinol 2015, 54(1):R15–R29.

[17] Eisermann K, Fraizer G: The androgen receptor and VEGF: mechanisms of androgen-regulated angiogenesis in prostate cancer. Cancers (Basel) 2017,9(4):E32.

[18] Schweizer MT, Yu EY: AR-Signaling in human malignancies: prostate cancer and beyond. Cancers (Basel), 2017, 9(1):E7.

[19] Kannel W.B., Hjortland M.C., McNamara P.M. et al. Menopause and risk of cardiovascular disease: the Framingham study. Ann. Intern. Med. 1976; 85 :447-452

[20] Edward Morris. The menopause and postreproductive health, Gynaecology by ten teachers, 2017, 20th edition, cha. 8; 171-94.

[21] Wild S., Pierpoint T., McKeigue P., Jacobs H.S. Cardiovascular disease in women with polycystic ovary syndrome at long-term follow-up: a retrospective cohort study. Clin. Endocrinol. (Oxf). 2000; 52 :595-600.

[22] Orshal J.M., Khalil R.A. Gender, sex hormones, and vascular tone. Am. J. Physiol. Regul. Integr. Comp. Physiol. 4. 2004; 286: R233– R249.

[23] Mendelsohn M.E., Rosano G.M. Hormonal regulation of normal vascular tone in males. Circ. Res. 2003; 93: 1142-1145.

[24] Mendelsohn M.E., Karas R.H. Molecular and cellular basis of cardiovascular gender differences. Science 2005; 308: 1583-1587.

[25] Crews J.K., Khalil R.A. Gender-specific inhibition of Ca2+ entry mechanisms of arterial vasoconstriction by sex hormones. Clin. Exp. Pharmacol. Physiol. 1999; 26 :707-715.

[26] Kanashiro C.A., Khalil R.A. Gender-related distinctions in protein kinase C activity in rat vascular smooth muscle. Am. J. Physiol. Cell Physiol. 2001; 280 :C34– C45.

[27] Mendelsohn M.E., Karas R.H. The protective effects of estrogen on the cardiovascular system. N. Engl. J. Med. 1999;340 :1801-1811.

[28] Mendelsohn M.E. Protective effects of estrogen on the cardiovascular system. Am. J. Cardiol. 2002; 89: 12E– 18E.

[29] Mendelsohn M.E. Genomic and nongenomic effects of estrogen in the vasculature. Am. J. Cardiol. 2002; 90: 3F– 6F

[30] Collins P., Rosano G.M., Sarrel P.M. et al. 17 Beta-estradiol attenuates acetylcholine-induced coronary arterial constriction in women but not men with coronary heart disease. Circulation 1995; 92 :24-30.

[31] Chambliss K.L., Yuhanna I.S., Anderson R.G., Mendelsohn M.E., Shaul P.W. ER b has non-genomic action in caveolae. Mol. Endocrinol. 2002; 16: 938-946.

[32] Chen Z., Yuhanna I.S., Galcheva-Gargova Z., Karas R.H., Mendelsohn M.E., Shaul P.W. Estrogen receptor alpha mediates the nongenomic activation of endothelial nitric oxide synthase by estrogen. J. Clin. Invest. 1999; 103 :401-406.

[33] Pare G., Krust A., Karas R.H. et al. Estrogen receptor-α mediates the protective effects of estrogen against vascular injury. Circ. Res. 2002; 90 :1087-1092.

[34] Hodgin J.B., Krege J.H., Reddick R.L. et al. Estrogen receptor alpha is a major mediator of 17beta-estradiol's atheroprotective effects on lesion size in Apoe−/− mice. J. Clin. Invest. (2001) 107 333-340.

[35] Zhu Y., Bian Z., Lu P. et al. Abnormal vascular function and hypertension in mice deficient in estrogen receptor β. Science 2002; 295: 505-508.

[36] Hodges Y.K., Tung L., Yan X.D., Graham J.D., Horwitz K.B., Horwitz L.D. Estrogen receptors alpha and beta: prevalence of estrogen

receptor beta mRNA in human vascular smooth muscle and transcriptional effects. Circulation 2000;101 :1792-1798.

[37] Nakamura Y., Suzuki T., Sasano H. Estrogen actions and in situ synthesis in smooth muscle cells and their correlation with atherosclerosis. J. Steroid Biochem. Mol. Biol. 2005; 93: 263-268.

[38] Post W.S., Goldschmidt-Clermont P.J., Wilhide C.C. et al. Methylation of the estrogen receptor gene is associated with aging and atherosclerosis in the cardiovascular system. Cardiovasc. Res. 1999; 43: 985-991.

[39] Vitale C., Mercuro G., Cerquetani E. et al. Time since menopause influences the acute and chronic effect of estrogens on endothelial function. Arterioscler. Thromb. Vasc. Biol. 2008;28 :348-352.

[40] Volterrani M., Rosano G., Coats A., Beale C., Collins P. Estrogen acutely increases peripheral blood flow in postmenopausal women. Am. J. Med. 1995;99 :119-122.

[41] Rosano G.M., Gebara O., Sheiban I. et al. Acute administration of 17beta-estradiol reduces endothelin-1 release during pacing-induced ischemia. Int. J. Cardiol. 2006 ;116: 34-39.

[42] Adamopoulos S., Rosano G.M., Ponikowski P. et al. Impaired baroreflex sensitivity and sympathovagal balance in syndrome X. Am. J. Cardiol. 1998; 82: 862-868

[43] Sudhir K., Chou T.M., Messina L.M. et al. Endothelial dysfunction in a man with disruptive mutation in oestrogen-receptor gene. Lancet 1997; 349: 1146-1147.

[44] Sudhir K., Chou T.M., Chatterjee K. et al. Premature coronary artery disease associated with a disruptive mutation in the estrogen receptor gene in a man. Circulation 1997; 96 :3774-3777.

[45] Carani C., Qin K., Simoni M. et al. Effect of testosterone and of estradiol in a man with aromatase deficiency. N. Engl. J. Med. 1997 ;337: 91-95.

[46] Smith E.P., Boyd J., Frank G.R. et al. Estrogen resistance caused by a mutation in the estrogen-receptor gene in a man. N. Engl. J. Med. 1994 ;331: 1056-1061.

[47] Lew R., Komesaroff P., Williams M., Dawood T., Sudhir K. Endogenous estrogens influence endothelial function in young men. Circ. Res. 2003; 93: 1127-1133.

[48] Kneale B.J., Chowienczyk P.J., Brett S.E., Coltart D.J., Ritter J.M. Gender differences in sensitivity to adrenergic agonists of forearm resistance vasculature. J. Am. Coll. Cardiol. 2000 ;36 :1233-1238.

[49] Giralt D, Domingues-Montanari S, Mendioroz M, Ortega L, Maisterra O, Perea-Gainza M, Delgado P, Rosell A, Montaner J. The gender gap in stroke: A meta-analysis. Acta Neurol Scand. 2012;125:83-90.

[50] Regitz-Zagrosek V, Oertelt-Prigione S, Prescott E, Franconi F, Gerdts E, Foryst-Ludwig A, Maas AH, Kautzky-Willer A, Knappe-Wegner D, Kintscher U, Ladwig KH, Schenck-Gustafsson K, Stangl V. Gender in cardiovascular diseases: Impact on clinical manifestations, management, and outcomes. Eur Heart J. 2016;37:24-34.

[51] Lloyd-Jones DM, Evans JC, Levy D. Hypertension in adults across the age spectrum: Current outcomes and control in the community. JAMA. 2005;294:466-472

[52] Lakoski S.G., Brosnihan B., Herrington D.M. Hormone therapy, C-reactive protein, and progression of atherosclerosis: data from the Estrogen Replacement on Progression of Coronary Artery Atherosclerosis (ERA) trial. Am. Heart J. 2005; 150 :907-911.

[53] Hodis H.N., Mack W.J., Azen S.P. et al. Women's Estrogen-Progestin Lipid-Lowering Hormone Atherosclerosis Regression Trial Research Group Hormone therapy and the progression of coronary-artery atherosclerosis in postmenopausal women. N. Engl. J. Med. 2003; 349 :535-545.

[54] Manson J.E., Allison M.A., Rossouw J.E. et al. Estrogen therapy and coronary-artery calcification. N. Engl. J. Med. 2007;356 :2591-2602.

[55] Mendelsohn M.E., Karas R. HRT and the young at heart. N. Engl. J. Med. 2007; 21: 2639-2641

[56] Arnal J.F., Scarabin P.Y., Tremollieres F., Laurell H., Gourdy P. Estrogens in vascular biology and disease: where do we stand today? Curr. Opin. Lipidol. 2007;18 :554-560.

[57] Mikkola T.S., Clarkson T.B. Estrogen replacement therapy, atherosclerosis, and vascular function. Cardiovasc. Res. 2002 ;53: 605-619.

[58] Adam, W (1943) Ostrogene erzeugen Hypertrombinamie. Zbl Gynak 67:551-554

[59] Wu F.C., Von Eckardstein A. Androgens and coronary artery disease. Endocr. Rev. 2003 ;24 :183-217.

[60] Yildiz O., Seyrek M. Vasodilating mechanisms of testosterone. Exp. Clin. Endocrinol. Diabetes 2007;115: 1-6.

[61] Von Eckardstein A., Wub F.C.W. Testosterone and atherosclerosis. Growth Horm. IGF Res. 2003; 13: S72– S84.

[62] English K.M.J.R., Jones T.H., Morice A.H., Channer K.S. Testosterone acts as a coronary vasodilator by a calcium antagonistic action. J. Endocrinol. Invest. 2002; 25:455-458.

[63] Jones R.D., Hugh Jones T., Channer K.S. The influence of testosterone upon vascular reactivity. Eur. J. Endocrinol. 2004; 151: 29-37.

[64] McCrohon J.A., Death A.K., Nakhla S. et al. Androgen receptor expression is greater in macrophages from male than from female donors. A sex difference with implications for atherogenesis. Circulation 2000; 101: 224-226

[65] McCredie R.J., McCrohon J.A., Turner L., Griffiths K.A., Handelsman D.J., Celermajer D.S. Vascular reactivity is impaired in genetic females taking high dose androgens. J. Am. Coll. Cardiol. 1998; 32:1331-1335.

[66] Worboys S., Kotsopoulos D., Teede H., McGrath B., Davis S.R. Evidence that parenteral testosterone therapy may improve endothelium-dependent and -independent vasodilation in postmenopausal women already receiving estrogen. J. Clin. Endocrinol. Metab. 2001; 86:158-161.

[67] Alexandersen P., Haarbo J., Byrjalsen I., Lawaetz H., Christiansen C. Natural androgens inhibit male atherosclerosis: a study in castrated, cholesterol-fed rabbits. Circ. Res. 1999; 84:813-819.

[68] Rosano G.M.C., Leonardo F., Pagnotta P. et al. Acute anti-ischemic effect of testosterone in men with coronary artery disease. Circulation (1999) :1666-1670.

[69] Phillips G.B., Pinkernell B.H., J ing T.Y. The association of hypotestosteronemia with coronary artery disease in men. Arterioscler. Thromb. 1994 ;14 :701-706.

[70] Dahlgren E., Janson P.O., Johansson S., Lapidus L., Oden A. Polycystic ovary syndrome and risk for myocardial infarction.Evaluated from a risk factor model based on a prospective population study of women. Acta Obstet. Gynecol. Scand.(1992) Dec;71(8):599-604.

[71] Tikkanen M.J., Vihma V., Jauhiainen M. et al. Lipoprotein-associated estrogens. Cardiovasc. Res. 2002;56:184-188.

[72] Chikani G., Zhu W., Smart E.J. et al. Lipids: potential regulators of nitric oxide generation. Am. J. Physiol. Endocrinol. Metab. 2004; 287:E386– E389.

[73] Hergenc G., Schulte H., Assmann G., Von Eckardstein A. Associations of obesity markers, insulin, and sex hormones with HDL-cholesterol levels in Turkish and German individuals. Atherosclerosis 1999; 145 :147-156.

[74] Tchernof A., Labrie F., Belanger A., Despres J.P. Obesity and metabolic complications: contribution of dehydroepiandrosterone and other steroid hormones. J. Endocrinol. (Suppl.) 1996; 150 :S155– S164.

[75] Tsai E.C., Boyko E.J., Leonetti D.L., Fujimoto W.Y. Low serum testosterone level as a predictor of increased visceral fat in Japanese-American men. Int. J. Obes. Relat. Metab. Disord. 2000 ;24: 485-491.

[76] Isidori A.M., Giannetta E., Greco E.A. et al. Effects of testosterone on body composition, bone metabolism and serum lipid profile in middle-aged men: a meta-analysis. Clin. Endocrinol. (Oxf). 2005; 63 :280-293.

[77] Tan K.C., Shiu S.W., Pang R.W., Kung A.W. Effects of testosterone replacement on HDL subfractions and apolipoprotein A-I containing lipoproteins. Clin. Endocrinol. (Oxf) 1998; 48 :187-194.

[78] Khaw K.T., Barrett-Connor E. Lower endogenous androgens predict central adiposity in men. Ann. Epidemiol. 1992; 2: 675-682.

[79] Poehlman E.T., Toth M.J., Gardner A.W. Changes in energy balance and body composition at menopause: a controlled longitudinal study [retraction in: Sox HC. Ann. Intern. Med. 2003; 139: 702]. Ann. Intern. Med. 1995; 123: 673-675.

[80] Carr M.C. The emergence of the metabolic syndrome with menopause. J. Clin. Endocrinol. Metab. 2003 ;88 :2404-2411.

[81] Tchernof A., Poehlman E.T., Despres J.P. Body fat distribution, the menopause transition, and hormone replacement therapy. Diabetes Metab. 2000; 26 :12-20.

[82] Simon D., Charles M.A., Naohul K., Orssaud G. Association between plasma testosterone and cardiovascular risk factors in healthy adult men. The Telecom Study. J. Clin. Endocrinol. Metab. 1997; 82 :682-685.

[83] Barrett-Connor E. Lower endogenous androgen levels dyslipidaemia in men with NIDDM. Ann. Intern. Med. 1992 ;117 :807-811.

[84] Kapoor D., Malkin C.J., Channer K.S., Jones T.H. Androgens, insulin resistance and vascular disease in men. Clin. Endocrinol. (Oxf) ,2005 ;63: 239-250.

[85] Anderson G.L., Limacher M., Assaf A.R. et al. Effects of conjugated equine estrogen in postmenopausal women with hysterectomy: the Women's Health Initiative randomized controlled trial. JAMA 2004;291 :1701-1712.

[86] Katznelson L., Finkelstein J.S., Schoenfeld D.A. et al. Increase in bone density and lean body mass during testosterone administration in men

with acquired hypogonadism. J. Clin. Endocrinol. Metab. 1996; 81 :4358-4365.

[87] Ferrannini E., Natali A., Capaldo B. et al. Insulin resistance, hyperinsulinemia, and blood pressure: role of age and obesity. European Group for the Study of Insulin Resistance (EGIR). Hypertension 1997; 30: 1144-1149.

[88] B. Lawrence Riggs.The mechanisms of estrogen regulation of bone resorption.The Journal of Clinical Investigation, November 2000, Volume 106, Number 10:1203-4.

[89] Riggs, B.L., Khosla, S., and Melton, L.J., III. 1998.A unitary model for involutional osteoporosis estrogen deficiency causes both type I and type IIosteoporosis in postmenopausal women and contributes to bone loss in aging men. J. BoneMiner. Res. 13:763-773.

[90] Manolagas, S.C. 2000. Birth and death of bone cells: basic regulatory mechanisms and implications for the pathogenesis and treatment of osteoporosis. Endocr. Rev. 21:115-137.

[91] Pacifici, R. 1996. Estrogen, cytokines, and pathogenesisof postmenopausal osteoporosis. J. Bone Miner. Res. 11:1043-1051

[92] Cenci, S., et al. 2000. Estrogen deficiency induces bone loss by enhancing T cell production of TNFa. J. Clin. Invest. 106:1229-1237

[93] Mikihito Hayashi, Tomoki Nakashima, Noriko Yoshimura, Kazuo Okamoto, Sakae Tanaka, Hiroshi Takayanagi, Autoregulation of Osteocyte Sema3A Orchestrates Estrogen Action and Counteracts Bone Aging, Cell Metabolism 2019; 29: 627-637

[94] Susan Stevenson, Julie Thornton, Effect of estrogens on skin aging and the potential role of SERMs.Clinical Interventions in Aging 2007:2(3): 283-297

[95] Thornton MJ. 2002. The biological actions of estrogens on skin. Exp Dermatol 11: 487-502.

[96] Thornton MJ. 2005. Oestrogen functions in skin and skin appendages. Expert Opin Ther Targets, 9: 617-29.

[97] Ashcroft GS, Ashworth JJ. 2003. Potential role of estrogens in wound healing Am. J. Clin. Dermatol, 4: 737-43.

[98] Dunna SF, Finlay AY. 1989. Psoriasis: improvement during and worsening after pregnancy. Br J Dermatol, 120: 584.

[99] Boyd AS, Morris LF, Phillips CM, et al. 1996. Psoriasis and pregnancy hormone and immune system interaction. Int J Dermatol, 35: 169-72.

[100] Raychaudhuri SP, Navare T, Gross J, et al. 2003. Clinical course of psoriasis during pregnancy. Int J Dermatol, 42: 518-20.

[101] Weinstock MA. 1994. Epidemiologic investigation of nonmelanoma skin cancer mortality: the Rhode Island Follow-Back Study. J Invest Dermatol, 102: 6S–9S.

[102] Tsukahara K, Moriwaki S, Ohuchi A, et al. 2001. Ovariectomy accelerates photoaging of rat skin. Photochem Photobiol, 73: 525-31.

[103] Tsukahara K, Nakagawa H, Moriwaki S, et al. 2004. Ovariectomy is sufficient to accelerate spontaneous skin ageing and to stimulate ultraviolet irradiation-induced photoageing of murine skin. Br J Dermatol, 151: 984-94.

[104] Urano R, Sakabe K, Seiki K, et al. 1995. Female sex hormone stimulates

cultured human keratinocyte proliferation and its RNA- and proteinsyntheticactivities. J Dermatol Sci, 9: 176-84.

[105] Miller JG, Mac Neil S. 1997. Gender and cutaneous melanoma. Br J Dermatol 136: 657-65.

[106] Dae Kyung Kim, MD and Michael B Chancellor, MD. Is Estrogen for Urinary Incontinence Good or Bad, Rev Urol. 2006 Spring; 8(2): 91-92.

[107] Iosif CS, Batra S, Ek A, Astedt B (1981) Estrogen receptors in the human female lower urinary tract. Am J Obstet Gyneco I141: 817-820.

[108] Blakeman PJ, Hilton P, Bulmer IN (1996a) Mapping estrogen and progesterone receptors throughout the female lower urinary tract. Neurourol Urodyn 15: 324-325.

[109] Ingelman-Sundberg A, Rosen J, Gustafsson SA, Carlstrom K (1981) Cytosol estrogen receptors in urogenital tissues in stress incontinent women. Acta Obstet Gynecol Scand 60: 585-586

[110] Smith P, Heimer G, Lindskog M, Ulmsten U (1993) Oestradiol releasing vaginal ring for treatment of postmenopausal urogenital atrophy. Maturitas 16:145-154.

[111] Blakeman PJ, Hilton P, Bulmer IN (1996b) Estrogen status and cell cycle activity in the female lower urinary tract. Neurourol Urodyn 15: 325-326.

[112] Samsioe G, Jansson I, Meelstron D, Svanborg A (1985) Occurrence, nature and treatmentof urinary incontinence in a 70year old female population. Maturitas 7: 335-342.

[113] Smith PJB (1976) The effect of estrogens on bladder function in the female. In Management of the menopause and post menopausal years. MTP, Lancaster, pp 291-298.

[114] Semmens JP, Tsai CC, Semmens EC, Loadholt HB (1985) Effects of estrogen therapy on vaginal physiology during menopause. Obstet Gyneco I66:15-18.

[115] McCallin PF, Taylor ES, Whitehead RW (1950) A study of the changes in the urinary sediment during the menstrual cycle. Am J Obstet Gyneco I60: 64-74

[116] Soloman C, Panagotopoulos P, Oppenheim A (1958) The use of urinary sediment as an aid in endocrinological disorders in the female. Am J Obstet Gynecol 76: 56-60

[117] Van Geelen 1M, Doesburg WH, Thomas CMG, Martin CB Jr (1981) Urodynamic studies in the normal menstrual cycle: the relationship between hormonal changes during the menstrual cycle and the urethral pressure profile. Am J Obstet Gynecol 141: 384-392

[118] Cutner A, Carey A, Cardozo LD (1992) Lower urinary tract symptoms in early pregnancy J Obstet Gynaecol 12: 75-78

[119] Stanton SL, Kerr-Wilson R, Harris VG (1980) The incidence of urological symptoms in normal pregnancy. Br J Obstet Gynaecol 87: 897-900.

[120] Cutner A, Burton G, Cardozo LD et al. (1991) Does progesterone cause an irritable bladder? Int Urogynecol J Pelvic Floor Dysfunct 98: 1181-1183.

[121] Blakeman PJ, Hilton P, Bulmer IN (1997) Androgen receptors in the female lower urinary tract. Int Urogynecol J Pelvic Floor Dysfunct 8: S54.

[122] Abrams P, Blaivas JG, Stanton SL et al. (1990) The standardisation of terminology of lower urinary tract function. Br J Obstet Gynaecol 97:1-16.

[123] Gangar KF, Vyas S, Whitehead M, Crook D, Meire H, Campbell S (1991)

Plasticity index in the internal carotid artery in relation to transdermal oestradiol and time since menopause. Lancet 338: 839-842.

[124] Jackson S, Vyas S (1998) A double-blind, placebo controlled study of postmenopausal estrogen replacement therapy and carotid artery pulsatility index. Br J Obstet Gynaecol 105:408-412

[125] Fantl JA, Cardozo LD, McClish DK (1994) Estrogen therapy in the management of urinary incontinence in postmenopausal women: a meta-analysis. First report of the Hormones and Urogenital Therapy Committee. Obstet Gyneco I83: 12-18

[126] Sultana CJ, Walters MD (1995) Estrogen and urinary incontinence in women. Maturitas 20:129-138

[127] Walter S, Wolf H, Barlebo H et al. (1978) Urinary incontinence in postmenopausal women treated with estrogens. Urol Int 33: 135-143

[128] Samsioe G, Jansson I, Meelstron D, Svanborg A (1985) Occurrence, nature and treatment of urinary incontinence in a 70year old female population. Maturitas 7: 335

[129] Raz R, Stamm WE (1993) A controlled trial of intravaginal estriol in postmenopausal women with recurrent urinary tract infections. N Engl J Med 329: 753-756.

[130] Eric Bachman, Thomas G. Travison, Shehzad Basaria, Maithili N. Davda, Wen Guo, Michelle Li, John Connor Westfall, Harold Bae, Victor Gordeuk, Shalender Bhasin. Testosterone Induces Erythrocytosis via Increased Erythropoietin and Suppressed Hepcidin: Evidence for a New Erythropoietin/Hemoglobin Set Point. The Journals of Gerontology: Series A, Volume 69, Issue 6, June 2014, Pages 725-735

[131] Ronald E. Allen, Kenneth C. Masak, Pamela K. McAllister, Robert A. Merkel Effect of Growth Hormone, Testosterone and Serum Concentration on Actin Synthesis in Cultured Satellite Cells. Journal of Animal Science, Volume 56, Issue 4, April 1983, Pages 833-837

[132] MacLusky NJ, Clark AS, Naftolin F, Goldman-Rakic PC (1987) Estrogen formation in the mammalian brain: possible role of aromatase in sexual differentiation of hippocampus and neocortex. Steroids 50:459-474

[133] McEwen BS, Liederberg I, Chaptal C, Krey LC (1977) Aromatization: important for sexual differentiation of the neonatal rat brain. Horm Behav 9:249-263

[134] Baulieu E, Schumacher M (2000). "Progesterone as a neuroactive neurosteroid, with special reference to the effect of progesterone on myelination". Steroids. 65 (10-11): 605-12.

[135] Woolley CS, McEwen BS (1993) Roles of estrogen and progesterone in regulation of hippocampal dendritic spine density during the estrous cycle in the rat. J Comp Neuro I336: 293-306

[136] Jordan Marrocco, PhD and Bruce S. McEwen, PhD, Sex in the brain: hormones and sex differences, Dialogues Clin Neurosci. 2016 Dec; 18(4): 373-383

[137] Paganini-Hill A, Henderson VW (1994) Estrogen deficiency and risk of Alzheimer's disease in women. Am J Epidem 140: 256-261.

[138] Henderson VW, Paganini-Hill A, Emanuel CK, Dunn ME, Buckwalter JG (1994) Estrogen replacement therapy in older women: comparisons between Alzheimer's disease cases and

nondemented control subjects. Arch Neurol 51: 896-900;

[139] Tang M-X, Jacobs D, Stern Y, Marder K, Schofield P, Gurland B, Andrews H, Mayeux R (1996) Effect of estrogen during menopause on risk and age at onset of Alzheimer's disease. Lancet 348: 429-432

[140] James W. Simpkins, Evelyn Perez, and Meharvan Singh. The Potential for Estrogens in Preventing Alzheimer's Disease and Vascular Dementia, Ther Adv Neurol Disord. 2009 Jan; 2(1): 31-49

[141] Yang Hyun Lee, Jungho Cha, Seok Jong Chung, Han Soo Yoo, Young H. Sohn, Byoung Seok Ye and Phil Hyu Lee. Beneficial effect of estrogen on nigrostriatal dopaminergic neurons in drug-naïve postmenopausal Parkinson's disease Scientific Reports volume 9, Article number: 10531 (2019)

[142] Henderson VW, Paganini-Hill A. 1994. Oestrogens and Alzheimer's disease. Annu Prog Repord Med 2: 1-21.

[143] McCullough LD, Blizzard K, Simpson ER, Oz OK, Hurn PD. 2003. Aromatase cytochrome P 450 and extragonadal estrogen play a role in ischemic neuroprotection. J Neurosci 23: 8701-8705

[144] Nakamura NH, Rosell DR, Akama KT, McEwen BS. 2004. Estrogen and ovariectomy regulate mRNA and protein of glutamic acid decarboxylases and cation-chloride cotransporters in the adult rat hippocampus. Neuroendocrinology 80: 308-323

[145] Ledoux VA, Smejkalova T, May RM, Cooke BM, Woolley CS. 2009. Estradiol facilitates the release of neuropeptide Y to suppress hippocampus-dependent seizures. J Neurosci 29: 1457-1468

[146] Nilsen J, Brinton RD. 2004. Mitochondria as therapeutic targets of estrogen action in the central nervous system. Curr Drug Targets CNS Neurol Disord 3: 297-313.

[147] Hojo Y, Hattori T-a, Enami T, Furukawa A, Suzuki K, et al. 2003. Adult male rat hippocampus synthesizes estradiol from pregnenolone by cytochromes P45017alpha and P 450 aromatase localized in neurons. Proc Natl Acad Sci U S A 101: 865-870

[148] Hajszan T, Milner TA, Leranth C. 2007. Sex steroids and the dentate gyrus. Prog Brain Res 163: 399-415

[149] Pike CJ, Nguyen T-VV, Ramsden M, Yao M, Murphy MP, Rosario ER. 2008. Androgen cell signaling pathways involved in neuroprotective actions. Horm Behav 53: 693-705.

[150] Romeo RD, McCarthy JB, Wang A, Milner TA, McEwen BS. 2005a. Sex differences in hippocampal estradiol-induced N-methyl-D-aspartic acid binding and ultrastructural localization of estrogen receptor-alpha. Neuroendocrinology 81: 391-399

[151] Romeo RD, Staub D, Jasnow AM, Karatsoreos IN, Thornton JE, McEwen BS. 2005b. Dihydrotestosterone increases hippocampal N-methyl-D-aspartate binding but does not affect choline acetyltransferase cell number in the forebrain or choline transporter levels in the CA1 region of adult male rats. Endocrinology 146: 2091-2097

[152] King WJ, Greene GL. Monoclonal antibodies localize oestrogen receptor in the nuclei of target cells. Nature. 1984; 307: 745-747.

[153] McCarthy MM, Auger AP, Bale TL, De Vries GJ, Dunn GA, Forger NG, Murray EK, Nugent BM, Schwarz JM,

Wilson ME. The epigenetics of sex differences in the brain. J Neurosci. 2009; 29: 12815-12823.

[154] Grossman CJ (1984) Regulation of the immune system by sex steroids. Endocr Rev 5:435-455

[155] Grossman CJ (1985) Interactions between the gonadal steroids and the immune system. Science 227:257-261

[156] Baral E, Nagy E, Berczi I (1996) The effect of tamoxifen on the immune response. In Kellen JA (ed) Tamoxifen. Beyond the anti estrogen. Birkhiiuser, Boston, MA, USA, P 137

[157] Mosselman S, Polman J, Dijkema R (1996) ER beta: identification and characterization of a novel human estrogen receptor. FEBS Lett 392: 49-53

[158] Zuckerman SH, Bryan-Poole N, Evans GF, Short L, Glasebrook AL (1995) In vivo modulation of murine tumor necrosis factor and interleukin-6 during endotoxemia by estrogen agonists and antagonists. Immunology 86:18-24

[159] Zuckerman SH, Ahmari SE, Bryan-Poole N, Evans GF, Short L, Glasebrook AL (1996) Estriol: a potent regulator of TNF and IL-6 expression in murine model of endotoxemia. Inflammation 20: 581-597

[160] Stein B, Young MX (1995) Repression of the interleukin-6 promoter by estrogen receptor is mediated by NF-TCB and C/EBP, B. Mol Cell Bioi 15:4971-4979

[161] Ghosh SK, Zhang DH, Ray A (1997) Repression of interleukin-6 gene expression by 17 f3-estradiol: inhibition of the DNA-binding activity of the transcription factors NF-IL6 and NF-Jd3 by the estrogen receptor. FEBS Lett 409: 78-85

[162] Lee BY, Huynh T, Prichard LE, McGuire J, Polan ML (1995) Gonadal steroids modulate Interleukin-l receptor antagonist mRNA expression in cultured human monocytes Biochem Biophys Res Commun 209:279-285

[163] Wang Y, Campbell HD, Young IG (1993) Sex hormones and dexamethasone modulate Interleukin-5 gene expression in T lymphocytes. J Steroid Biochem Mol Bioi 44: 203

[164] Bamberger AM, Erdmann I, Bamberger CM, Jenatschke SS, Schulte HM (1997) Transcriptional regulation of the human 'leukemia inhibitory factor' gene: modulation by glucocorticoids and estradiol. Mol Cell Endocrino I127: 71-79

[165] Wira CR, Rossoll RM (1995) Antigen presenting cells in the female reproductive tract influence of the estrus cycle and antigen presentation by uterine epithelial and stromal cells. Endocrinology 136: 4526-4534

[166] Sorachi K, Kumagai S, Sugita M, Yodoi J, Imura H (1993) Enhancing effect of 17f3 estradiol on human NK cell activity. Immunol Lett 36: 31-36

[167] Screpanti I, Felli MP, Toniato E, Meco D, Martinotti S, Frati L, Santoni A, Gulio A (1991) Enhancement of natural killer-cell susceptibility of human breast cancercells by estradiol and v-Ha-ras oncogene. Int J Cancer 47: 445-449

[168] Albertini MR, Gibson DFC, Robinson SP, Howard SP, Tans KJ, Lindstrom MJ Robinson RR, Tormey DC, Jordan YC, Sondel PM (1992) Influence of estradiol and tamoxifen on susceptibility of human breast cancer cell lines to lysis by lymphokine activated killer cells. J Immunother 11: 30-39

[169] Muller D, Chen M, Vikingsson A, Hildeman D, Pederson K (1995)

Estrogen influences CD4+ T-Iymphocyte activity in vitro in J3z-microglobulin-deficient mice. Immunology 86:162-167

[170] Ito I, Hayashi T, Yamada K, Kuzuya M, Naito M, Iguchi A (1995) Physiological concentrations of estradiol inhibits polymorphonuclear leucocyte chemotaxis via a receptor mediated mechanism. Life Sci 56: 2247-2253

[171] Berczi I, Nagy E (1997) Hormones as immune modulating agents. In: Krezina TF (ed) Immune modulating agents. Marcel Dekker, Inc. New York, NY, USA, p 75

[172] Berczi I (1986) Gonadotropins and sex hormones. In: Berczi I (ed) Pituitary function and immunity. CRC Press, Boca Raton, FL, USA, P 185.

[173] Berczi I, Baragar FD, Chalmers 1M, Keystone EC, Nagy E, Warrington RJ (1993) Hormonesin self tolerance and autoimmunity: a role in the pathogenesis of rheumatoid arthritis? Autoimmunity 16: 45-56

[174] Cutolo M, Sulli A, Barone A, Seriolo B, Accardo S (1993) Macrophages, synovial tissue and rheumatoid arthritis. Clin Exp Rheumatoll 1: 331-339

[175] Lahita RG (1996) The basis of gender effects in the connective tissue diseases. An Med Interne Paris 147:241-247

[176] Wilder RL (1996) Adrenal and gonadal steroid hormone deficiency in the pathogenesis of rheumatoid arthritis. J Rheumatol Supp I44: 10-12

[177] Sana Shabbir, Assad Hafeez, and Muhammad Jawad Khan Estrogen shields women from COVID-19 complications by reducing ER stress, Med Hypotheses. 2020 Oct; 143: 110148.

Chapter 2

Nociceptive TRP Channels and Sex Steroids

Óscar Enciso-Pablo, Karina Angélica Méndez-Reséndiz, Tamara Rosenbaum and Sara Luz Morales-Lázaro

Abstract

Proteins belonging to Transient Receptor Potential (TRP) family are nonselective cation channels that play an essential role in mammalian physiology, functioning as transducers of several environmental signals including those of chemical, thermal and mechanical natures. A subgroup of these receptors is expressed in sensory neurons where they are activated by noxious stimuli and are key players of pain responses in the organism. Some TRP channels are molecular targets for the classical and non-classical effects of sex steroids. This chapter will describe the close relationship between nociceptive TRP channels and sex steroids as well as their impact on nociception and pain-related responses.

Keywords: TRP channels, nociception, steroids, pain, sensory neurons

1. Introduction

The somatosensory system is a complex network of neurons and peripheral receptors that encodes specific information about the state of organisms and their environment, providing them with the ability to detect harmful stimuli [1–3].

According to the International Association for the Study of Pain (IASP), the neuronal process encoding noxious stimuli is known as nociception. A subpopulation of high-threshold sensory neurons known as nociceptors mediates this process by detecting harmful signals from chemical and physical nature **Figure 1** [1, 4]. Nociceptors are neurons with a peripheral axonal branch that innervates cutaneous, articular and visceral afferents, and a central axonal branch that innervates the dorsal horn of the spinal cord. The cell bodies of mammalian nociceptors are located in the dorsal root ganglia (DRG) and in the trigeminal ganglia (TG) and they are classified as medium and small diameter neurons. The axons of these nociceptors are classified as Aδ- and C-fibers depending on their diameter, degree of myelinization, conduction speed and the type of sensory stimuli that they transmit [1, 4, 5].

The Aδ-fibers are characterized by 2–6 μm diameters, are myelinated and present a relatively fast conduction speed between 5 and 30 m/s. The central branch of these fibers reaches the superficial laminae of the dorsal horn. These nociceptor fibers allow the conduction of cold, pressure and heat signals [5].

Remarkably, C-fibers are the ones to mainly establish nociceptive innervation. These are unmyelinated axons with a diameter of 0.4 to 1.2 μm and a conduction speed between 0.5 and 2 m/s. C-fibers innervate laminae I and II of the dorsal horn

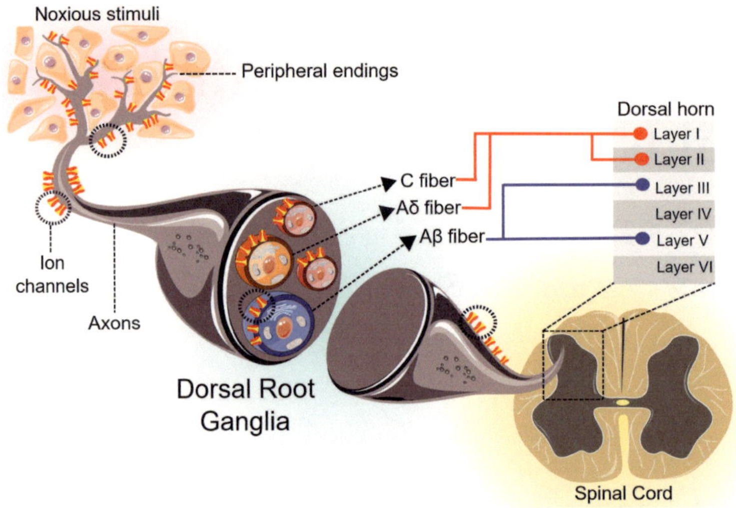

Figure 1.
Nociception. Harmful stimuli are transduced along the terminal axon of specialized pseudounipolar neurons (nociceptors), which are classified as unmyelinated C fibers (red) and thinly myelinated Aδ fibers (orange); myelinated Aβ fibers (blue) transduce innocuous stimuli. The cell bodies of these peripheral sensory neurons are located in the dorsal root ganglia and trigeminal ganglia. Nociceptors innervate the epidermis and viscera, transducing noxious stimuli through the activation of several ion channels such as members of the TRP family. Finally, the information is transmitted to second order neurons located in the dorsal horn: C fibers and Aδ fibers mainly establish contact with neurons from layers I and II, while tactile Aβ fibers end mainly in layers III and V.

of the spinal cord and are activated in a polymodal fashion by mechanical, thermal (noxious cold or heat) and chemical stimuli [4, 5].

Diverse injurious stimuli detected by nociceptors are transformed into electrical activity, a process known as transduction where thermal, mechanical, or chemical signals are converted into ion flux through the activation of specialized ion channels [1]. In this way, noxious signals trigger fluctuations in the electrochemical gradient of nociceptors leading to membrane depolarization and subsequent action potentials, as a direct consequence of changes in the activation of ion channels expressed in the nociceptors [6]. Action potentials reach second-order neurons housed in the superficial laminae of the dorsal horn that project towards the spinothalamic and/or spinoparabrachial tracts contributing to the perception of noxious stimuli [2, 3, 7].

The study of the impact of sex steroids on the processing of noxious stimuli has been relevant to our understanding of the underlying differences between females and males. In the last decades, growing evidence related to sexual dimorphism in the perception of harmful signals and the development of pain conditions has been highlighted [8]. Several studies in humans using mechanical, chemical, electrical, or thermal stimuli have suggested that women have more sensitivity to some noxious stimuli than men [8–11]. However, other contrasting reports have concluded that there is no difference in nociception between genders [12, 13]. Even though these differences are still not clear, the most reasonable explanation pinpoints sex steroids as the most relevant effectors. For example, some conditions such as headache, back and temporomandibular pain increase with pubertal development in girls, where the gonadal steroids produce crucial changes in women physiology [14]. Remarkably, differences in the perception of thermal stimuli between different sexes have also been reported, suggesting that women have greater sensitivity to heat than men [15]. In relation to this, an epidemiological study indicated that low testosterone concentrations in women are associated with an increase in the sensation of cold [16], clearly suggesting that steroids influence nociception.

2. Nociceptive TRP channels

The functional properties of nociceptors are critically regulated by the activity of ion channels expressed in their plasma membrane. Some of these channels belong to the Transient Receptor Potential (TRP) family that play vital roles as detectors of a wide range of biological signals. Some TRP channels are crucial receptors within nociceptors since they function as molecular machinery to transduce several noxious sensory stimuli [17].

In mammals, the TRP family consists of 27 members grouped into 6 subfamilies based on their sequence homology as follows: TRPC (canonical), TRPV (vanilloid), TRPM (melastatin), TRPP (polycystin), TRPML (mucolipin) and TRPA (ankyrin) subfamilies. A seventh group is the TRPN (no mechanoreceptor) subfamily which is not found in mammals, although it is found in the fruit fly, in *C. elegans* and zebrafish [18]. These receptors are nonselective cation channels that show an overall tetrameric structure, with each monomer being a six-pass transmembrane (S1-S6) protein with a hydrophilic re-entrant loop between the last two transmembrane segments that give rise to the ion conduction pore in the tetrameric arrangement, **Figure 2**. These channels have cytosolic N- and C- termini which are highly variable between the different members of the TRP subfamilies [19].

Some TRP channels are expressed in nociceptors where they display essential roles in the transduction of several noxious stimuli. Among these nociceptive TRP channels are TRPA1, TRPV1–4, TRPM2–3 and TRPM8 [17] which are activated by noxious thermal, chemical and mechanical signals and hence they are important pain-mediators, **Table 1**.

The **TRPA1 channel**, originally described as a cold sensor [20], is activated by several external compounds such as isothiocyanates contained in natural products such as wasabi, horseradish and mustard oil. Other natural TRPA1 activators are allicin and cinnamaldehyde, compounds found in garlic and cinnamon, respectively, and acrolein is also an exogenously-found compound that activates this ion channel [21–24]. TRPA1's activation by temperature in humans is still controversial, since some reports have described that TRPA1 is an insensitive cold-channel [23, 24],

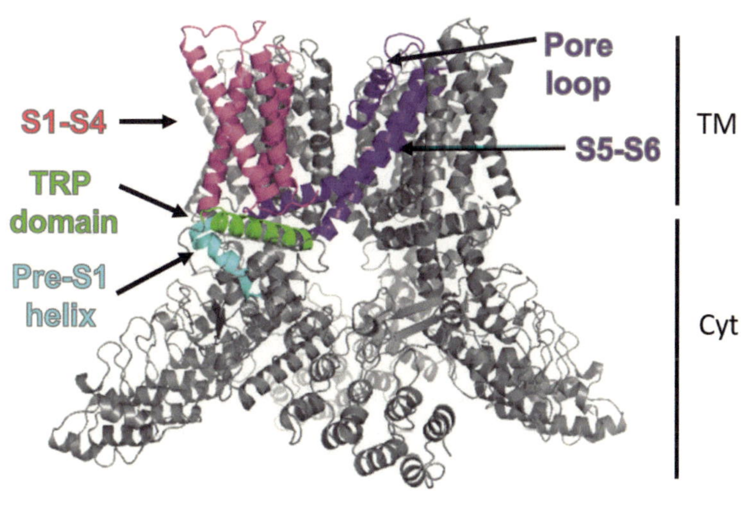

Figure 2.
Overall 3D-structure of a TRP channel. Tetrameric assemble for TRP channels. The colored domains represent conserved domains in these channels: Transmembrane domain (S1-S6); the re-entrant loop forms the ion conduction pore; the pre-S1 helix joins the N-terminal to the S1; TRP box localized in the C-terminus. TM and Cyt: transmembrane and cytosolic regions. (TRPV1 3D- structure, PDB: 3J5P).

Receptor	Temperature	Physical Stimulus	Natural Compounds	Endogenously-produced Compounds
TRPA1	<17°C and noxious heat	Stretch	Allicin, Cinnamaldehyde, Allylisothiocyanate	Androstenedione Lysophosphatidic acid
TRPV1	≥42°C	Osmolality (hyper) Stretch	Capsaicin, Allicin, Resiniferatoxin, Tetrahydrocannabinol	N-arachidonoyl dopamine, Protons Lysophosphatidic acid Arachidonic acid and lipoxygenase-derived products, Anandamide
TRPV2	≥52°C	Osmolality (hypo), Stretch, Shear stress	Cannabidiol	_
TRPV3	30–39°C	_	Camphor, Gingerol, Zingerone, Carvacrol, Eugenol, Thymol	Farnesyl pyrophospahate
TRPV4	30–43°C	Osmolality (hypo), Shear stress	Bisandrographolide A	5,6-epoxyeicosatrienoic acid
TRPM2	>35°C	_	_	Adenosine diphosphate ribose, H_2O_2
TRPM3	≥40°C	Osmolality (hypo)	—	Pregnenolone sulfate
TRPM8	10–28°C		Menthol, Eucalyptol	Artemin, Testosterone

Table 1.
Nociceptive TRP channels and their main activators.

while several experiments have strengthened its role as a cold sensor [21, 25–27]. Furthermore, it has also been reported that TRPA1 channel has a redundant role as a noxious heat sensor in the mouse [28]. Indeed, this channel is also indirectly activated by inflammatory mediators like bradykinins and directly by lysophosphatidic acid (LPA, a compound released during injury tissue) and some reactive species produced as the 4-hydroxynonenal [24, 29, 30]. Thus, TRPA1 activation by these endogenous mediators produces inflammatory pain.

Among nociceptive TRP channels some members of the **vanilloid receptors** (i.e., TRPV1–4 channels) are also included. They are activated by warm (TRPV3-V4) to noxious heat (TRPV1-V2) and by several chemical compounds and osmotic changes.

The most studied channel of the vanilloid subfamily is the **TRPV1 channel**, originally described as the capsaicin receptor, since it is specifically activated by this pungent compound found in chili peppers [31]. This channel is also activated by compounds such as allicin, resiniferatoxin (a toxin found in the cactus-like plant *Euphorbia resinifera*) and by animal toxins such as the double-knot (a peptide toxin from the Earth Tiger tarantula), among others [31–33]. Additionally, several reports have demonstrated that TRPV1 activation is achieved by extracellular acid and intracellular basic pHs and heat (≥42°C) [31]. Furthermore, TRPV1 activation is produced by diverse compounds released during inflammation and tissue injury, for example, some arachidonic acid- and lipoxygenase-derived products, LPA and anandamide [34–36]. The high expression of the TRPV1 channel in small and medium-diameter neurons and its polymodal activation through several endogenous noxious stimuli, highlight it as a portal to pain; thus, the understanding of its regulation is a promising field to develop new strategies in the research field of pain and analgesia.

The vanilloid subfamily contains two less studied than TRPV1 members: **TRPV2 and TRPV3** channels. The former is expressed in medium- and large DRG neurons, activated by temperatures with a threshold of 52°C [37] and by mechanical stretch and osmotic swelling [38]; exogenous compounds like some cannabinoids and endogenous lipids as lysophosphatidyl choline are also TRPV2 activators [39, 40]. Interestingly, the key role of TRPV2 as a noxious sensor is related to mechanical nociception in the somatosensory system, where it is required for the detection of noxious mechanical stimuli [41].

The TRPV3 channel is expressed in keratinocytes and co-expressed with TRPV1 channels in small-diameter sensory neurons. This channel is activated by temperatures between 30 and 39°C [42, 43] and camphor and cannabidiol are exogenous compounds that are also TRPV3 activators [44, 45]. Interestingly, it has been reported that polymorphisms found in the human *TRPV2* and *TRPV3* genes are associated to the susceptibility and severity to fibromyalgia, suggesting the role of these channels in chronic pain disorders [46].

The other vanilloid receptor playing a nociceptive role is the **TRPV4 channel**. This channel is activated by warm temperatures (~30–43°C) and hypotonicity [47–49]. Among the endogenous compounds that are TRPV4 activators are some derivates of arachidonic acid [50, 51]. Interestingly, this ion channel transduces osmotic stimuli inducing nociception and it is also an important mediator of the pruritogens effects of some compounds like serotonin [52, 53].

Finally, another TRP channels important to nociception are some members of the TRPM subfamily: TRPM2-M3 and TRPM8 channels. Although the **TRPM2 channel** is mainly expressed in immune cells, some expression has also been detected in neurons from DRG and TG [54, 55]. The TRPM2 channel is a warm thermo-sensor, since it is activated at 35°C [56]; other activators for this channel are adenosine 5′-diphosphoribose (ADPR) and H_2O_2 [57, 58]. The activation of this channel through the generation of reactive species (ROS) implicates it as an important mediator of pain perception during stress oxidative conditions, that prevail in some conditions as fibromyalgia and neuropathy diabetic [59, 60].

The **TRPM3 channel**, initially identified in β-pancreatic cells [61] has an important role as a sensor of noxious heat, since it is activated by temperatures ≥40°C [62]. The activation of this channel can modulate glucose-induced insulin secretion and also nociception [61, 62]. Its role in the latter is due to high expression in small-diameter sensory neurons from DRG and TG [62] where it also serves as a sensor of noxious chemical stimuli to produce painful responses [62, 63]. Remarkably, TRPM3 together with TRPA1 and TRPV1 channels, form a redundant trio of sensors that mediates noxious heat transduction and provide protection against burn damage [28].

The group of nociceptive TRP channels also comprises the **TRPM8 channel**, a cold-transducer receptor (10–28°C) which is activated by natural compounds as menthol [64, 65]. This ion channel is predominantly expressed in a subpopulation of small-diameter sensory neurons lacking TRPV1 expression [64, 65]. TRPM8 overactivation is related to cold allodynia and hypersensitivity, pain caused by an innocuous cold stimulus and pain produce by enhanced sensitivity to cold stimulus, respectively [66, 67]. Similarly, to other TRP channels, some endogenous compounds such as artemin induces pain through TRPM8 activation [66]. Curiously, a steroid such as testosterone directly binds to this channel and induces its activation [68].

Clearly, the activation of these nociceptive channels is closely related to acute or chronic pain development and interestingly, some of these channels are targets for sex steroids actions, as we will describe here.

2.1 Estrogens and nociceptive TRP channels

Estrogens influence sexual differentiation in women and they have other essential functions in different biological processes as regulators of the cardiovascular system, metabolism, bone resorption and neuronal physiology [69]. These sex steroids comprise estrone (E1) and 17β estradiol (E2) and estriol (E3) [70]. Similarly, to other steroids, these estrogen's actions are exerted by their interaction with specific nuclear receptors, the estrogen receptors alpha and beta (ERα and ERβ) that act as transcription factors to trigger gene regulation through a classical genomic pathway [71]. Furthermore, their actions also are through the activation of a membrane localized receptor, the G Protein-Coupled Estrogen Receptor 1 or GPER1 (previously named GPR30), establishing a non-classical pathway to regulate molecular targets [72, 73]. Several reports have suggested that estrogens influence some painful conditions like fibromyalgia, migraine, irritable bowel syndrome and temporomandibular disorder, all of which are conditions with major prevalence in women than in men [74–78].

Indeed, several experiments made in pain animal models have demonstrated the existence of sexual dimorphism in response to pain. For example, rats from a diabetic neuropathy model exhibited lower mechanical pain thresholds than males. This difference was abolished in gonadectomized animals, highlighting the sex-related differences in diabetic hypersensitivity [79].

These differences could be attributed to estrogen actions on different targets implicated in the transduction of noxious stimuli such as TRP channels, as will be described below.

A close relationship between estrogens and the TRPV1 channel has been demonstrated by several reports. Initially, it was stablished through behavioral assays that female rats exhibited increased capsaicin pain-related responses as compared to males. Furthermore, ovariectomized rats increased their pain threshold to capsaicin, which was reverted by replacement with E2 in these ovariectomized rats [80]. E2 effects on the TRPV1 nociception have also been evaluated during the rat estrous cycle, where the rats in the proestrus phase showed higher capsaicin-pain responses than the rats in estrus. This observation suggested that high E2 levels exhibited in the proestrus, positively regulate pain associated to TRPV1 activation [80]. These results have also been obtained evaluating the mechanical and thermal pain threshold during the mice estrous cycle, showing that mice in the proestrus displayed lower pain thresholds than the mice in estrus [81]. Remarkably, female TRPV1 knockout mice exhibited comparable mechanical and thermal pain thresholds during the proestrus and estrus [81], strongly suggesting that this channel has a pivotal role in the transduction of these noxious stimuli and that its activation is regulated by estrogen levels. A partial molecular mechanism through which estrogens regulate the capsaicin-evoked pain has been described. Initially, it was suggested that TRPV1 protein levels are downregulated in the DRG from the ERα and ERβ knockout mice-model [82], indicating that this ion channel is a molecular target for the effects of estrogen receptors, **Figure 3**. Furthermore, several reports have evidenced that TRPV1 mRNA levels are upregulated by E2. For example, primary cell cultures of rat TG or mice DRG neurons treated with E2 displayed increases in TRPV1 mRNA levels [81, 83]. This TRPV1 mRNA upregulation has also been observed in the hippocampus from ovariectomized rats treated with E2, heightening the allodynia displayed in a rat inflammatory temporomandibular model [84].

The upregulation on TRPV1 gene expression has been also evidenced in synoviocytes, osteoclast precursors and endometrium [85–87]. Furthermore, experiments performed in cultures of human sensory neurons treated with E2 have shown increases in TRPV1 mRNA levels and similar results were obtained when

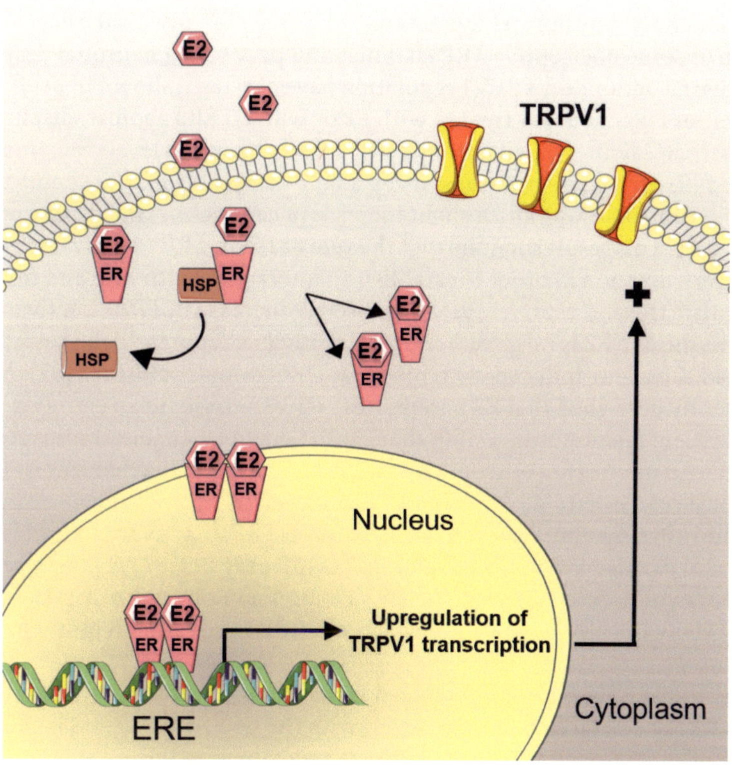

Figure 3.
Schematic representation of the estrogen classical genomic effect in the regulation of TRPV1 gene expression. The inactive estrogen receptors (ER) localized in the cytoplasm form a protein complex with the heat shock protein (HSP). Internalized 17β estradiol (E2) interacts with the ER, activating and targeting them to the nucleus where they recognize the estrogen response element (ERE), a specific sequence located in the target genes (i.e., TRPV1 gene), resulting in positive regulation of TRPV1 expression.

the sensory neurons were incubated with a specific agonist of the ERβ [81, 88]. The E2-dependent effects in the aforementioned cell systems were observed after 24 h of treatment, suggesting that E2 achieves its actions through the classical genomic pathway. This possibility is strengthened by the identification of a putative estrogen response element (ERE) located in the promoter region of the mouse *Trpv1* gene, implying that ERα could interact with this gene regulatory sequence to control TRPV1 gene transcription [89], **Figure 3**. These ERα bindings sites were also identified in the promoter sequences of the *Trpv3–6* genes pointing out that estrogens are regulators of the transcription of these genes [89]. Additionally, it has been determined that different areas of the brains of mice in the proestrus (where the estrogens levels are high) display augmented mRNA levels for the *Trpv2*, *v4* and *v6* genes [89]. In contrast, this report also showed that TRPV1 and TRPV5 mRNA levels are downregulated in the brain from mice in the proestrus [89].

Additionally, negative E2 effects on TRPV1 activation have been evidenced in ovariectomized rats, which displayed reduced production of gonadal estrogens and augmented neuronal mitochondrial oxidative stress [90]. This was demonstrated using primary cultures of hippocampal and DRG neurons from these rats, determining that the current densities produced through TRPV1 activation are augmented. A similar effect was observed for the TRPA1 and TRPM2 currents [90];

consequently, overactivation of these channels caused rises in cytosolic Ca^{2+} and triggered apoptotic dead of these neurons. These effects were prevented in cultures of neurons derived from ovariectomized rats treated with E2 suggesting that this steroid could have neuroprotective actions, avoiding Ca^{2+} overload caused by the activation of some nociceptive TRP channels and preventing neuronal death [90].

Negative E2 actions on TRPV1 regulation have also been shown in primary cultures of rat DRG neurons treated with E2 or with an ERβ agonist, displaying decreases in capsaicin-evoked currents while TRPV1 protein levels remained unchanged [91]. This effect was lost using a non-permeable E2 (E2 conjugated to bovine serum albumin) and a slight increase in capsaicin-evoked currents was observed [91]. This result suggests that the role of E2 on TRPV1 activation requires steroid internalization in order to establish an interaction with ERβ and to negatively regulate this ion channel [91]. The discrete increase in TRPV1 activation using the non-permeable E2 is in agreement with a previous report which showed that E2 potentiated capsaicin-induced currents in rat DRG primary cultures [92]. Moreover, it was recently described that E2 potentiates TRPV1 activity in an estrogen receptor independent fashion, suggesting that TRPV1 could be an ionotropic receptor for E2 [93]. An interesting outcome from these experimental evidences is that the changes observed in TRPV1 expression are achieved using low E2 concentrations (10–100 nM) [81, 83, 88]; however, the effects on TRPV1 activation need supraphysiological concentrations of the steroid (1–100 μM) [93, 94]. This suggests that low E2 concentrations could modify TRPV1 expression through a classical genomic pathway, whereas a non-classical E2 effect on TRPV1 activation requires high E2 concentrations.

Non-classical E2 actions are produced faster than the genomic effects and are mediated by the interaction of this steroid with the GPER1 [72, 73]. The interaction of E2 with this receptor triggers different signaling pathways, such as those of protein kinase A (PKA) and C (PKC) [72, 95], which could produce TRPV1 phosphorylation. The phosphorylated state of the channel decreases its activation threshold to several stimuli, a process known as sensitization [96]. For instance, a phosphorylated TRPV1 channel can be activated at innocuous heat (i.e., 37°C) [96, 97]. TRPV1 phosphorylation also regulates the channel's interaction with proteins like tubulin [98, 99], a protein association that is important to mediate mechanical gating of TRPV1 [100]. Interruption of the tubulin-TRPV1 complex through the TRPV1 phosphorylation on serine 800 (S800), decreases TRPV1 activation through osmotic stimuli [99, 100]. Interestingly, E2 through its association with GPER1, triggers the activation of PKCε signaling resulting in phosphorylation of TRPV1 in S800 and blocking the interaction of the channel with tubulin [99]; thus, E2 modifies microtubule-dependent TRPV1 mechanical pain sensitization.

The above data exemplify how TRPV1 is a target of classical and non-classical effects of estrogens, highlighting the estrogenic influence on nociception and pain mediated through the TRPV1 channel.

2.1.1 Estrogens upregulate TRPA1 and TRPV1 expression in endometriosis

Endometriosis is a debilitating chronic pelvic pain where the lining layer of the endometrium grows out of the uterus. This condition is highly estrogen-dependent and the lesion displays innervation of nociceptors co-expressing the TRPV1 and TRPA1 channels [101, 102]. Interestingly, mRNA levels for TRPA1 and TRPV1 are upregulated in the biopsies from women with endometriosis [88], thus it is feasible to consider that the overexpression of these channels could mediate the pain produced in this condition. The overexpression of these channels is likely to be through actions of estrogens, since they play a crucial role in the development of this anomalous pelvic condition. Particularly, it has been demonstrated that female rats treated with diethylstilbestrol, a non-selective estrogen receptor agonist, exhibited upregulation in the TRPV1 and TRPA1 mRNA levels [86] and this expression was found in endometrial cells. Moreover, cultured primary endometrial cells treated with this non-selective agonist also displayed increased TRPA1 and TRPV1 mRNA levels, whereas the treatment with E2 (which is a highly selective agonist of the ERα) only induced the upregulation of the TRPV1 mRNA levels [86]. The data suggests that these nociceptive TRP channels are regulated by the classical effects of estrogen receptors; additionally, these results showed the expression of these channels in non-neuronal cells from the rat endometria. TRPA1 and TRPV1 gene expression also has been demonstrated in human endometria from healthy women; furthermore, endometria samples from women suffering deep infiltrating endometriosis (one of the most severe forms of this condition) exhibit higher TRPV1 and TRPA1 expression, as compared to healthy women [103].

Additionally, it has been reported that hydroxylated estrogens (catechol estrogens) directly activate the TRPA1 channel [104]. This was evidenced using TRPA1-expressing HEK293 cells and whole-cell patch-clamp recordings that showed that 2-hydroxy-estrone (a catechol-estrogen) evoked currents through activation of TRPA1, similarly to another agonist for this channel, cinnamaldehyde. Thus, this hydroxylated estrogen acts as an endogenous agonist for this nociceptive channel [104]. Although, the physiological role of this activation has been demonstrated for insulin secretion in β-pancreatic cells, it would be interesting to explore if the excessive production of catechol-estrogens in endometriosis (as it has been previously reported [105]) affects the function of the TRPA1 channel expressed in endometrial cells and in the free nerve terminals surrounding this area. The expression of these channels in endometrial cells could represent a therapeutic alternative to relieve the main symptoms related to this painful condition; thus, it would be relevant to deepen the studies about the functional roles of TRP channels in these non-neuronal cells.

In addition to the above described evidence, the roles of TRPA1 and TRPV1 in endometriosis have been recently strengthened through the establishment of a mouse endometriosis model [106]. The endometriosis-like lesions induced in these animals displayed the presence of nerve fibers and inflammatory cells around the lesions. Remarkably, theses nerve fibers showed expression of TRPA1 and TRPV1 channels [106]. Furthermore, DRG neurons isolated from mice with induced endometriosis exhibited higher Ca^{2+} influx levels than neurons from sham animals, and this effect was through the activation of TRPA1 or TRPV1 channels [106]. The upregulation of these nociceptive channels could be directly associated with spontaneous abdominal pain observed in mice with endometriosis. Interestingly, the treatment of these mice with a synthetic androgen (danazol) or an aromatase inhibitor (letrozole), which are estrogen reducing agents, substantially relieved the spontaneously induced endometriosis pain [106]. These data reinforce the crucial role of estrogens in the development of endometriosis and highlight the importance of the TRPA1 and TRPV1 channels as molecular pain mediators in this debilitating form of abdominal pain.

2.2 Nociceptive TRP channels that are targeted by androgen actions

Androgens are steroids that influence the development of male characteristics and they are produced in the gonads (testicles and ovaries) and adrenal glands [107]. The main endogenously produced androgens are testosterone, androstenedione, dehydroepiandrosterone (DHEA) and dihydrotestosterone (DHT) [108]. Similarly, to other steroids, testosterone and DHT act as ligands for a specific protein, such as the androgen receptor (AR), while other androgens are weak ligands of the AR. This receptor regulates the expression of several target genes through a classical genomic pathway; furthermore, AR modifies cell physiology through non-classical and non-genomic effects [109].

Indeed, some androgens produce fast- non-genomic effects by interacting with other proteins like some TRP channels and modulating their function. For example, through whole-cell recording electrophysiological experiments, DHEA was shown to decrease capsaicin-dependent currents in dissociated DRG neurons [110]. DHEA effects seem to be direct and specific on TRPV1 channel activation, since with the use of a DHEA stereoisomer the inhibition of channel activation was no longer observed. Additionally, testosterone reduced the activation of TRPV1 to a lesser extent than DHEA [110]. This suggested the presence of a DHEA-binding site in the TRPV1 channel, which should be extracellularly localized, since the steroid was applied to the surface of the neurons during the electrophysiological recordings [110]. However, this remains undetermined and it is possible that DHEA has an antinociceptive role by inhibiting this channel.

The above data exemplified the rapid non-genomic effects of DHEA on TRPV1 activation. Additionally, testosterone seems to negatively regulate the expression of this channel, suggesting that TRPV1 is also a target for the classical actions of androgens. Supporting evidence for this was obtained in dissected TG from castrated male rats with orofacial myositis (induced by the Complete Freund's adjuvant) [111]. The trigeminal TRPV1 mRNA and protein levels from this rat model were upregulated. Interestingly, TRPV1 expression is unaffected in the TG from castrated rats subjected to testosterone replacement [111], suggesting that testosterone prevents the increase in TRPV1 expression, although the molecular mechanism for this regulation is still unknown.

The TRPA1 channel is another molecular target for the non-classical effects of androgens. As a first approach, it was demonstrated that synthetic aromatase inhibitors evoked currents through TRPA1 channels in isolated DRG neurons; however, these compounds were unable to produce currents in DRG neurons from TRPA1 knockout mice, suggesting specific actions of the aromatase inhibitors on the activation of this channel [112]. Indeed, it was demonstrated that the aromatase inhibitors produced pain-like behavior in mice, a conduct not displayed in the TRPA1 knockout mice [112]. Since these compounds increase the levels of androstenedione in plasma, the effects of this androgen on TRPA1 activation have also been studied [113]. The results showed that androstenedione produces currents in mouse DRG neurons that are partially dependent on TRPA1 activation [113]. Furthermore, remanent androstenedione currents were abolished in the presence of the TRPV1 antagonist capsazepine, suggesting that this androgen could activate nociceptive TRPA1 and TRPV1 channels. Although, androstenedione is unable to cause acute pain-like behavior in mice, the animals exhibited mechanical allodynia 30 to 120 min after its intradermal injection into their paws, an effect that was abolished with a TRPA1 antagonist [113]. These data indicate that androstenedione could act as a pain sensitizing molecule leading to the activation of TRPA1.

Finally, the TRPM8 channel is also regulated by androgens. Interestingly, this channel is a target for the classical and nonclassical actions of testosterone. Initial evidence showed that TRPM8 is an androgen-responsive gene since testosterone treatment in some prostate cancer cell lines produced upregulation in the TRPM8 mRNA levels [114, 115]. TRPM8 expression also increases in the urogenital tract from orchiectomized rats supplemented with testosterone, suggesting that this steroid positively regulates TRPM8 gene expression [116]. Bioinformatic gene analysis showed that the TRPM8 gene contains putative sites for the androgen receptor interaction (androgen response elements, ARE) in its promoter sequence. Through chromatin-immunoprecipitation assays, it was confirmed that androgens receptors bind to these AREs located near the start transcription site of the TRPM8 gene [117]. These data indicated that androgens regulate TRPM8 gene expression in a classical genomic fashion.

The TRPM8 channel also acts as an ionotropic testosterone receptor due to direct interaction with this ion channel, resulting in its activation [68, 118]. Experiments have shown that the TRPM8 channel and the androgen receptor compete for testosterone and dihydrotestosterone because activation of TRPM8 by these androgens is lost when both receptors are co-expressed [68]. An extracellularly-located testosterone binding site in the TRPM8 channel has been suggested [68], and by using molecular docking simulation we have identified an additional intracellular testosterone pocket located between the firts intracellular loop (pre-S1) and the transmembrane segments 1 and 2 (S1-S2) of the TRPM8 protein [119]. This analysis has also shown that an H-bond is formed between testosterone and an arginine located in the TRP box, similar to the H-bond established between testosterone and an arginine in the aromatase enzyme [119]. The similarity in the testosterone pockets of the aromatase and the TRPM8 proteins could suggest that this is a functional binding site for TRPM8 through which activation by this steroid could be achieved in a non-classical and fast fashion. Interestingly, it has been demonstrated that topic testosterone application on humans produced cold- and pain-sensation; the women resulted more sensitized to the testosterone effects than men [68], suggesting a sexual dimorphism in testosterone-produced nociception through TRPM8 activation.

A third non-classical mechanism for TRPM8 regulation by testosterone has been demonstrated in DRG neurons where the androgen receptor and TRPM8 channels form a protein complex in the plasma membrane [120]. High testosterone concentrations (100 nM) inhibit TRPM8 channel activation and the androgen receptor is translocated to the nucleus [120], **Figure 4**. The evaluation of the TRPM8-mediated cold perception performed in castrated mice or rats revealed a decrease in their threshold for mild-cold perception; interestingly, testosterone

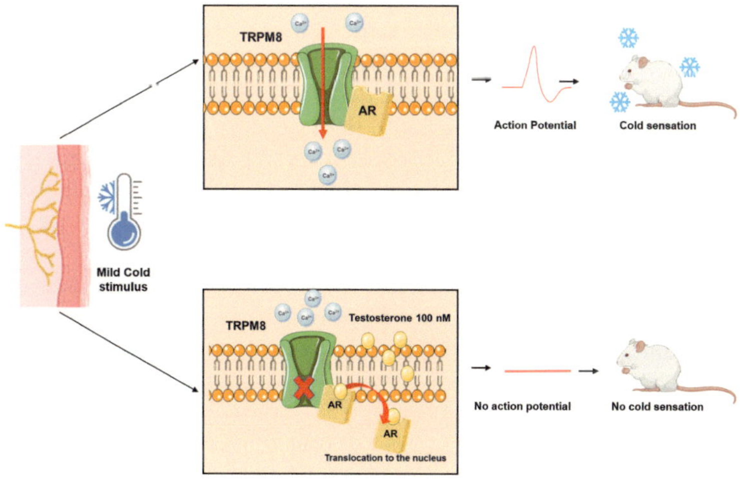

Figure 4.
Testosterone regulates the TRPM8-mediated mild-cold sensitivity. The mild-cold stimulus is transduced through the TRPM8 channel located in the cell surface of DRG neurons where it forms a protein complex with the androgen receptor (AR) (upper panel). A high concentration of testosterone (100 nM) decreases activation of the TRPM8 channel and produces translocation of the AR to the nucleus. The physiological consequence of this is the loss of the mild cold sensation (lower panel).

supplementation in these animals inhibited cold perception (temperatures between 16 and 18°C) [120]. This result would suggest that testosterone confers endurance to TRPM8-mediated mild cold perception, which could explain the underlying molecular mechanism for the cold sensation experienced by women presenting lower levels of testosterone [16].

2.3 Progesterone downregulates TRPV1 and TRPV4 channels expression

Progesterone is a steroid indispensable to the maintenance of pregnancy and it also plays important roles in the cardiovascular, immune, nervous systems and in the bones [121]. Progesterone is produced by the granulosa cells and the corpus luteum in the ovaries and, during pregnancy, the placenta is the major source of this steroid. Additionally, progesterone is produced in the nervous system, adrenal glands and testes [122]. The effects of progesterone are produced through nuclear receptors A and B (PRA/B), activating the classical genomic pathway to regulate gene expression. Furthermore, this steroid exerts a non-classical pathway through the activation of several membrane receptors (mPR) and other receptors as the progesterone receptor membrane components 1 and 2 (PGRMC1/2) and by the Sigma-1 Receptor (Sig-1R) [123, 124].

It has been demonstrated that progesterone regulates the expression of some TRP channels; for example, TRPV4 gene expression is negatively regulated by classical genomic progesterone effects [125]. Initial evidence for this was observed in epithelial and vascular cell lines and a recent report showed a correlation between TRPV4 expression and progesterone levels during the menstrual cycle, demonstrating that during the luteal phase when progesterone reaches its highest levels, TRPV4 expression is downregulated in human endometrial biopsies [126]. Furthermore, it has also been reported that TRPV4 expression is downregulated by a synthetic progestin (levonorgestrel) in a human Fallopian tubal epithelial cell line and mouse oviducts which could affect the transport of fertilized oocytes causing ectopic pregnancy [127].

Our group has determined that progesterone impacts on nociception by regulating the expression of TRPV1 channels [128]. Interestingly, this regulation is through a non-classical mechanism that requires an intermediate protein, the Sig-1R, which is a dynamic chaperone mainly localized in the endoplasmic reticulum and that can also be mobilized to the plasma membrane and nuclear envelope [129]. Progesterone decreases the levels of channels localized in the cell surface in HEK293 cells transfected with TRPV1 cDNA [128]. But how does progesterone produce this effect? Our results have shown that this is achieved by disrupting a protein complex formed between TRPV1 channels and the Sig-1R and by affecting the proper folding of TRPV1. Consequently, the channels are degraded by the proteasomal pathway and capsaicin-evoked currents are reduced [128]. The TRPV1 downregulation through progesterone actions was also observed in primary cultures of DRG neurons and we also demonstrated that during mice pregnancy when there are high progesterone levels, the threshold to capsaicin-dependent pain-like behaviors are augmented in comparison to non-pregnant mice, suggesting that progesterone confers protection to pain produced through activation of TRPV1 [128]. This work exemplified the antinociceptive actions that progesterone exerts through the decrease in the levels of TRPV1 channels localized in the plasma membrane of nociceptors and by the reduction of the transduction of harmful signals through this ion channel. Moreover, it has also been reported that progesterone disrupts the protein complex formed between Sig-1R and the TRPA1 and TRPM8 channels [130], suggesting that this steroid could impact the nociception through these nociceptive TRP channels.

3. Conclusion

Nociception is a neuronal process that protects against injurious stimuli that can be endogenously produced during inflammation or tissue injury processes. The transduction of these signals requires the activation of ion channels such as some members of the TRP family. In this chapter we have described how sex steroids influence nociception by regulating some of the TRP channels important for this neuronal process. Here we have described the data showing that estrogens and their nuclear receptors (ERα/β) positively regulate the expression of the TRPV1 and TRPA1 genes through a classical genomic pathway. The reports above discussed also show that progesterone and its nuclear receptors (PRA/B) negatively regulate TRPV4 gene expression.

We have also compiled and discussed the evidence about androstenedione's and testosterone's non-classical effects in the regulation of the activation of TRPA1 and TRPM8 ion channels directly. We have suggested a testosterone binding-pocket in the TRPM8 channel and we have also pinpointed an androstenedione binding-pocket in the C-terminal and pre-S1 regions of TRPV1 and TRPA1 channels [119].

These observations strengthen the notion that androgens act as direct molecular regulators of some nociceptive ion channels function, playing dual roles as nociceptive and antinociceptive molecules. For example, androstenedione has nociceptive actions on TRPA1 and TRPV1 activation and testosterone at low concentrations (picomolar range) can produce cold sensation through the TRPM8 channel, while high testosterone levels could improve resilience to cold sensation inhibiting the currents through TRPM8. Finally, the literature here reviewed shows that the nonclassical sex steroid effects are mediated by membrane receptors or even chaperones such as the Sig-1R, affecting signaling pathways and/or protein stability. This last finding exemplifies the antinociceptive effects of progesterone by which this hormone reduces the transduction of noxious stimuli mediated by TRPV1 channel activation. These data open a research field in which we will deepen our knowledge in the role of molecular sexual dimorphism and the interplay between nociceptive TRP channels and sex steroids.

Acknowledgements

Funding: Este trabajo fue apoyado por el FORDECYT-PRONACES (FORDECYT-PRONACES/64392/2020) del Consejo Nacional de Ciencia y Tecnología. También recibió apoyo de la Dirección General de Asuntos del Personal Académico (DGAPA)-Programa de Apoyo a Proyectos de Investigación e Innovación Tecnológica (PAPIIT) IN206819 y de los Estímulos a Investigaciones Médicas Miguel Alemán Valdés.

Conflict of interest

The authors declare no conflict of interest.

Notes/thanks/other declarations

Ó.E.P and K.A.M.R contributed equally to this work. This work comprises the MSc thesis work of Ó.E.P. from the Programa de Maestría y Doctorado en Ciencias Bioquímicas at the Universidad Nacional Autónoma de México and the PhD thesis work of K.A.M.R. student from the Programa de Doctorado en Ciencias Biomédicas at the Universidad Nacional Autónoma de México. We thank Alejandra Llorente for her administrative support.

Author details

Óscar Enciso-Pablo, Karina Angélica Méndez-Reséndiz, Tamara Rosenbaum and Sara Luz Morales-Lázaro*
Department of Cognitive Neuroscience, Institute of Cellular Physiology, UNAM, México City, México

*Address all correspondence to: saraluzm@ifc.unam.mx

References

[1] Tracey, W.D., Jr. *Nociception.* Curr Biol. 2017. 27(4): p. R129-R133. 10.1016/j.cub.2017.01.037

[2] Basbaum, A.I., et al. *Cellular and molecular mechanisms of pain.* Cell. 2009. 139(2): p. 267-84. 10.1016/j.cell.2009.09.028

[3] Woolf, C.J. and Q. Ma. *Nociceptors--noxious stimulus detectors.* Neuron. 2007. 55(3): p. 353-64. 10.1016/j.neuron.2007.07.016

[4] Armstrong, S.A. and M.J. Herr, *Physiology, Nociception*, in *StatPearls*. 2020: Treasure Island (FL).

[5] Dubin, A.E. and A. Patapoutian. *Nociceptors: the sensors of the pain pathway.* J Clin Invest. 2010. 120(11): p. 3760-72. 10.1172/JCI42843

[6] Waxman, S.G. and G.W. Zamponi. *Regulating excitability of peripheral afferents: emerging ion channel targets.* Nat Neurosci. 2014. 17(2): p. 153-63. 10.1038/nn.3602

[7] Todd, A.J. *Neuronal circuitry for pain processing in the dorsal horn.* Nat Rev Neurosci. 2010. 11(12): p. 823-36. 10.1038/nrn2947

[8] Fillingim, R.B., et al. *Sex, gender, and pain: a review of recent clinical and experimental findings.* J Pain. 2009. 10(5): p. 447-85. 10.1016/j.jpain.2008.12.001

[9] Bartley, E.J. and R.B. Fillingim. *Sex differences in pain: a brief review of clinical and experimental findings.* Br J Anaesth. 2013. 111(1): p. 52-8. 10.1093/bja/aet127

[10] Cairns, B.E. *The influence of gender and sex steroids on craniofacial nociception.* Headache. 2007. 47(2): p. 319-24. 10.1111/j.1526-4610.2006.00708.x

[11] Hashmi, J.A. and K.D. Davis. *Deconstructing sex differences in pain sensitivity.* Pain. 2014. 155(1): p. 10-3. 10.1016/j.pain.2013.07.039

[12] Racine, M., et al. *A systematic literature review of 10 years of research on sex/gender and experimental pain perception - part 1: are there really differences between women and men?* Pain. 2012. 153(3): p. 602-18. 10.1016/j.pain.2011.11.025

[13] Racine, M., et al. *A systematic literature review of 10 years of research on sex/gender and pain perception - part 2: do biopsychosocial factors alter pain sensitivity differently in women and men?* Pain. 2012. 153(3): p. 619-35. 10.1016/j.pain.2011.11.026

[14] LeResche, L., et al. *Relationship of pain and symptoms to pubertal development in adolescents.* Pain. 2005. 118(1-2): p. 201-9. 10.1016/j.pain.2005.08.011

[15] Lue, Y.J., et al. *Thermal pain tolerance and pain rating in normal subjects: Gender and age effects.* Eur J Pain. 2018. 22(6): p. 1035-1042. 10.1002/ejp.1188

[16] Gotmar, A., et al. *Symptoms in peri- and postmenopausal women in relation to testosterone concentrations: data from The Women's Health in the Lund Area (WHILA) study.* Climacteric. 2008. 11(4): p. 304-14. 10.1080/13697130802249769

[17] Mickle, A.D., A.J. Shepherd, and D.P. Mohapatra. *Sensory TRP channels: the key transducers of nociception and pain.* Prog Mol Biol Transl Sci. 2015. 131: p. 73-118. 10.1016/bs.pmbts.2015.01.002

[18] Clapham, D.E., L.W. Runnels, and C. Strubing. *The TRP ion channel family.* Nat Rev Neurosci. 2001. 2(6): p. 387-96. 10.1038/35077544

[19] Rosasco, M.G. and S.E. Gordon, *TRP Channels: What Do They Look Like?*, in *Neurobiology of TRP Channels*, T.L.R. Emir, Editor. 2017: Boca Raton (FL). p. 1-9.

[20] Story, G.M., et al. *ANKTM1, a TRP-like channel expressed in nociceptive neurons, is activated by cold temperatures.* Cell. 2003. 112(6): p. 819-29. 10.1016/s0092-8674(03)00158-2

[21] Bandell, M., et al. *Noxious cold ion channel TRPA1 is activated by pungent compounds and bradykinin.* Neuron. 2004. 41(6): p. 849-57. 10.1016/s0896-6273(04)00150-3

[22] Bautista, D.M., et al. *Pungent products from garlic activate the sensory ion channel TRPA1.* Proc Natl Acad Sci U S A. 2005. 102(34): p. 12248-52. 10.1073/pnas.0505356102

[23] Jordt, S.E., et al. *Mustard oils and cannabinoids excite sensory nerve fibres through the TRP channel ANKTM1.* Nature. 2004. 427(6971): p. 260-5. 10.1038/nature02282

[24] Bautista, D.M., et al. *TRPA1 mediates the inflammatory actions of environmental irritants and proalgesic agents.* Cell. 2006. 124(6): p. 1269-82. 10.1016/j.cell.2006.02.023

[25] Fajardo, O., et al. *TRPA1 channels mediate cold temperature sensing in mammalian vagal sensory neurons: pharmacological and genetic evidence.* J Neurosci. 2008. 28(31): p. 7863-75. 10.1523/JNEUROSCI.1696-08.2008

[26] Karashima, Y., et al. *TRPA1 acts as a cold sensor in vitro and in vivo.* Proc Natl Acad Sci U S A. 2009. 106(4): p. 1273-8. 10.1073/pnas.0808487106

[27] Moparthi, L., et al. *Human TRPA1 is intrinsically cold- and chemosensitive with and without its N-terminal ankyrin repeat domain.* Proc Natl Acad Sci U S A. 2014. 111(47): p. 16901-6. 10.1073/pnas.1412689111

[28] Vandewauw, I., et al. *A TRP channel trio mediates acute noxious heat sensing.* Nature. 2018. 555(7698): p. 662-666. 10.1038/nature26137

[29] Trevisani, M., et al. *4-Hydroxynonenal, an endogenous aldehyde, causes pain and neurogenic inflammation through activation of the irritant receptor TRPA1.* Proc Natl Acad Sci U S A. 2007. 104(33): p. 13519-24. 10.1073/pnas.0705923104

[30] Kittaka, H., et al. *Lysophosphatidic acid-induced itch is mediated by signalling of LPA5 receptor, phospholipase D and TRPA1/TRPV1.* J Physiol. 2017. 595(8): p. 2681-2698. 10.1113/JP273961

[31] Caterina, M.J., et al. *The capsaicin receptor: a heat-activated ion channel in the pain pathway.* Nature. 1997. 389(6653): p. 816-24. 10.1038/39807

[32] Bohlen, C.J., et al. *A bivalent tarantula toxin activates the capsaicin receptor, TRPV1, by targeting the outer pore domain.* Cell. 2010. 141(5): p. 834-45. 10.1016/j.cell.2010.03.052

[33] Salazar, H., et al. *A single N-terminal cysteine in TRPV1 determines activation by pungent compounds from onion and garlic.* Nat Neurosci. 2008. 11(3): p. 255-61. 10.1038/nn2056

[34] Hwang, S.W., et al. *Direct activation of capsaicin receptors by products of lipoxygenases: endogenous capsaicin-like substances.* Proc Natl Acad Sci U S A. 2000. 97(11): p. 6155-60. 10.1073/pnas.97.11.6155

[35] Nieto-Posadas, A., et al. *Lysophosphatidic acid directly activates TRPV1 through a C-terminal binding site.* Nat Chem Biol. 2011. 8(1): p. 78-85. 10.1038/nchembio.712

[36] Zygmunt, P.M., et al. *Vanilloid receptors on sensory nerves mediate the vasodilator action of anandamide.* Nature. 1999. 400(6743): p. 452-7. 10.1038/22761

[37] Caterina, M.J., et al. *A capsaicin-receptor homologue with a high threshold for noxious heat.* Nature. 1999. 398(6726): p. 436-41. 10.1038/18906

[38] Muraki, K., et al. *TRPV2 is a component of osmotically sensitive cation channels in murine aortic myocytes.* Circ Res. 2003. 93(9): p. 829-38. 10.1161/01.RES.0000097263.10220.0C

[39] De Petrocellis, L., et al. *Effects of cannabinoids and cannabinoid-enriched Cannabis extracts on TRP channels and endocannabinoid metabolic enzymes.* Br J Pharmacol. 2011. 163(7): p. 1479-94. 10.1111/j.1476-5381.2010.01166.x

[40] Monet, M., et al. *Lysophospholipids stimulate prostate cancer cell migration via TRPV2 channel activation.* Biochim Biophys Acta. 2009. 1793(3): p. 528-39. 10.1016/j.bbamcr.2009.01.003

[41] Katanosaka, K., et al. *TRPV2 is required for mechanical nociception and the stretch-evoked response of primary sensory neurons.* Sci Rep. 2018. 8(1): p. 16782. 10.1038/s41598-018-35049-4

[42] Smith, G.D., et al. *TRPV3 is a temperature-sensitive vanilloid receptor-like protein.* Nature. 2002. 418(6894): p. 186-90. 10.1038/nature00894

[43] Xu, H., et al. *TRPV3 is a calcium-permeable temperature-sensitive cation channel.* Nature. 2002. 418(6894): p. 181-6. 10.1038/nature00882

[44] De Petrocellis, L., et al. *Cannabinoid actions at TRPV channels: effects on TRPV3 and TRPV4 and their potential relevance to gastrointestinal inflammation.* Acta Physiol (Oxf). 2012. 204(2): p. 255-66. 10.1111/j.1748-1716.2011.02338.x

[45] Moqrich, A., et al. *Impaired thermosensation in mice lacking TRPV3, a heat and camphor sensor in the skin.* Science. 2005. 307(5714): p. 1468-72. 10.1126/science.1108609

[46] Park, D.J., et al. *Polymorphisms of the TRPV2 and TRPV3 genes associated with fibromyalgia in a Korean population.* Rheumatology (Oxford). 2016. 55(8): p. 1518-27. 10.1093/rheumatology/kew180

[47] Guler, A.D., et al. *Heat-evoked activation of the ion channel, TRPV4.* J Neurosci. 2002. 22(15): p. 6408-14. 20026679

[48] Liedtke, W., et al. *Vanilloid receptor-related osmotically activated channel (VR-OAC), a candidate vertebrate osmoreceptor.* Cell. 2000. 103(3): p. 525-35. 10.1016/s0092-8674(00)00143-4

[49] Watanabe, H., et al. *Heat-evoked activation of TRPV4 channels in a HEK293 cell expression system and in native mouse aorta endothelial cells.* J Biol Chem. 2002. 277(49): p. 47044-51. 10.1074/jbc.M208277200

[50] Berna-Erro, A., et al. *Structural determinants of 5′,6′-epoxyeicosatrienoic acid binding to and activation of TRPV4 channel.* Sci Rep. 2017. 7(1): p. 10522. 10.1038/s41598-017-11274-1

[51] Watanabe, H., et al. *Anandamide and arachidonic acid use epoxyeicosatrienoic acids to activate TRPV4 channels.* Nature. 2003. 424(6947): p. 434-8. 10.1038/nature01807

[52] Akiyama, T., et al. *Involvement of TRPV4 in Serotonin-Evoked Scratching.* J Invest Dermatol. 2016. 136(1): p. 154-160. 10.1038/JID.2015.388

[53] Alessandri-Haber, N., et al. *Hypotonicity induces TRPV4-mediated nociception in rat.* Neuron. 2003. 39(3): p. 497-511. 10.1016/s0896-6273(03)00462-8

[54] Matsumoto, K., et al. *Role of transient receptor potential melastatin 2 (TRPM2) channels in visceral nociception and hypersensitivity.* Exp Neurol.

2016. 285(Pt A): p. 41-50. 10.1016/j.expneurol.2016.09.001

[55] Vandewauw, I., G. Owsianik, and T. Voets. *Systematic and quantitative mRNA expression analysis of TRP channel genes at the single trigeminal and dorsal root ganglion level in mouse.* BMC Neurosci. 2013. 14: p. 21. 10.1186/1471-2202-14-21

[56] Togashi, K., et al. *TRPM2 activation by cyclic ADP-ribose at body temperature is involved in insulin secretion.* EMBO J. 2006. 25(9): p. 1804-15. 10.1038/sj.emboj.7601083

[57] Perraud, A.L., et al. *ADP-ribose gating of the calcium-permeable LTRPC2 channel revealed by Nudix motif homology.* Nature. 2001. 411(6837): p. 595-9. 10.1038/35079100

[58] Wehage, E., et al. *Activation of the cation channel long transient receptor potential channel 2 (LTRPC2) by hydrogen peroxide. A splice variant reveals a mode of activation independent of ADP-ribose.* J Biol Chem. 2002. 277(26): p. 23150-6. 10.1074/jbc.M112096200

[59] Sozbir, E. and M. Naziroglu. *Diabetes enhances oxidative stress-induced TRPM2 channel activity and its control by N-acetylcysteine in rat dorsal root ganglion and brain.* Metab Brain Dis. 2016. 31(2): p. 385-93. 10.1007/s11011-015-9769-7

[60] Yuksel, E., et al. *Involvement of TRPM2 and TRPV1 channels on hyperalgesia, apoptosis and oxidative stress in rat fibromyalgia model: Protective role of selenium.* Sci Rep. 2017. 7(1): p. 17543. 10.1038/s41598-017-17715-1

[61] Wagner, T.F., et al. *Transient receptor potential M3 channels are ionotropic steroid receptors in pancreatic beta cells.* Nat Cell Biol. 2008. 10(12): p. 1421-30. 10.1038/ncb1801

[62] Vriens, J., et al. *TRPM3 is a nociceptor channel involved in the detection of noxious heat.* Neuron. 2011. 70(3): p. 482-94. 10.1016/j.neuron.2011.02.051

[63] Held, K., et al. *Activation of TRPM3 by a potent synthetic ligand reveals a role in peptide release.* Proc Natl Acad Sci U S A. 2015. 112(11): p. E1363-72. 10.1073/pnas.1419845112

[64] Peier, A.M., et al. *A TRP channel that senses cold stimuli and menthol.* Cell. 2002. 108(5): p. 705-15. 10.1016/s0092-8674(02)00652-9

[65] Bautista, D.M., et al. *The menthol receptor TRPM8 is the principal detector of environmental cold.* Nature. 2007. 448(7150): p. 204-8. 10.1038/nature05910

[66] Lippoldt, E.K., et al. *Artemin, a glial cell line-derived neurotrophic factor family member, induces TRPM8-dependent cold pain.* J Neurosci. 2013. 33(30): p. 12543-52. 10.1523/JNEUROSCI.5765-12.2013

[67] Xing, H., et al. *TRPM8 mechanism of cold allodynia after chronic nerve injury.* J Neurosci. 2007. 27(50): p. 13680-90. 10.1523/JNEUROSCI.2203-07.2007

[68] Asuthkar, S., et al. *The TRPM8 protein is a testosterone receptor: II. Functional evidence for an ionotropic effect of testosterone on TRPM8.* J Biol Chem. 2015. 290(5): p. 2670-88. 10.1074/jbc.M114.610873

[69] Barkhem, T., S. Nilsson, and J.A. Gustafsson. *Molecular mechanisms, physiological consequences and pharmacological implications of estrogen receptor action.* Am J Pharmacogenomics. 2004. 4(1): p. 19-28. 10.2165/00129785-200404010-00003

[70] Gruber, C.J., et al. *Production and actions of estrogens.* N Engl J Med. 2002. 346(5): p. 340-52. 10.1056/NEJMra000471

[71] Yasar, P., et al. *Molecular mechanism of estrogen-estrogen receptor signaling.*

Reprod Med Biol. 2017. 16(1): p. 4-20. 10.1002/rmb2.12006

[72] Hammes, S.R. and E.R. Levin. *Extranuclear steroid receptors: nature and actions.* Endocr Rev. 2007. 28(7): p. 726-41. 10.1210/er.2007-0022

[73] Revankar, C.M., et al. *A transmembrane intracellular estrogen receptor mediates rapid cell signaling.* Science. 2005. 307(5715): p. 1625-30. 10.1126/science.1106943

[74] Buse, D.C., et al. *Sex differences in the prevalence, symptoms, and associated features of migraine, probable migraine and other severe headache: results of the American Migraine Prevalence and Prevention (AMPP) Study.* Headache. 2013. 53(8): p. 1278-99. 10.1111/head.12150

[75] van Oosterhout, W.P.J., et al. *Female sex hormones in men with migraine.* Neurology. 2018. 91(4): p. e374-e381. 10.1212/WNL.0000000000005855

[76] Lovell, R.M. and A.C. Ford. *Global prevalence of and risk factors for irritable bowel syndrome: a meta-analysis.* Clin Gastroenterol Hepatol. 2012. 10(7): p. 712-721 e4. 10.1016/j.cgh.2012.02.029

[77] Wan, B., et al. *Gender-Stratified Prevalence of Psychiatric and Pain Diagnoses in a Primary Care Patient Sample with Fibromyalgia.* Pain Med. 2019. 20(11): p. 2129-2133. 10.1093/pm/pnz084

[78] Bagis, B., et al. *Gender difference in prevalence of signs and symptoms of temporomandibular joint disorders: a retrospective study on 243 consecutive patients.* Int J Med Sci. 2012. 9(7): p. 539-44. 10.7150/ijms.4474

[79] Joseph, E.K. and J.D. Levine. *Sexual dimorphism in the contribution of protein kinase C isoforms to nociception in the streptozotocin diabetic rat.* Neuroscience. 2003. 120(4): p. 907-13. 10.1016/s0306-4522(03)00400-7

[80] Lu, Y.C., et al. *17Beta-estradiol mediates the sex difference in capsaicin-induced nociception in rats.* J Pharmacol Exp Ther. 2009. 331(3): p. 1104-10. 10.1124/jpet.109.158402

[81] Payrits, M., et al. *Estradiol Sensitizes the Transient Receptor Potential Vanilloid 1 Receptor in Pain Responses.* Endocrinology. 2017. 158(10): p. 3249-3258. 10.1210/en.2017-00101

[82] Cho, T. and V.V. Chaban. *Expression of P2X3 and TRPV1 receptors in primary sensory neurons from estrogen receptors-alpha and estrogen receptor-beta knockout mice.* Neuroreport. 2012. 23(9): p. 530-4. 10.1097/WNR.0b013e328353fabc

[83] Yamagata, K., et al. *Estrogens Exacerbate Nociceptive Pain via Up-Regulation of TRPV1 and ANO1 in Trigeminal Primary Neurons of Female Rats.* Endocrinology. 2016. 157(11): p. 4309-4317. 10.1210/en.2016-1218

[84] Wu, Y.W., et al. *17-Beta-estradiol enhanced allodynia of inflammatory temporomandibular joint through upregulation of hippocampal TRPV1 in ovariectomized rats.* J Neurosci. 2010. 30(26): p. 8710-9. 10.1523/JNEUROSCI.6323-09.2010

[85] Chen, F., et al. *Estrogen inhibits RANKL-induced osteoclastic differentiation by increasing the expression of TRPV5 channel.* J Cell Biochem. 2014. 115(4): p. 651-8. 10.1002/jcb.24700

[86] Pohoczky, K., et al. *Estrogen-dependent up-regulation of TRPA1 and TRPV1 receptor proteins in the rat endometrium.* J Mol Endocrinol. 2016. 56(2): p. 135-49. 10.1530/JME-15-0184

[87] Wu, Y.W., et al. *Synovial TRPV1 is upregulated by 17-beta-estradiol and involved in allodynia of inflamed temporomandibular joints in female rats.* Arch Oral Biol. 2015. 60(9): p. 1310-8. 10.1016/j.archoralbio.2015.05.011

[88] Greaves, E., et al. *Elevated peritoneal expression and estrogen regulation of nociceptive ion channels in endometriosis.* J Clin Endocrinol Metab. 2014. 99(9): p. E1738-43. 10.1210/jc.2014-2282

[89] Kumar, S., et al. *Transient receptor potential vanilloid 1-6 (Trpv1-6) gene expression in the mouse brain during estrous cycle.* Brain Res. 2018. 1701: p. 161-170. 10.1016/j.brainres.2018.09.005

[90] Yazgan, Y. and M. Naziroglu. *Ovariectomy-Induced Mitochondrial Oxidative Stress, Apoptosis, and Calcium Ion Influx Through TRPA1, TRPM2, and TRPV1 Are Prevented by 17beta-Estradiol, Tamoxifen, and Raloxifene in the Hippocampus and Dorsal Root Ganglion of Rats.* Mol Neurobiol. 2017. 54(10): p. 7620-7638. 10.1007/s12035-016-0232-5

[91] Xu, S., et al. *17beta-estradiol activates estrogen receptor beta-signalling and inhibits transient receptor potential vanilloid receptor 1 activation by capsaicin in adult rat nociceptor neurons.* Endocrinology. 2008. 149(11): p. 5540-8. 10.1210/en.2008-0278

[92] Chen, S.C., T.J. Chang, and F.S. Wu. *Competitive inhibition of the capsaicin receptor-mediated current by dehydroepiandrosterone in rat dorsal root ganglion neurons.* J Pharmacol Exp Ther. 2004. 311(2): p. 529-36. 10.1124/jpet.104.069096

[93] Ramirez-Barrantes, R., et al. *TRPV1-Estradiol Stereospecific Relationship Underlies Cell Survival in Oxidative Cell Death.* Front Physiol. 2020. 11: p. 444. 10.3389/fphys.2020.00444

[94] Chen, S.C. and F.S. Wu. *Mechanism underlying inhibition of the capsaicin receptor-mediated current by pregnenolone sulfate in rat dorsal root ganglion neurons.* Brain Res. 2004. 1027(1-2): p. 196-200. 10.1016/j.brainres.2004.08.053

[95] DeLeon, C., D.Q.-H. Wang, and C.K. Arnatt. *G Protein-Coupled Estrogen Receptor, GPER1, Offers a Novel Target for the Treatment of Digestive Diseases.* 2020. 11(843). 10.3389/fendo.2020.578536

[96] Lopshire, J.C. and G.D. Nicol. *The cAMP transduction cascade mediates the prostaglandin E2 enhancement of the capsaicin-elicited current in rat sensory neurons: whole-cell and single-channel studies.* J Neurosci. 1998. 18(16): p. 6081-92.

[97] Joseph, J., et al. *Phosphorylation of TRPV1 S801 Contributes to Modality-Specific Hyperalgesia in Mice.* J Neurosci. 2019. 39(50): p. 9954-9966. 10.1523/JNEUROSCI.1064-19.2019

[98] Goswami, C., T.B. Hucho, and F. Hucho. *Identification and characterisation of novel tubulin-binding motifs located within the C-terminus of TRPV1.* J Neurochem. 2007. 101(1): p. 250-62. 10.1111/j.1471-4159.2006.04338.x

[99] Goswami, C., et al. *Estrogen destabilizes microtubules through an ion-conductivity-independent TRPV1 pathway.* J Neurochem. 2011. 117(6): p. 995-1008. 10.1111/j.1471-4159.2011.07270.x

[100] Prager-Khoutorsky, M., A. Khoutorsky, and C.W. Bourque. *Unique interweaved microtubule scaffold mediates osmosensory transduction via physical interaction with TRPV1.* Neuron. 2014. 83(4): p. 866-78. 10.1016/j.neuron.2014.07.023

[101] Liu, J., et al. *The expression and functionality of transient receptor potential vanilloid 1 in ovarian endometriomas.* Reprod Sci. 2012. 19(10): p. 1110-24. 10.1177/1933719112443876

[102] McKinnon, B.D., et al. *Inflammation and nerve fiber interaction in endometriotic pain.* Trends Endocrinol Metab. 2015. 26(1): p. 1-10. 10.1016/j.tem.2014.10.003

[103] Bohonyi, N., et al. *Local upregulation of transient receptor*

potential ankyrin 1 and transient receptor potential vanilloid 1 ion channels in rectosigmoid deep infiltrating endometriosis. Mol Pain. 2017. 13: p. 1744806917705564. 10.1177/1744806917705564

[104] Ma, W., et al. *Catechol estrogens stimulate insulin secretion in pancreatic beta-cells via activation of the transient receptor potential A1 (TRPA1) channel.* J Biol Chem. 2019. 294(8): p. 2935-2946. 10.1074/jbc.RA118.005504

[105] Hevir, N., M. Ribic-Pucelj, and T. Lanisnik Rizner. *Disturbed balance between phase I and II metabolizing enzymes in ovarian endometriosis: a source of excessive hydroxy-estrogens and ROS?* Mol Cell Endocrinol. 2013. 367(1-2): p. 74-84. 10.1016/j.mce.2012.12.019

[106] Fattori, V., et al. *Nonsurgical mouse model of endometriosis-associated pain that responds to clinically active drugs.* Pain. 2020. 161(6): p. 1321-1331. 10.1097/j.pain.0000000000001832

[107] Mooradian, A.D., J.E. Morley, and S.G. Korenman. *Biological actions of androgens.* Endocr Rev. 1987. 8(1): p. 1-28. 10.1210/edrv-8-1-1

[108] Schiffer, L., W. Arlt, and K.H. Storbeck. *Intracrine androgen biosynthesis, metabolism and action revisited.* Mol Cell Endocrinol. 2018. 465: p. 4-26. 10.1016/j.mce.2017.08.016

[109] Bennett, N.C., et al. *Molecular cell biology of androgen receptor signalling.* Int J Biochem Cell Biol. 2010. 42(6): p. 813-27. 10.1016/j.biocel.2009.11.013

[110] Chen, F., et al. *Partial agonist/antagonist properties of androstenedione and 4-androsten-3beta,17beta-diol.* J Steroid Biochem Mol Biol. 2004. 91(4-5): p. 247-57. 10.1016/j.jsbmb.2004.04.009

[111] Bai, X., X. Zhang, and Q. Zhou. *Effect of Testosterone on TRPV1 Expression in a Model of Orofacial Myositis Pain in the Rat.* J Mol Neurosci. 2018. 64(1): p. 93-101. 10.1007/s12031-017-1009-7

[112] Fusi, C., et al. *Steroidal and non-steroidal third-generation aromatase inhibitors induce pain-like symptoms via TRPA1.* Nat Commun. 2014. 5: p. 5736. 10.1038/ncomms6736

[113] De Logu, F., et al. *TRPA1 Mediates Aromatase Inhibitor-Evoked Pain by the Aromatase Substrate Androstenedione.* Cancer Res. 2016. 76(23): p. 7024-7035. 10.1158/0008-5472.CAN-16-1492

[114] Bidaux, G., et al. *Evidence for specific TRPM8 expression in human prostate secretory epithelial cells: functional androgen receptor requirement.* Endocr Relat Cancer. 2005. 12(2): p. 367-82. 10.1677/erc.1.00969

[115] Zhang, L. and G.J. Barritt. *Evidence that TRPM8 is an androgen-dependent Ca2+ channel required for the survival of prostate cancer cells.* Cancer Res. 2004. 64(22): p. 8365-73. 10.1158/0008-5472.CAN-04-2146

[116] Yang, Z., et al. *Effect of surgical castration on expression of TRPM8 in urogenital tract of male rats.* Mol Biol Rep. 2012. 39(4): p. 4797-802. 10.1007/s11033-011-1271-7

[117] Asuthkar, S., et al. *TRPM8 channel as a novel molecular target in androgen-regulated prostate cancer cells.* Oncotarget. 2015. 6(19): p. 17221-36. 10.18632/oncotarget.3948

[118] Asuthkar, S., et al. *The TRPM8 protein is a testosterone receptor: I. Biochemical evidence for direct TRPM8-testosterone interactions.* J Biol Chem. 2015. 290(5): p. 2659-69. 10.1074/jbc.M114.610824

[119] Mendez-Resendiz, K.A., et al. *Steroids and TRP Channels: A Close Relationship.* Int J Mol Sci. 2020. 21(11). 10.3390/ijms21113819

[120] Gkika, D., et al. *Testosterone-androgen receptor: The steroid link inhibiting TRPM8-mediated cold sensitivity.* FASEB J. 2020. 10.1096/fj.201902270R

[121] Taraborrelli, S. *Physiology, production and action of progesterone.* Acta Obstet Gynecol Scand. 2015. 94 Suppl 161: p. 8-16. 10.1111/aogs.12771

[122] Goletiani, N.V., D.R. Keith, and S.J. Gorsky. *Progesterone: review of safety for clinical studies.* Exp Clin Psychopharmacol. 2007. 15(5): p. 427-44. 10.1037/1064-1297.15.5.427

[123] Garg, D., et al. *Progesterone-Mediated Non-Classical Signaling.* Trends Endocrinol Metab. 2017. 28(9): p. 656-668. 10.1016/j.tem.2017.05.006

[124] Maurice, T., C. Gregoire, and J. Espallergues. *Neuro(active)steroids actions at the neuromodulatory sigma1 (sigma1) receptor: biochemical and physiological evidences, consequences in neuroprotection.* Pharmacol Biochem Behav. 2006. 84(4): p. 581-97. 10.1016/j.pbb.2006.07.009

[125] Jung, C., et al. *The progesterone receptor regulates the expression of TRPV4 channel.* Pflugers Arch. 2009. 459(1): p. 105-13. 10.1007/s00424-009-0706-7

[126] De Clercq, K., et al. *Functional expression of transient receptor potential channels in human endometrial stromal cells during the luteal phase of the menstrual cycle.* Hum Reprod. 2015. 30(6): p. 1421-36. 10.1093/humrep/dev068

[127] Li, C., et al. *TRPV4 is involved in levonorgestrel-induced reduction in oviduct ciliary beating.* J Pathol. 2019. 248(1): p. 77-87. 10.1002/path.5233

[128] Ortiz-Renteria, M., et al. *TRPV1 channels and the progesterone receptor Sig-1R interact to regulate pain.* Proc Natl Acad Sci U S A. 2018. 115(7): p. E1657-E1666. 10.1073/pnas.1715972115

[129] Hayashi, T. and T.P. Su. *Sigma-1 receptor chaperones at the ER-mitochondrion interface regulate Ca(2+) signaling and cell survival.* Cell. 2007. 131(3): p. 596-610. 10.1016/j.cell.2007.08.036

[130] Cortes-Montero, E., et al. *Ligands Exert Biased Activity to Regulate Sigma 1 Receptor Interactions With Cationic TRPA1, TRPV1, and TRPM8 Channels.* Front Pharmacol. 2019. 10: p. 634. 10.3389/fphar.2019.00634

Section 2

Androgens

Chapter 3

Androgens' Effects across the Lifespan in Men and Animal Models

Cheryl A. Frye, Jennifer K. Torgersen, Vincent F. Lembo and Kelly Drew

Abstract

The clinical literature and recent studies in our laboratory using rodent models demonstrate that there are individual differences in androgens' pleiotropic effects across the lifespan that need to be better understood. The question to address that challenges the field is that levels of androgens (current and/or prior) may not drive differing responses to androgens. The clinical example of Post-finasteride Syndrome, in which side-effects persist long after treatment is discontinued, supports investigations of this novel question relating to long-term effects of androgen manipulations, independent of existing levels of androgens.

Keywords: steroids, neurosteroids, testosterone, 3a-Androstanediol, post-finasteride syndrome, traumatic brain injury

1. Introduction

Androgens have well-known trophic actions on the reproductive, nervous, skeletal, and cardiovascular systems throughout the lifespan. A focus in behavioral neuroendocrinology has been on understanding dose-dependency, brain targets, cellular mechanisms of testosterone (T) and its metabolites for reproduction through androgen receptors. Research has challenged the existing paradigm about androgen action,

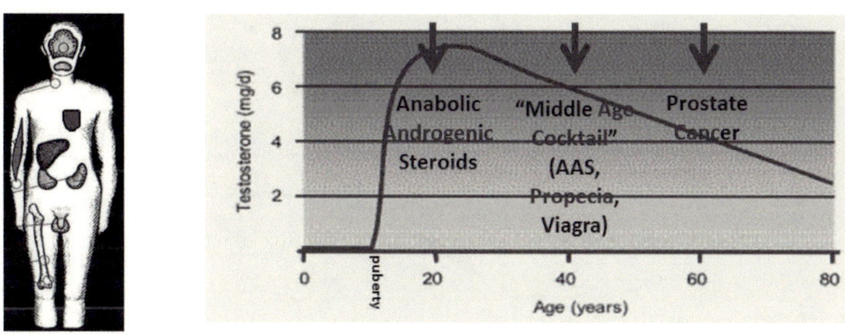

Figure 1.
Androgens target brain, heart, muscle, liver, kidneys, adrenals, testes, penis, bones (left) and (right) changes in androgens across the lifespan with a decade by decade decline naturally or by points indicated by arrows with pharmacological interventions or disease [1].

as well as taking a novel approach to understand how these trophic actions in the brain occur in relation to growth in the body (reproductive organs). Given androgens' pervasive trophic effects from early development throughout adulthood, unique studies are discussed that impact our understanding of androgens' actions (**Figure 1**).

2. Actions of androgens

2.1 Disparate effects and mechanisms of androgens may be meaningful

Androgens have profound effects on physiological and psychological function. This is apparent throughout the lifespan and with normal development as well as in pathological situations. In early development, androgens lay the framework for sex differences in reproductive tissues and brain circuitry and behavior. At puberty, typical diurnal secretion of androgens in males is initiated. The main circulating androgen is T, which can be aromatized into estradiol and 5α-reduced to dihydrotestosterone (DHT). DHT is further converted to 5α-androstane,3α,17β-diol (3α-diol) by 3α-hydroxysteroid dehydrogenase. These different androgens have varied effects and mechanisms that will be discussed throughout this paper (**Figure 2**).

2.2 Patterns of androgens and effects in men

Men experience a decade-by-decade decline in androgens, with marked androgen deficiency typically observed in the 6th–8th decade of life [1]. This shift in balance of androgens and estrogens can contribute to some of the adverse physiological effects observed in aging, such as reduced muscle mass, osteoporosis, and gynecomastia, as well as increase risk of prostate pathologies. The brain is also adversely affected by these changes as evidenced by memory impairments, reduced libido, and an increased risk for depression among some men. As such, many older men turn to androgen-based therapies to ameliorate these symptoms. However, androgen-based therapies may increase risk for unwanted proliferation in the prostate, as well as other physical and psychological side effects. Moreover, men are often reported to use androgen replacement therapies even in their 4th decade or earlier, suggesting that some men may be particularly sensitive to even modest androgen decline, or trophic effects of synthetic androgens (e.g. anabolic steroids).

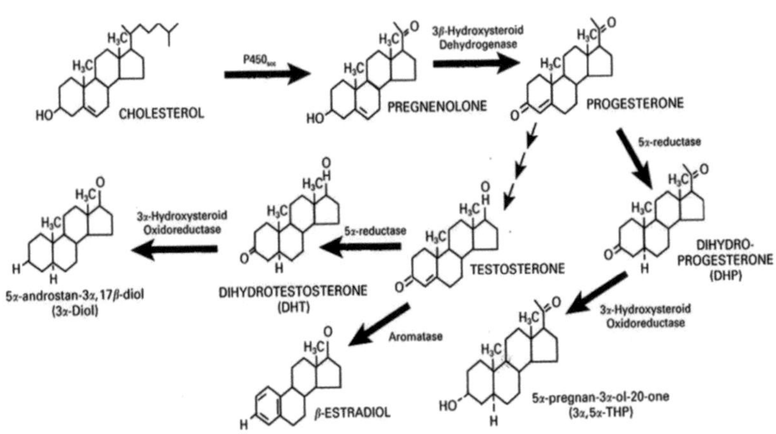

Figure 2.
Metabolism- depicts T metabolism via aromatase to estradiol and 5α-reductase and 3α-hydroxysteroid oxidoreductase to dihydrotestosterone and 3α-diol.

A serious concern is that such treatments have potential to increase risk for prostate pathologies and other unwanted effects for brain function.

2.3 Disparate effects and mechanisms of androgens may be meaningful

Some men use treatments, such as finasteride, a 5α-reductase inhibitor, to manipulate trophic effects of androgens (e.g. alopecia, benign prostatic hyperplasia) and to reduce side effects of synthetic androgens. There can be long-term effects of such treatment. Finasteride use has been linked to sexual dysfunctions and mental side effects, including depression, even months after its use is discontinued ("Post-finasteride Syndrome") [2–4]. The individual differences in response to androgens, as well as their manipulations, are not understood but will be discussed herein. Foci will be on androgen receptor-independent effects and mechanisms (estrogen receptor β- ERβ; brain derived neurotrophic factor- BDNF) of 5α-reductase manipulations and the T metabolite (3α-diol) for driving trophic effects in the brain that may be parsed from such effects in peripheral targets (prostate) (**Figure 3**).

2.4 Novel targets of androgens and why they may be meaningful

Individual differences in responses to androgens may be attributed in part to current and past exposure to androgens and/or their manipulation, and subsequent actions at ERβ and BDNF. To address this challenging question of individual differences in responses to androgens, a unique strain and species comparison approach has been utilized. Rat and mouse models with different androgen load, androgen replacement, and 5α-reductase inhibition have been utilized. Social/reproductive, cognitive, and affective behavior, androgen levels, and indices of growth (BDNF, prostate weight) has been measured to model age- and androgen manipulation-related changes in physical and psychological function. One-rate limiting step to elucidating better treatment options for androgen-related pathologies is to have animal models that mimic the human condition and can be used to systematically address question about persistent effects of androgens in the brain and peripheral targets. These studies address questions of clinical importance with substantial depth and breadth for human health, given the pervasive nature of androgens' lifelong effects throughout the body.

2.5 The normative role of androgens for physiological and psychological processes

Androgens have well-known growth-enhancing effects to regulate development and functional aspects of the reproductive, central nervous system, skeletal, and cardiovascular systems throughout the lifespan (thru the lifespan that include patterns of androgen secretion. Supported by early investigations in the field [5], the capacity of androgens that are secreted from the testes during early pre- or peri-natal development may "organize" the central nervous system, including the

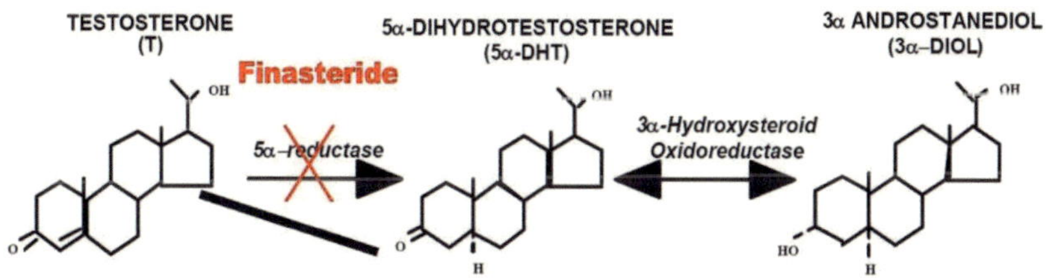

Figure 3.
Mechanism of action of finasteride.

neural control of post-pubertal patterns of androgen release, as well as sensitivity of specific brain structures to androgens in adulthood for behaviors. From birth until sexual maturation, androgen levels are typically low. At puberty, androgen levels increase and remain high until midlife when androgen levels begin to decline. Many of the targets of androgens have been highlighted by changes in the tissues' functions with decline in androgens. Among people, this is often assessed by determining age-related changes in function. Unlike the precipitous decline in ovarian function with reproductive senescence that is observed among women, men experience a decade-by-decade decline in androgens. **Figure 4** displays the data from Handelsman et al. 1995 and show the decline in these hormones with age [6]. This decline is termed "andropause" and, although the nature of the decline in steroids is different from that observed during the menopause of women, both situations have clear symptomology associated with steroid decline at this time. For example, decline in bioactive androgens in men with aging is associated with diminished libido, fatigue, decreased muscle mass, osteoporosis, depression, and/or cognitive dysfunctions. Given the aging population and robust effect that androgens have on physiological and psychological function, there is now great interest in the role of androgen-based therapies to obviate some of these symptoms. Moreover, there are younger populations that are using synthetic androgens, such as illicit anabolic androgenic steroids (AAS), with or without other drugs to alter steroid metabolism (finasteride). A serious concern that limits the use of steroid-based treatments in men is their potential to increase risk for prostate pathologies as well as psychological effects (**Figure 5**).

2.6 Typical approach to understanding the normative effects of androgens – sex differences, seasonal and correlational effects

In behavioral neuroendocrinology, to determine the role of a hormone for a behavioral process, an approach is to assess endogenous changes in hormones,

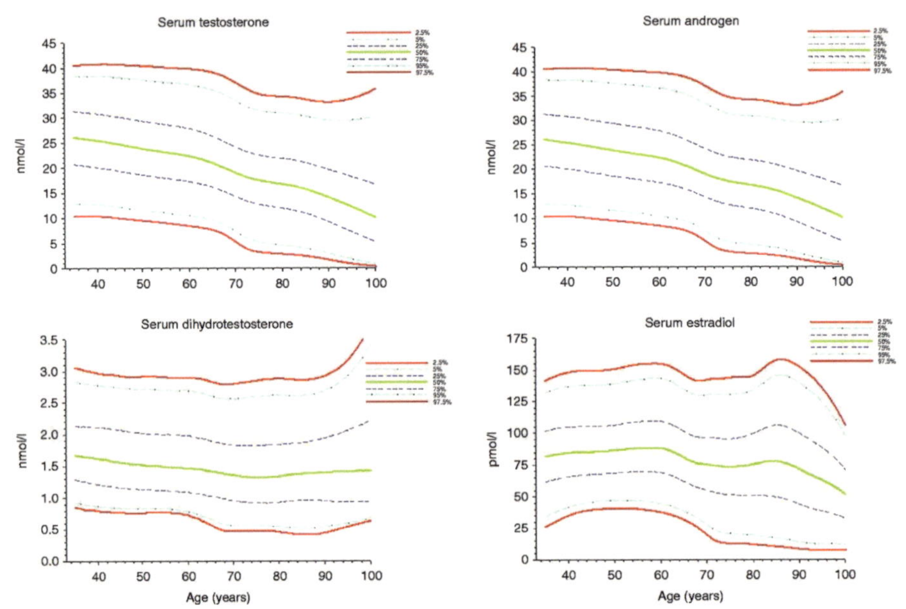

Figure 4.
Plot of smoothed age-specific population centiles (97.5, 95, 75, 50, 25, 5, and 2.5%) for serum testosterone (nmol/l; upper left), DHT (nmol/l; lower left), androgen (nmol/l; right top), and E_2 *(pmol/l; right lower) in 10897 samples from men aged over 35 years from population-based studies in three Australian cities (Adelaide, Perth, and Sydney) using LC–MS steroid measurements from a single lab with data analyses using GAMLSS modeling. A full color version of this figure is available at http://dx.doi.org/10.1530/EJE-15-0380.*

Symptoms of Testosterone Deficiency Among Men

Physical:
- Decreased body hair
- Decreased muscle strength and mass
- Development of breast tissue
- Hot flashes, sweats
- Sleep disturbances and fatigue
- Osteoporosis/ height loss

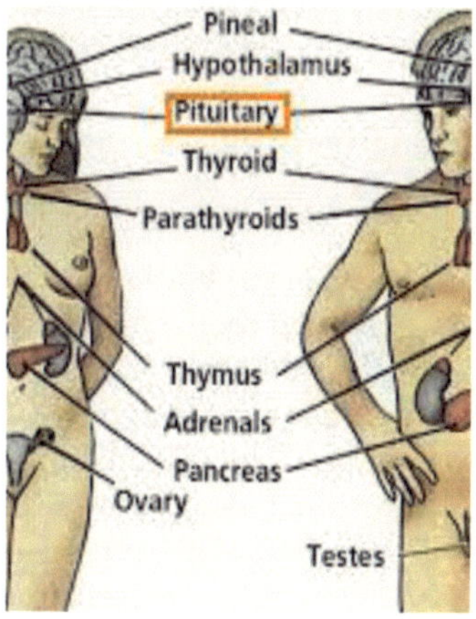

Cardiometabolic:
- Increased body mass and abdominal obesity
- Metabolic syndrome
- Insulin resistance and type 2 diabetes

Sexual:
- Delayed puberty
- Hypogonadism (small testes)
- Decreased frequency of sexual thoughts and desire, and sexual activity
- Decreased or absent morning/nighttime erections
- Erectile Dysfunction and/or infertility

Psychological:
- Changes in mood
- Greater lability
- Anger, irritability, sadness, depression
- Overall sense of poor well-being and health
- Poor cognitive function
- Reduced concentration, spacail performance, and verbal memory

Figure 5.
Summary of effects of loss of androgens among men https://www.guidelinesinpractice.co.uk/mens-health/testosterone-deficiency-treat-men-who-have-bothersome-symptoms/454121.articleSigns and symptoms.

extirpation of the hormone (i.e. surgical removal of the gonads), and replacement back of a hormone. Endogenous changes are used to assess the extent to which levels of the hormone in question vary with the behavioral endpoint of interest. This is usually assessed in males by investigating behaviors and androgens that vary from: 1) females (which typically have lower levels of androgens), 2) by season (e.g. seasonal breeders), and 3) across the lifespan (post-pubertal, with androgen decline in advanced aging). One example of this type of investigation would be assessments of reproductively relevant behavior, such as aggression, among a seasonal breeder, such as a deer. Male, but not female, deer begin to grow antlers (which have utility for aggressive responding in this species) during mating season post-puberty. Aggressive behavior among male deer coincides with peak levels of androgens and is reduced during non-breeding season associated with androgens levels at nadir.

2.7 Typical approach to understanding the normative effects of androgens

To begin to assess the causative role of the hormone in this behavior, the second and third approaches of extirpation and replacement are utilized; extirpation should remove the hormone and result in abolishment of the behavior and then replacement back of this hormone should reinstate the behavior. A classic example of this approach is the Berthold experiment. Although this experiment predates basic knowledge that hormones existed, it had been known for centuries in agriculture that there are clear behavioral differences in male animals when their testes were removed. Dr. Berthold is credited with completing the first systematic study (1849) of extirpation and replacement of the testes (which we now know are a main source of circulating androgens) to investigate secondary sex characteristics and reproductive behaviors of roosters. Roosters were castrated and reductions in appetitive and consummatory aspects of mating, as well as secondary sex characteristics, were abolished. This was reversed when roosters were implanted with testes. Dr. Berthold hypothesized that these changes in behavior and phenotype were due to a substance in the testes (rather than actions via nerves in the body, which was the prevailing notion at the time).

In summary, although these methods to understand effects of hormonal variations, extirpation, and replacement have a long history and have clearly contributed to our understanding of the relationship between hormones and a hormone-mediated behavior, there is also individual differences in the responses of individuals that need to be better understood. The relationship between a behavior and hormone levels may not be linear, and this relationship may be mediated by individual experience (i.e. current/prior androgen exposure), a response first noted over 60 years ago [7].

2.8 Typical approach to understanding the normative effects of androgens

Actions of T metabolites may account for some of T's functional effects. T, the primary androgen secreted from the testes, travels in circulation to the brain (as well as many other target organs) and then can be metabolized by enzymes to other neuroactive metabolites. T can be aromatized into estradiol (E_2) and 5α-reduced to DHT (**Figure 6**). DHT is metabolized to 5α-androstane,3α,17β-diol (3α-diol). A consideration in understanding the effects of androgens is novel sources of androgens beyond metabolism. The traditional idea is that neuroactive metabolites such as 3α-diol are formed following secretion of T from the testes, which is then converted by 5α-reductase and 3α-HSD in androgen sensitive targets, such as the brain.

2.9 The brain is an endocrine organ and can produce androgens

These enzymes as well as others are critical for *de novo* production of androgens in the brain (termed "neurosteroidogenesis) from precursors, such as cholesterol, pregnanolone, and progesterone. The biosynthetic pathway for neurosteroid production involves many recognized factors, including the 18kDA translocator protein (see **Figure** 7): TSPO, a.k.a. peripheral-type benzodiazepine receptor), the steroidogenic acute regulatory (StAR) protein, cytochrome P450-dependent C27 side chain cleavage enzymes (P450scc), 3β-hydroxysteroid dehydrogenase (3β-HSD),

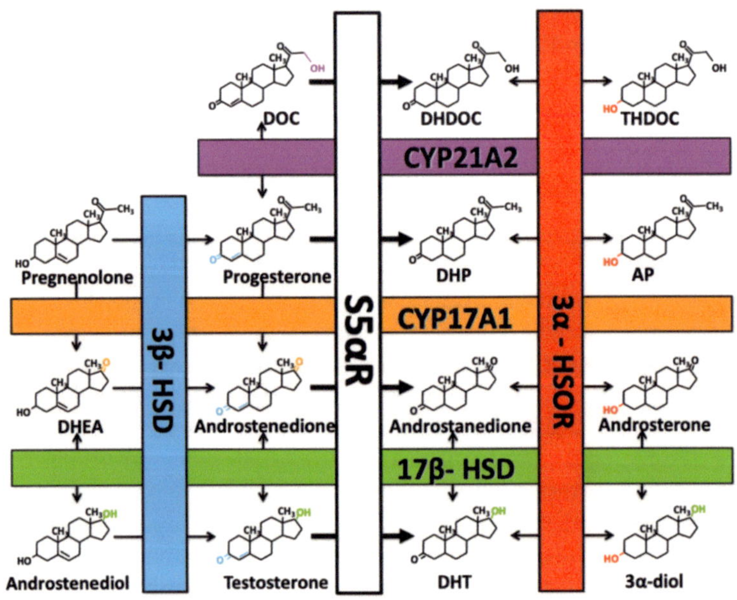

Figure 6.
Metabolic pathways for formation of testosterone and its metabolites in the brain, figure provided by and modified from colleague Marco Bortelatto.

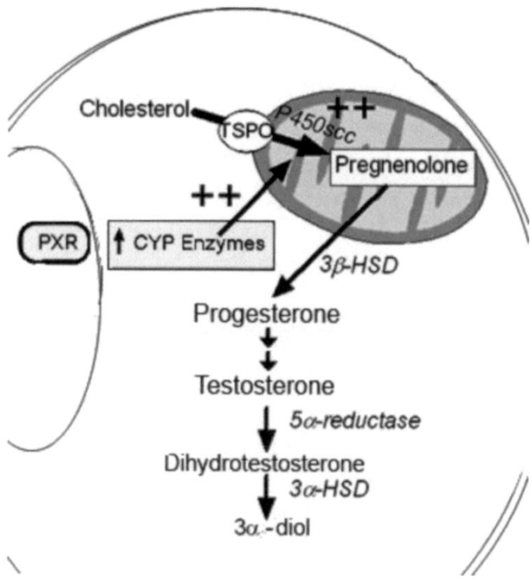

Figure 7.
Neurosteroidogenesis- formation of 3α-diol from cholesterol.

5α-reductase, and 3α-HSD. TSPO and StAR have actions to transport cholesterol (a requisite precursor for all steroids) into the mitochondria. In the mitochondria, cholesterol is oxidized by P450scc to form pregnanolone, which is then metabolized by 3β-HSD to progesterone. Progesterone can then be metabolized to form T. A pathway to form 3α-diol from T involves sequential actions of 5α-reductase (an irreversible action that forms DHT) and then 3α-hydroxysteroid 3α-HSD. Most recently, we have been investigating the pregnane xenobiotic receptor (PXR) as a novel target for neurosteroid production [8].

2.10 ERβ and $GABA_A$ receptors as targets for androgens in brain

Here we focus on two novel targets of androgens for trophic effects, estrogen receptor beta (ERβ) and $GABA_A$ receptors. Androgen metabolites act at a variety of targets to influence psychological (affective, cognitive) and physiological processes (prostate). High physiological androgens are associated with improved affective and cognitive performance; castration (gonadectomy- GDX) increases anxiety-like behavior, and detriments in their cognitive abilities and effects can be reversed with administration of T [9–14]. These studies using the typical approach assessed these effects in young male rodents (with comparable lifetime exposure to

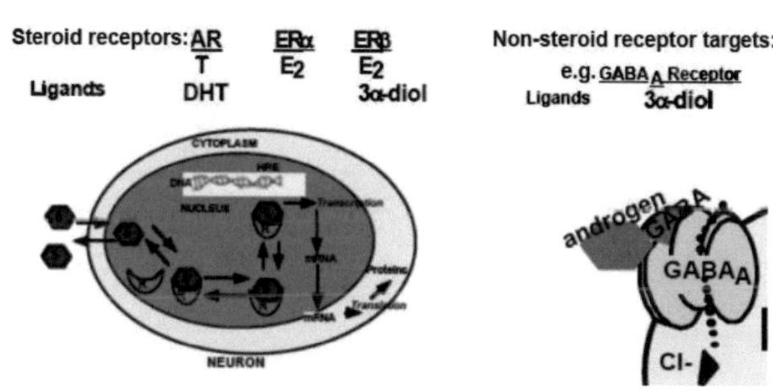

Figure 8.
Receptor targets of androgens.

androgens). Aged male rodents do not have improved cognitive or affective performance when administered T, compared to their younger counterparts; this effect was associated with a reduced capacity for producing 3α-diol [14]. 3α-diol may be similarly effective, if not more so, than administration of T alone for decreasing anxiety behavior of GDX rats [12, 13]. Blocking formation of 3α-diol through administration of indomethacin can reverse these beneficial effects of androgens on affect and cognition [12, 13, 15]. An important consideration in understanding the role androgens is their different mechanisms of action. See **Figure 8.**

2.11 The brain has multiple targets for androgens

3α-diol has novel mechanisms of action. T and DHT bind to androgen receptors (ARs), and some of the proliferative effects of androgens on the prostate may be through this mechanism. However, it seems that non-AR mechanisms of other T metabolites may be important for cognitive and/or affective behavior. 3α-diol has actions via ERβ and $GABA_A$ receptors [16–20] (**Figure 8**). E_2 readily binds to cognate ERα and ERβ, and can enhance benign prostatic hyperplasia and adenocarcinoma, likely via actions at ERα, not ERβ, but this is not completely understood. Indeed, androgens' and estrogens' (anti)proliferative effects may depend in part upon tissue type and actions at ERs subtypes, ERα and ERβ, which are differentially distributed across the body and brain. In the prostate, ERβ is highly expressed in epithelial cells. Although ERα is localized in the stroma, ERα also has been found in premalignant and malignant epithelium of the prostate. In the brain, ERβ expression predominates in hippocampus and cortex, regions involved in cognition and affect. ERβ knockout mice have prostate hyperplasia in aging, suggesting a potential inhibitory role of ERβ for prostate growth [21, 22]. However, the stress reducing, cognitive and affective behavior enhancing effects likely occur through actions at ERβ as male mice or rats have greater responses to androgens that have actions at ERβ and ERβ knockout mice show reductions in these cognitive and affective responses [17]. Mice with the tfm mutation, rendering ARs non-functional, respond better than do wildtype mice to administration of 3α-diol for anti-depressive behavior in the forced swim test (**Figure 9**). Thus, trophic effects of androgens in the brain and body may be dissociable and involve different targets beyond the traditional target of androgens, the ARs.

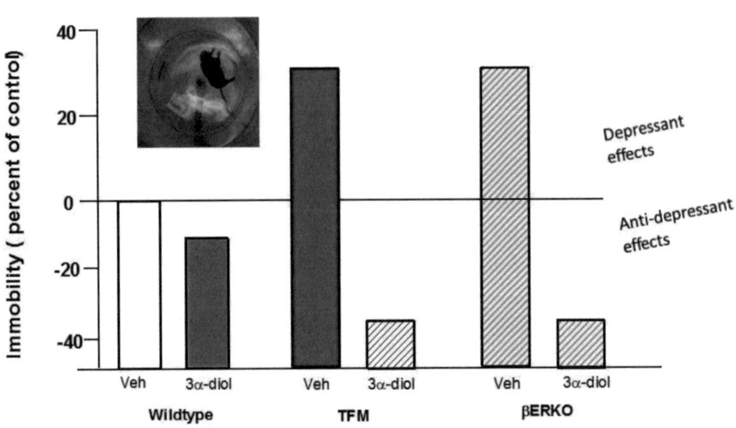

Figure 9.
Tfm and ERβ knockout mice show more depressive-like behavior than do wildtype mice, an effect that can be reversed by administration of 3α-diol in the forced swim.

2.12 BDNF as another novel mechanism for individual differences in responses to androgens

In addition to mechanisms of androgens in the brain and body through ERβ, the proposed project will investigate brain-derived neurotrophic factor (BDNF) as a target for these trophic actions. BDNF is a neurotrophin that is abundantly expressed in many central nervous system regions, most notably in regions of interest in the proposed studies for their involvement in cognitive, affective, and reproductive function (prefrontal cortex, hippocampus, and hypothalamus). BDNF is considered a marker of brain plasticity owing to its role in synaptic reorganization, neurogenesis, and dendritic branching and spine formation as well as cognitive and affective processes. Moreover, there is growing evidence for the role of gonadal hormones for regulating BDNF, namely, estradiol [23]. Less is known about the role of androgens for BDNF, but there is some evidence for sex differences, regimen, and region/cell-specific effects of androgens for BDNF. For instance, it has been argued that T produces tonic suppression of BDNF levels in mossy fibers of the hippocampus among adult male rats (but the opposite occurs with estradiol among female rats [24]. Indeed, among male rats that do not show GDX-induced decrements in cognitive performance, there is increased BDNF in mossy fibers of the hippocampus [25]. Enriched environment increases testosterone and BDNF levels in the grossly-dissected hippocampus of female, more so than male rats, compared to rats living under typical lab conditions [26]. However, among male mice, GDX decreased levels of BDNF in pyramidal neurons in the CA1 area, an effect prevented by T replacement [27]. Physiological dosing of T produced antidepressant effects that were mitigated when the BDNF target, extracellular signal-regulated kinase 2, is blocked [28]. We propose that some effects of T for BDNF may be related to its metabolite, 3α-diol. We have found that hippocampus levels of BDNF are reduced among mice with knockout of ERβ, coincident with lower 3α-diol levels (**Figure 8**). These findings indicate the role of androgens for BDNF is not linear, and there are gender, regimen, and target-specific effects (**Figure 10**).

2.13 Differential responses to androgens

Variations in the levels of T and its metabolites, may influence affect and/or cognition in men. Men who have higher endogenous levels of T have a lower incidence of depression [29]. Conversely, young hypogonadal men, with low endogenous T and DHT levels, are more likely to be diagnosed with an anxiety or depressive disorder, and exhibit decreased performance in cognitive tasks [30, 31].

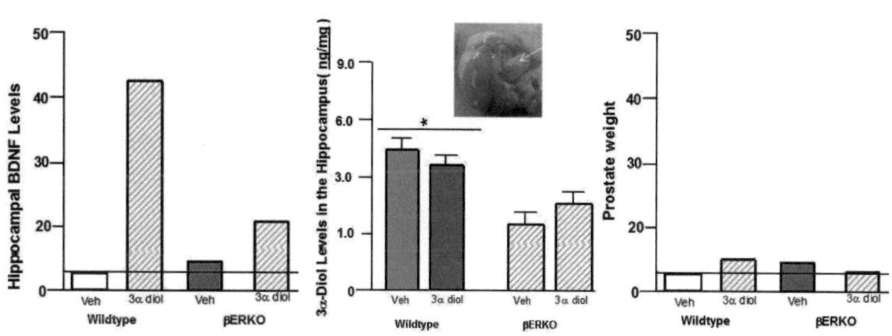

Figure 10.
3α-diol administration increases BDNF levels, but not prostate weight, among wildtype mice, irrespective of 3α-diol levels in the hippocampus. Among ERβ knockout mice, 3α-diol levels are lower and there is reduced BDNF in the hippocampus (but no change in prostate weight).

Treatment for these men includes T replacement, which can increase positive, and decrease negative, mood, while improving cognition [32]. However, a different pattern is apparent with use of androgens, such as AAS, among some eugonadal men. AAS are the synthetic variants of T. They are abused by growing numbers of individuals in this country ranging from adolescents, seeking to improve their appearance, to professional athletes attempting to elevate their performance. The costs associated with AAS abuse are substantial. For the individual, AAS abuse is associated with many adverse physical and behavioral consequences. There can be dramatic cognitive and mood changes that are observed among some users of AAS ("'roid rage") and other serious, permanent side effects: kidney and liver damage, liver cancer, heart disease, and hypertension, suppression of T production, testicular atrophy, and gynecomastia. In adolescent males, AAS abuse can hasten the onset of adulthood, promote early baldness, limit stature, and cause premature growth plate closing. Together, these data suggest that there are individual differences in response to androgens that may be related to current hormonal state and/or age.

2.14 Aging and androgens

In aged men, there is a decade-by- decade decline in levels of androgens and an increase in bioavailable estrogens, with marked androgen deficiency most typically observed in the 6th–8th, even 9th, decade of life [33]. However, this shift in balance of androgens and estrogens can contribute to some of the adverse physiological effects observed in aging (termed "andropause"), such as reduced muscle mass, osteoporosis, and gynecomastia, as well as increase risk of prostate pathologies (from benign prostate hyperplasia to prostate carcinoma). The brain is also adversely affected by these changes and there are increased memory impairments, reduced libido/sex drive, and an increased risk for depression. As such, many men turn to androgen-based therapies to replace back androgens to ameliorate these symptoms. Clinical studies have demonstrated that administration of T to some aged men reinstates their affective and cognitive performance [34–36]. Despite the notion that marked androgen deficiency is most common after 60 years of age among men, men are often reported to use androgen replacement therapies even in their 4th decade, suggesting that some men may be particularly sensitive to decline or age-related changes in androgens, but this is not clear.

2.15 Prostate health and androgens

T and its metabolites have trophic effects on the prostate in addition to other reproductive structures of males from early development. Among older men, decline in androgens, and an increase in estrogens, may underlie risk for prostate proliferation. Indeed, treatments for prostate cancer include those that alter androgen levels (releasing hormone or metabolism inhibitors) [37] and/or actions (androgen receptor antagonists). DHT binds with a higher affinity than does T to ARS [36], and DHT is highly active in prostate, where it may cause proliferation [38]. Because of this, 5α-reductase inhibitors have been used as a treatment for BPH and prostate cancer [39–41]. As prostate cancer progresses, carcinomas can become steroid-insensitive and metastasize, leaving no effective treatments. Moreover, there can be side effects of such androgen manipulations. For instance, men have a slightly decreased sex drive with finasteride, which can be reversed upon treatment cessation [42], among most individuals. There is a clinical situation where there is a prolonged response to such androgen manipulations, even when the therapy has ceased, that is informing present studies (below).

2.16 Post-finasteride syndrome

The 5α-reductase inhibitor, finasteride, whose mechanism of action can be seen in **Figure 11**, is approved for treatment of benign prostate hyperplasia and male pattern baldness (androgenic alopecia). It also has off-label use among men using AAS to decrease side effects of AAS or block detection of AAS with drug tests. Effects of finasteride treatment to persistently reduce levels of DHT and 3α-diol glucoronidate have been reported among older men assessed over a years (~75 reduction from baseline; [43]. Benefits of finasteride for benign prostate hyperplasia and alopecia generally occur after chronic administration (6+ months) and subside when the treatment is discontinued [44, 45]. However, a more recent report suggests that there are individual differences in response to finasteride for alopecia. In this study, men were treated with finasteride and hair growth assessed over 10 years. Men that had the greatest increase in hair growth were those who had started treatment over 30 years of age, suggesting those that had experienced longer decline in hair growth were most responsive to the treatment. Additionally, subjects that had the greatest amount of hair growth in the first year were those same subjects who had the greatest overall hair growth over the period of the study [46]. Together, these

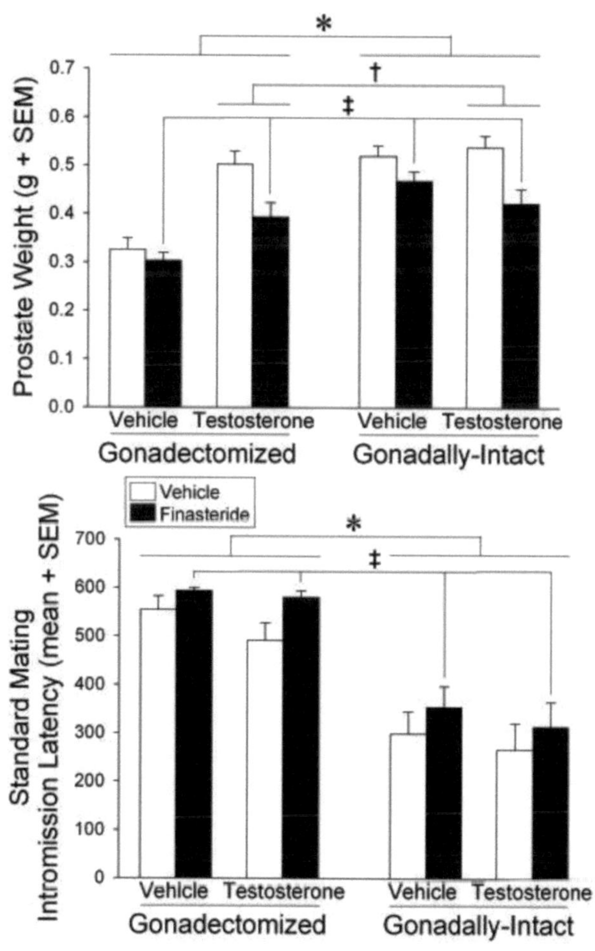

Figure 11.
*Prostate weight (top) and the latency to intromit in standard mating paradigm (bottom) among gonadectomized (GDX) or gonadally-intact male rats implanted with vehicle, testosterone, and/or finasteride. * indicates main effect of gonadal condition; † indicates main effect of T condition; ‡ indicates main effect of inhibitor condition,* p < 0.05.

results suggest that there are individual differences in response to manipulation of 5α-reductase by finasteride. Additionally, there is evidence of individual differences in response to finasteride when considering side effects of this treatment.

The known side effects of finasteride include sexual dysfunction (e.g. loss of libido, impotence, ejaculatory or erectile dysfunction), gynecomastia, changes in cognition, and affect (including depression, which was added to the product package insert by Merck in 2010). Of particular interest is that there are side effects after finasteride is discontinued. For example, there are reports of persistent sexual dysfunction following discontinuation of finasteride [4, 46–48]. Additionally, former users of finasteride report sexual dysfunction and have high scores on the Beck Depression Inventory more than 3 months after cessation of finasteride use [2, 3]. In this study, 75% of men (61 total in the study) showing persistent sexual dysfunction following finasteride discontinuation had symptoms of depression (assessed by Beck Depression Inventory) over 3 months later. It is assumed in these individuals that endogenous androgen levels have normalized, so the question remains regarding potential mechanisms of these long-term changes in behavioral responses. A recent publication has shown that there seems to be a reduced capacity for neuroactive steroid production (as measured in cerebrospinal fluid or plasma) of individuals with side effects following discontinuation of finasteride for alopecia [49]. Studies in patients at risk for prostate cancer prescribed finasteride demonstrate increased testosterone and decreased DHT and 3α-diol glucuronide (mainly produced in the liver) in circulation [43], in addition to differences in cholesterol profile [49]. Whether levels coincide with symptoms is not understood. We have collected pilot data in support of this idea in male rats. In this study, male rats were GDX or gonadally-intact and were administered T or vehicle chronically in conjunction with finasteride or vehicle. Rats that were GDX, compared to intact rats, had lower circulating T and DHT levels, smaller prostates and longer latencies to initiate sexual contacts with a female (as to be expected). T-replacement increased plasma T and prostate mass. Similar to GDX, finasteride decreased prostate weight and inhibited sexual behavior (**Figure 11**). A preliminary finding in this study was that the finasteride treatment had variable effects to reduce the 5α-reduced metabolite, DHT, and that the levels determined do not seem to coincide with the behavioral patterns observed. As such, the present proposal is informed by the clinical literature and preliminary results in our laboratory using an animal model. Thus, of clinical relevance is consideration of long-term effects of androgen manipulations that extend beyond the treatment period. We propose, such as with post-finasteride syndrome, that there may be long-term consequences of changing androgen milieu that may be independent of specific levels of androgens at a particular time.

One factor that seems to be linking the individual differences in responses to androgens is related to different current and/or prior exposure to androgens, rather than linear effects of androgen levels for the response; additionally, effects of androgens may be via novel targets, ERβ, BDNF or $GABA_A$ activity. Studies will be challenging the current notion in field of behavioral neuroendocrinology that behavioral effects are not just due to the levels at the time the behaviors are assessed, but that there can be persistent effects beyond this. Testing this hypothesis is also a challenge to pharmacology in that effects/side effects should subside when the drug is discontinued. Proposed work is a challenge to the insular nature of science in that assessments of androgens will not only be in the brain/behavior, but also an investigation of brain effects in context of body (e.g. prostate growth/sex behavio4). Overall, to address this question about long-term consequences of changing androgen milieu that may be independent of specific levels of androgen concentrations at a particular time and novel cellular targets for these effects, is a transformative approach to the problem that must be taken.

Recently, the chemist who began making Viagra has appeared in daytime TV shows such as Dr. Oz and Dr. Phil. He has made a great deal of money for himself and his company, so much so that he feels guilty because Viagra is based on L-Arginine, which increases blood flow to all cells of the body. This was effective for ED and could be used by most people except those with risk for hypertension, heart attack, and stroke, and is readily available at low to no cost in pharmacies groceries stories. The investigator knew this, he only needed to figure out how to more specifically increase the blood flow and also had to increase not just consummatory (bigger and longer erections) aspects of behavior, but motivational (increase sex drive, sexual confidence, energy) which L-argnine itself did not do. Through my extensive pharmacological training and knowledge of naturopathic medicine, I suggest the use of Boron rather than L-Arginine so that blood flow would be more directed to the penis rather than the whole body, preventing potential side effects of heart attack, stroke, etc. Orchic could be added because it has a beneficial effect on mood patterns to reduce stress and promote relaxation. Saw palmetto is well known Asia to enhance energy, strength and stamina. Nettle extract is a known aphrodisiac that can also help boost testosterone levels. Biopterin is used to more rapidly enter target sites and boost energy, stamina, and sexual motivation. My colleague gave up most of the formula that increases testosterone and nitric oxide production in the penis and results in improved libido, sexual motivation, sexual confidence, and sexual performance. Within days there were multiple substances on the market, most of which were a supplement similar to this. It is unclear what the long-term consequences are going to be of this supplement, however it may well be a solution to using finasteride for hair growth and it may help those with post finasteride syndrome as part of their recovery on sexual side effects and ahedonia. Like all good cooks, who occasionally have memory lapses, I did not include a key naturopathic ingredient in our original formula. We do however hope to have our product patented out and on the market soon, aimed at the target audiences indicated above and hitting targets that are not just based upon ED or consummatory aspects of finasteride syndrome but also will have beneficial aspects of drive and motivation (regulated by dopamine) and impulse control regulated by the inputs on the A8, A9, A10 dopamine cell bodies (GABA, GLUTAMATE), and other drive desire aspects to socialize (oxytoxin) [50].

Author details

Cheryl A. Frye[1,2,3*], Jennifer K. Torgersen[1], Vincent F. Lembo[2] and Kelly Drew[3]

1 The State University of New York at Albany, Psychology, Biology, Neuroscience and Life Science Programs, Albany, NY, USA

2 Comprehensive Neuropsychological Services, Albany, NY, USA

3 Alaska INBRE / University of Alaska, Fairbanks, Alaska

*Address all correspondence to: cafrye@albany.edu

References

[1] M Travison TG, Morley JE, Araujo AB, O'Donnell AB, McKinlay JB. The relationship between libido and testosterone levels in aging men. J Clin Endocrinol Metab. 2006 Jul;91(7):2509-13. doi: 10.1210/jc.2005-2508. Epub 2006 May 2. PMID: 16670164.c

[2] Irwig MS. Persistent sexual side effects of finasteride: could they be permanent? J Sex Med. 2012 Nov;9(11):2927-32. doi: 10.1111/j.1743-6109.2012.02846.x. Epub 2012 Jul 12. PMID: 22789024.

[3] Irwig MS. Depressive symptoms and suicidal thoughts among former users of finasteride with persistent sexual side effects. J Clin Psychiatry. 2012 Sep;73(9):1220-3. doi: 10.4088/JCP.12m07887. Epub 2012 Aug 7. PMID: 22939118.

[4] Traish AM, Hassani J, Guay AT, Zitzmann M, Hansen ML. Adverse side effects of 5α-reductase inhibitors therapy: persistent diminished libido and erectile dysfunction and depression in a subset of patients. J Sex Med. 2011 Mar;8(3):872-84. doi: 10.1111/j.1743-6109.2010.02157.x. Epub 2010 Dec 22. PMID: 21176115.

[5] Phoenix CH, Goy RW, Gerall AA, Young WC (1959) Organizing action of prenatally administered testosterone propionate on the tissues mediating mating behavior in the female guinea pig. Endocrinology 65:163-196. 10.1210/endo-65-3-369. PMID: 14432658.

[6] Handelsman DJ, Yeap B, Flicker L, Martin S, Wittert GA, Ly LP. Age-specific population centiles for androgen status in men. Eur J Endocrinol. 2015 Dec;173(6):809-17. doi: 10.1530/EJE-15-0380. Epub 2015 Sep 18. PMID: 26385186.

[7] Grunt JA, Young WC. Consistency of sexual behavior patterns in individual male guinea pigs following castration and androgen therapy. J Comp Physiol Psychol. 1953 Apr;46(2):138-44. doi: 10.1037/h0053840. PMID: 13044875.

[8] Frye CA, Paris JJ, Walf AA, Rusconi JC. Effects and Mechanisms of 3α,5α,-THP on Emotion, Motivation, and Reward Functions Involving Pregnane Xenobiotic Receptor. Front Neurosci. 2012 Jan 19;5:136. doi: 10.3389/fnins.2011.00136. PMID: 22294977; PMCID: PMC3261425.

[9] Bitran D, Kellogg CK, Hilvers RJ. Treatment with an anabolic-androgenic steroid affects anxiety-related behavior and alters the sensitivity of cortical GABAA receptors in the rat. Horm Behav. 1993 Dec;27(4):568-83. doi: 10.1006/hbeh.1993.1041. PMID: 8294123.

[10] Ceccarelli I, Scaramuzzino A, Aloisi AM. Effects of gonadal hormones and persistent pain on non-spatial working memory in male and female rats. Behav Brain Res. 2001 Aug 27;123(1):65-76. doi: 10.1016/s0166-4328(01)00195-4. PMID: 11377730.

[11] Frye CA, Seliga AM. Testosterone increases analgesia, anxiolysis, and cognitive performance of male rats. Cogn Affect Behav Neurosci. 2001 Dec;1(4):371-81. doi: 10.3758/cabn.1.4.371. PMID: 12467088.

[12] Frye CA, Edinger KL. Testosterone's metabolism in the hippocampus may mediate its anti-anxiety effects in male rats. Pharmacol Biochem Behav. 2004 Jul;78(3):473-81. doi: 10.1016/j.pbb.2004.04.019. PMID: 15251256.

[13] Edinger KL, Frye CA. Testosterone's analgesic, anxiolytic, and cognitive-enhancing effects may be due in part to actions of its 5alpha-reduced metabolites in the hippocampus. Behav Neurosci. 2004 Dec;118(6):1352-64. doi:

10.1037/0735-7044.118.6.1352. PMID: 15598144.

[14] Frye CA, Edinger KL, Lephart ED, Walf AA. 3alpha-androstanediol, but not testosterone, attenuates age-related decrements in cognitive, anxiety, and depressive behavior of male rats. Front Aging Neurosci. 2010 Apr 8;2:15. doi: 10.3389/fnagi.2010.00015. PMID: 20552051; PMCID: PMC2874398.

[15] Frye CA, Edinger KL, Seliga AM, Wawrzycki JM. 5alpha-reduced androgens may have actions in the hippocampus to enhance cognitive performance of male rats. Psychoneuroendocrinology. 2004 Sep;29(8):1019-27. doi: 10.1016/j.psyneuen.2003.10.004. PMID: 15219653.

[16] Edinger KL, Frye CA. Androgens' effects to enhance learning may be mediated in part through actions at estrogen receptor-beta in the hippocampus. Neurobiol Learn Mem. 2007 Jan;87(1):78-85. doi: 10.1016/j.nlm.2006.07.001. Epub 2006 Aug 14. PMID: 16904920; PMCID: PMC3633449.

[17] Frye CA, Bloom MS, Wersinger S. The 50th anniversary of the discovery of the estrogen receptor--conversations about hormones then and now. Physiol Behav. 2010 Feb 9;99(2):147-8. doi: 10.1016/j.physbeh.2009.11.001. Epub 2009 Nov 13. PMID: 19914266.

[18] Gee KW. Steroid modulation of the GABA/benzodiazepine receptor-linked chloride ionophore. Mol Neurobiol. 1988 Winter;2(4):291-317. doi: 10.1007/BF02935636. PMID: 2855977.

[19] Handa RJ, Pak TR, Kudwa AE, Lund TD, Hinds L. An alternate pathway for androgen regulation of brain function: activation of estrogen receptor beta by the metabolite of dihydrotestosterone, 5alpha-androstane-3beta,17beta-diol. Horm Behav. 2008 May;53(5):741-52. doi: 10.1016/j.yhbeh.2007.09.012. Epub 2007 Dec 11. PMID: 18067894; PMCID: PMC2430080.

[20] Pak TR, Chung WC, Lund TD, Hinds LR, Clay CM, Handa RJ. The androgen metabolite, 5alpha-androstane-3beta, 17beta-diol, is a potent modulator of estrogen receptor-beta1-mediated gene transcription in neuronal cells. Endocrinology. 2005 Jan;146(1):147-55. doi: 10.1210/en.2004-0871. Epub 2004 Oct 7. PMID: 15471969.

[21] Couse JF, Korach KS. Estrogen receptor null mice: what have we learned and where will they lead us? Endocr Rev. 1999 Jun;20(3):358-417. doi: 10.1210/edrv.20.3.0370. Erratum in: Endocr Rev 1999 Aug;20(4):459. PMID: 10368776.

[22] Jarred RA, McPherson SJ, Bianco JJ, Couse JF, Korach KS, Risbridger GP. Prostate phenotypes in estrogen-modulated transgenic mice. Trends Endocrinol Metab. 2002 May-Jun;13(4):163-8. doi: 10.1016/s1043-2760(02)00575-1. PMID: 11943560.

[23] Pluchino N, Russo M, Santoro AN, Litta P, Cela V, Genazzani AR. Steroid hormones and BDNF. Neuroscience. 2013 Jun 3;239:271-9. doi: 10.1016/j.neuroscience.2013.01.025. Epub 2013 Feb 1. PMID: 23380505.

[24] Scharfman HE, MacLusky NJ. Differential regulation of BDNF, synaptic plasticity and sprouting in the hippocampal mossy fiber pathway of male and female rats. Neuropharmacology. 2014 Jan;76 Pt C(0 0):696-708. doi: 10.1016/j.neuropharm.2013.04.029. Epub 2013 May 6. PMID: 23660230; PMCID: PMC3769475.

[25] Skucas VA, Duffy AM, Harte-Hargrove LC, Magagna-Poveda A, Radman T, Chakraborty G, Schroeder CE, MacLusky NJ, Scharfman HE. Testosterone depletion in adult male rats increases mossy fiber transmission, LTP, and sprouting in area CA3 of hippocampus. J Neurosci.

2013 Feb 6;33(6):2338-55. doi: 10.1523/JNEUROSCI.3857-12.2013. PMID: 23392664; PMCID: PMC3711621.

[26] Bakos J, Hlavacova N, Rajman M, Ondicova K, Koros C, Kitraki E, Steinbusch HW, Jezova D. Enriched environment influences hormonal status and hippocampal brain derived neurotrophic factor in a sex dependent manner. Neuroscience. 2009 Dec 1;164(2):788-97. doi:10.1016/j.neuroscience.2009.08.054. Epub 2009 Aug 29. PMID: 19723563.

[27] Li M, Masugi-Tokita M, Takanami K, Yamada S, Kawata M. Testosterone has sublayer-specific effects on dendritic spine maturation mediated by BDNF and PSD-95 in pyramidal neurons in the hippocampus CA1 area. Brain Res. 2012 Nov 12;1484:76-84. doi: 10.1016/j.brainres.2012.09.028. Epub 2012 Sep 23. PMID: 23010313.

[28] Carrier N, Kabbaj M. Extracellular signal-regulated kinase 2 signaling in the hippocampal dentate gyrus mediates the antidepressant effects of testosterone. Biol Psychiatry. 2012 Apr 1;71(7):642-51. doi: 10.1016/j.biopsych.2011.11.028. Epub 2012 Jan 20. PMID: 22265242; PMCID: PMC3307821.

[29] Earls F. Sex differences in psychiatric disorders: origins and developmental influences. Psychiatr Dev. 1987 Spring;5(1):1-23. PMID: 3601929

[30] Howell S, Shalet S. Testosterone deficiency and replacement. Horm Res. 2001;56 Suppl 1:86-92. doi: 10.1159/000048142. PMID: 11786693.

[31] Kaminetsky JC. Testosterone therapy in hypogonadal men. Introduction. Clin Cornerstone. 2005;7 Suppl 4:S5-7. doi: 10.1016/s1098-3597(05)80090-0. PMID: 16651206.

[32] Zitzmann M. Testosterone and the brain. Aging Male. 2006 Dec;9(4):195-9. doi: 10.1080/13685530601040679. PMID: 17178554.

[33] Morley JE, Kaiser FE, Sih R, Hajjar R, Perry HM 3rd. Testosterone and frailty. Clin Geriatr Med. 1997 Nov;13(4):685-95. PMID: 9354749.

[34] Alexander GM, Swerdloff RS, Wang C, Davidson T, McDonald V, Steiner B, Hines M. Androgen-behavior correlations in hypogonadal men and eugonadal men. II. Cognitive abilities. Horm Behav. 1998 Apr;33(2):85-94. doi: 10.1006/hbeh.1998.1439. PMID: 9647934.

[35] Delhez M, Hansenne M, Legros JJ. Andropause and psychopathology: minor symptoms rather than pathological ones. Psychoneuroendocrinology. 2003 Oct;28(7):863-74. doi: 10.1016/s0306-4530(02)00102-6. PMID: 12892654.

[36] Janowsky JS. Thinking with your gonads: testosterone and cognition. Trends Cogn Sci. 2006 Feb;10(2):77-82. doi: 10.1016/j.tics.2005.12.010. Epub 2006 Jan 4. PMID: 16386941.

[37] Roselli CE, Salisbury RL, Resko JA. Genetic evidence for androgen-dependent and independent control of aromatase activity in the rat brain. Endocrinology. 1987 Dec;121(6):2205-10. doi: 10.1210/endo-121-6-2205. PMID: 3678147.

[38] Tindall DJ, Rittmaster RS. The rationale for inhibiting 5alpha-reductase isoenzymes in the prevention and treatment of prostate cancer. J Urol. 2008 Apr;179(4):1235-42. doi: 10.1016/j.juro.2007.11.033. Epub 2008 Feb 20. Erratum in: J Urol. 2008 Jun;179(6):2490. PMID: 18280514; PMCID: PMC2667246

[39] Brufsky A, Fontaine-Rothe P, Berlane K, Rieker P, Jiroutek M, Kaplan I, Kaufman D, Kantoff P. Finasteride and flutamide as potency-sparing androgen-ablative therapy for advanced adenocarcinoma of the prostate. Urology. 1997

Jun;49(6):913-20. doi: 10.1016/s0090-4295(97)00091-5. PMID:

[40] Fleshner NE, Trachtenberg J. Combination finasteride and flutamide in advanced carcinoma of the prostate: effective therapy with minimal side effects. J Urol. 1995 Nov;154(5):1642-5; discussion 1645-6. PMID: 7563310.

[41] Marks LS, Partin AW, Dorey FJ, Gormley GJ, Epstein JI, Garris JB, Macairan ML, Shery ED, Santos PB, Stoner E, deKernion JB. Long-term effects of finasteride on prostate tissue composition. Urology. 1999 Mar;53(3):574-80. PMID: 10096387.

[42] Amory JK, Anawalt BD, Matsumoto AM, Page ST, Bremner WJ, Wang C, Swerdloff RS, Clark RV. The effect of 5alpha-reductase inhibition with dutasteride and finasteride on bone mineral density, serum lipoproteins, hemoglobin, prostate specific antigen and sexual function in healthy young men. J Urol. 2008 Jun;179(6):2333-8. doi: 10.1016/j.juro.2008.01.145. Epub 2008 Apr 18. PMID: 18423697;PMCID: PMC2684818.

[43] Stanczyk FZ, Azen CG, Pike MC. Effect of finasteride on serum levels of androstenedione, testosterone and their 5α-reduced metabolites in men at risk for prostate cancer. J Steroid Biochem Mol Biol. 2013 Nov;138:10-6. doi: 10.1016/j.jsbmb.2013.02.015. Epub 2013 Mar 6. PMID: 23474436.

[44] Edwards JE, Moore RA. Finasteride in the treatment of clinical benign prostatic hyperplasia: a systematic review of randomised trials. BMC Urol. 2002 Dec 12;2:14. doi: 10.1186/1471-2490-2-14. Epub 2002 Dec 12. PMID: 12477383; PMCID: PMC140032.

[45] Leyden J, Dunlap F, Miller B, Winters P, Lebwohl M, Hecker D, Kraus S, Baldwin H, Shalita A, Draelos Z, Markou M, Thiboutot D, Rapaport M, Kang S, Kelly T, Pariser D, Webster G, Hordinsky M, Rietschel R, Katz HI, Terranella L, Best S, Round E, Waldstreicher J. Finasteride in the treatment of men with frontal male pattern hair loss. J Am Acad Dermatol. 1999 Jun;40(6 Pt 1):930-7. doi: 10.1016/s0190-9622(99)70081-2. PMID: 10365924.

[46] Irwig MS, Kolukula S. Persistent sexual side effects of finasteride for male pattern hair loss. J Sex Med. 2011 Jun;8(6):1747-53. doi: 10.1111/j.1743-6109.2011.02255.x. Epub 2011 Mar 18. PMID: 21418145.

[47] Rossi A, Cantisani C, Scarnò M, Trucchia A, Fortuna MC, Calvieri S. Finasteride, 1 mg daily administration on male androgenetic alopecia in different age groups: 10-year follow-up. Dermatol Ther. 2011 Jul-Aug;24(4):455-61. doi: 10.1111/j.1529-8019.2011.01441.x. PMID: 21910805.

[48] Melcangi RC, Caruso D, Abbiati F, Giatti S, Calabrese D, Piazza F, Cavaletti G. Neuroactive steroid levels are modified in cerebrospinal fluid and plasma of post-finasteride patients showing persistent sexual side effects and anxious/depressive symptomatology. J Sex Med. 2013 Oct;10(10):2598-603. doi: 10.1111/jsm.12269. Epub 2013 Jul 24. PMID: 23890183.

[49] Duskova M, Hill M, Starka L. Changes of metabolic profile in men treated for androgenetic alopecia with 1 mg finasteride. Endocr Regul. 2010 Jan;44(1):3-8. doi: 10.4149/endo_2010_01_3. PMID: 20151762.

[50] Godar SC, Cadeddu R, Floris G, Mosher LJ, Mi Z, Jarmolowicz DP, Scheggi S, Walf AA, Koonce CJ, Frye CA, Muma NA, Bortolato M. The Steroidogenesis Inhibitor finasteride reduces the response to both stressful and rewarding stimuli. Biomolecules. 9. DOI: 10.3390/biom9110749 PMID 31752360.

Chapter 4

Androgen Signaling in the Placenta

Agata M. Parsons Aubone, River Evans and Gerrit J. Bouma

Abstract

The placenta is a multifunctional, transitory organ that mediates transport of nutrients and waste, gas exchange, and endocrine signaling. In fact, placental secretion of hormones is critical for maintenance of pregnancy, as well as growth and development of healthy offspring. In this chapter, the role of androgens in placental development and function is highlighted. First, a brief summary will be provided on the different mammalian placental types followed by an overview of placental steroidogenesis. Next, the chapter will focus on genomic and non-genomic androgen signaling pathways. Finally, an overview will be provided on the current status of androgen signaling in the placenta during normal and abnormal pregnancies.

Keywords: pregnancy, placenta, testosterone, dihydrotestosterone, androgen receptor

1. Introduction

Establishing and maintaining pregnancy requires a finely regulated series of physiological events involving mother, fetus, and placenta. The essential role of steroid hormones in the production and maintenance of many of these changes is well characterized. For example, important effects of progesterone include preparation of the endometrium for implantation [1], modulation of the maternal immune response to tolerate the fetal allograft, maintenance of myometrial quiescence [2], and preparation of mammary glands for lactation. Estrogens appear to influence uterine blood flow and neovascularization, increase the expression of critical proteins that are involved in progesterone production and steroid metabolism and participate in preparation of mammary glands for lactation [3, 4]. Throughout pregnancy, levels of maternal circulating androgens, including testosterone (T), dihydrotestosterone (DHT), dehydroepiandrosterone (DHEA) and androstenedione (A4) increase, with concentrations three-fold higher by the third trimester when compared to non-pregnant levels in women [5]. Although T is a well-known precursor for estrogens (E2) synthesis, the placenta can both be a source and a target for androgens. The goal of this chapter is to summarize what is known about androgens and androgen receptor in pregnancy and compare it between species and between different types of placenta.

2. Placenta classification

The placenta is a multifunctional, transitory organ that mediates transport of nutrients and waste, gas exchange, and endocrine signaling. In fact, placental secretion of hormones is critical for maintenance of pregnancy, as well as growth and development of a healthy offspring. Despite fulfilling similar functions, there is a wide range of diversity in placental anatomo-histology among species.

During early embryogenesis, the first cells to differentiate are trophoblast cells, which form the chorion or fetal portion of the placenta. Villous trophoblast cells have two distinct cell populations; undifferentiated cytotrophoblast cells and differentiated syncytiotrophoblast tissue. The syncytiotrophoblast tissue is a continuous, multinucleated, specialized layer of epithelial cells, which covers the villous surface and is in direct contact with maternal blood. This layer is formed by fusion of cytotrophoblast cells.

Placental gross morphological classification is based on the shape and the area of contact between fetal and maternal tissue [6]. There are four commonly describe placental shapes among mammals:

1. **Diffuse placenta**, present in the horse and pig, has chorionic villi in contact with the uterine endometrium throughout the entire surface of the allantochorion, forming either folds (pig) or microcotyledons (horse).

2. **Cotyledonary placenta**, present in ruminants, is made up of multiple discrete areas of attachment called cotyledons, which are formed by the interaction between the fetal allantochorion and the maternal endometrium. The fetal side of this type of placenta is called cotyledons, the maternal side is called caruncles, and the cotyledon-caruncle complexes are known as placentomes.

3. **Zonary placenta**, present in carnivores such as dogs and cats, has the shape of a complete (dog and cat) or incomplete band (ferrets and raccoons) of tissue surrounding the chorionic sack.

4. **Discoid placenta**, present in rodents and primates, is formed by a collection of villi on a single (mice and human) or double (rabbit) disc.

In addition to the gross morphological classification, placentas are also categorized by histology (**Figure 1**) which is based on the different number of cell layers separating fetal from maternal circulation [7]. Before the placenta is formed, there are a total of six layers of tissue separating maternal and fetal blood. Three of these layers are fetal extraembryonic membranes in the chorioallantoic placenta of all mammals, all of which are components of the mature placenta. These three layers include endothelium lining allantoic capillaries, connective tissue in the form of chorioallantoic mesoderm, and chorionic epithelium, derived from trophoblast cells. There are also three layers on the maternal side, but the number of these layers which are retained after placentation varies greatly among species. The three potential maternal layers in a placenta are endothelium lining endometrial blood vessels, connective tissue of the endometrium, and endometrial epithelial cells.

Based on this degree of separation, or number of layers separating the fetal and maternal tissues, there are four different types of placenta (see **Figure 1**):

1. **Epitheliochorial placenta**, present in pig and horse, consists of all six layers separating maternal from fetal blood throughout gestation. The trophoblast cells make contact with the uterine epithelium forming microcotyledons (horse) or chorionic folds (pig). Microcotyledons contain highly vascularized chorionic villi that extend into elaborate invaginations of the endometrium. Chorionic folds are formed by the lining of the chorionic villi into the wrinkled surface of the uterine epithelium.

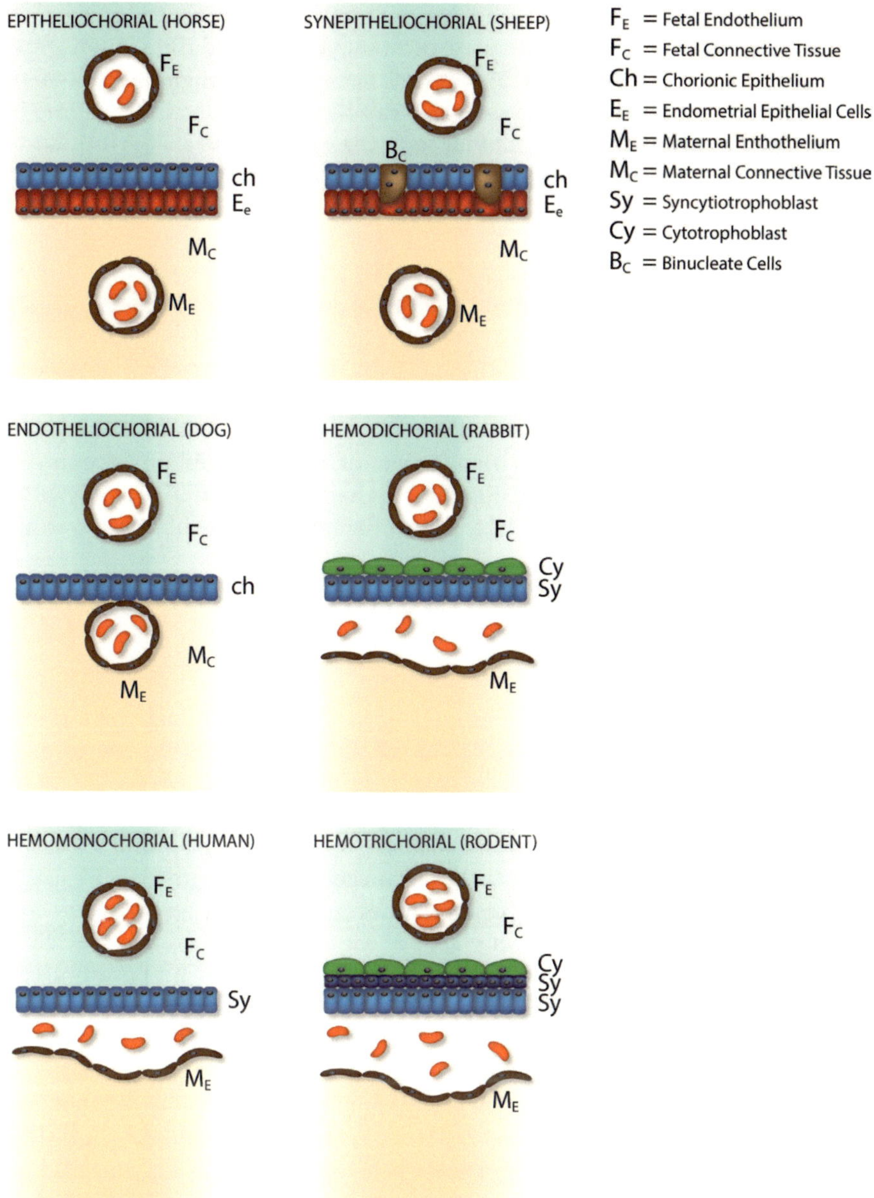

Figure 1.
Histological classification of the placenta.

2. **Synepitheliochorial placenta**, present in ruminants, contains the same layers as an epitheliochorial placenta. In this type of placenta, the uterine epithelium is modified by invasion and fusion of binucleate cells forming the syncytium, which contains embryonic and maternal nuclei. More recently, multinucleated trophoblast giant cells (TGC), formed by incomplete cytokinesis of mono-nucleated trophoblast cells, are believed to remove endometrial epithelial cells and fuse and contribute to the syncytial trophoblast layer [8].

3. **Endotheliochorial placenta**, present in carnivores (cats and dogs), is formed when the endometrial epithelium is disrupted during placentation, and fetal chorionic epithelial cells come in contact with maternal endothelial cells.

During implantation, cytotrophoblast cells surround the central third of the chorioallantois and proliferate to form a syncytium called the syncytiotrophoblast layer. The syncytiotrophoblast layer erodes through the endometrial epithelium and grows around maternal capillaries. Initially, the invading fetal cells are in the form of villi, but villi soon coalesce to form a labyrinthine-type placenta. For this reason, only four tissue layers separate the maternal from the fetal blood.

4. **Hemochorial placenta**, present in humans and rodents, is the most invasive form of placentation. Fetal chorionic epithelium is bathed in maternal blood because chorionic villi have invaded through endometrial epithelium and eroded through maternal endothelium. The number of trophoblast layers in contact with the maternal circulation shows variation between species. It is hemomonochorial in humans, with one layer of syncytiotrophoblast, and hemodichorial in primates, with one layer of syncytiotrophoblast upon one layer of cytotrophoblast cells. Finally, it is hemotrichorial in rodents with one layer of cytotrophoblast and two layers of syncytiotrophoblast separating maternal and fetal blood.

3. Placenta steroidogenesis

A key function of the placenta is the secretion of hormones. Like other steroid hormones, T is derived from cholesterol and the synthesis involves several enzymatic steps. The first and fundamental step in its biosynthesis involves the oxidative breakdown of the cholesterol side chain by the enzyme P450scc (side-chain cleavage), a mitochondrial cytochrome oxidase, resulting in the loss of six carbon atoms to give rise to pregnenolone. Only certain cell types in humans are capable of pregnenolone synthesis, including testicular Leydig cells, ovarian theca and corpus luteal cells, placental trophoblast cells, cells of the adrenal cortex, and specific cells in the brain, such as the pyramidal and granular neurons of the hippocampus and the Purkinje cells from the cerebellum [9]. The resulting pregnenolone is either converted to progesterone or 17 α-hydroxypregnenolone via 3β-hydroxysteroid dehydrogenase (HSD3B) or cytochrome P450 17A1 (CYP17A1), respectively. Progesterone is secreted into maternal circulation, and 17α-hydroxypregnenolone can be metabolized to DHEA via CYP17A1. DHEA is oxidized into A4 via HSD3B. A4 is then reduced to 5 α-androstenedione via 5 α-reductase (SRD5A). DHEA and A4 can be converted by 17 β-hydroxysteroid dehydrogenase into androstenediol and T, respectively. Subsequently, T is converted into DHT via 5 α-reductase (SRD5A). T and 5 α-androstenedione can further be metabolized to estrogens via aromatase (CYP19A1) [10]. A summarized overview of placental steroidogenesis is provided in **Figure 2**.

Androgens are synthesized in tissues where 17α-hydroxylase/17,20-lyase cytochrome P450 (P450c17) exists. This enzyme is located in different tissues such as fetal and maternal adrenal glands, fetal ovaries and testes, and the corpus luteum, depending on to the animal species. In non-pregnant woman, 50% of all DHEA is secreted by the adrenal glands, 20% from the ovarian theca and 30% is derived from metabolism of circulating DHEA sulfate [11]. Adrenal glands and ovaries produce equal amounts of A4, with the total daily production rate 1.4-6.2 mg/day [12]. 50% of T is synthesized in the ovaries and adrenals and the other half is produced from A4 in the peripheral tissues. Daily production rate of T in non-pregnant women is in the order of 0.1–0.4 mg/day. Finally, the conversion of T to

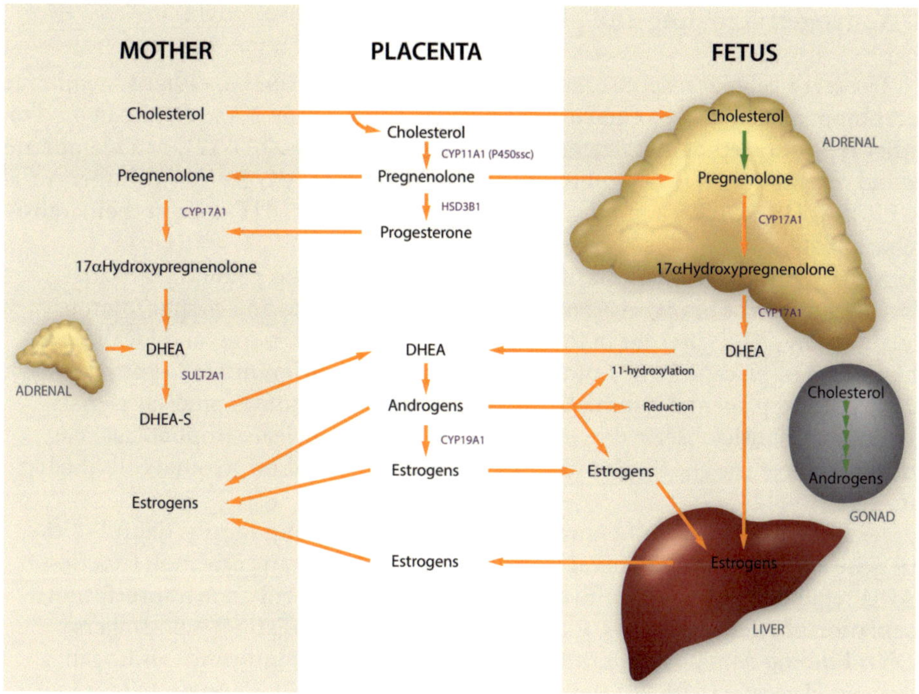

Figure 2.
Summarized overview of the functional interaction between the placental, maternal and fetal compartments for the biosynthesis of progesterone, estrogens and androgens by the human placenta. Progesterone is produced mainly from maternal cholesterol. Progesterone can be metabolized into DHEA by the maternal and fetal adrenal gland. DHEA can be converted into T. Subsequently, T can further be metabolized to estrogens via aromatase (CYP19A1). In horses, the placenta does not appear to express P450c17 and thus cannot convert de novo *c21 progestogens (pregnenolone and progesterone) to the c19 androgens (DEHA and A4). It is for this reason that the reaction occurs in the fetal adrenal.*

DHT occurs in peripheral tissues, such as ovaries and skin, with a daily production rating between 4.3 and 12.5 mg/day.

During pregnancy, an additional source of androgens comes from the fetus and placenta (**Figure 2**). Androgens are principally synthesized in the corpus luteum during early stages of gestation in rats and dogs and this function is taken over by the placenta in late stages of gestation in rats [13]. In sheep and goats, P450c17 is present in the placenta [14]. Some studies revealed that the absence of P450c17 in human and horse placentas results in negligible androgen synthesis [15]. However, protein and mRNA levels of CYP17A1 have been detected in primary human trophoblast cells and the human trophoblast cell line JEG-3 and trophoblast cells were able to generate testosterone *de novo* [16]. Placentas associated with a male fetus at term have increased expression of 5 α-reductase compared to a female fetus [17]. This enzyme is involved in reducing T to DHT, a potent androgen with a higher binding affinity to AR than T, suggesting the placenta may play a role in the hormonal differences between pregnancies between female and male fetuses.

In horses, the placenta does not appear to express P450c17 and thus cannot convert *de novo* c21 progestogens (pregnenolone and progesterone) to the c19 androgens (DEHA and A4). In this case, the fetal gonads are the main androgen source as estrogens precursor during mid to late gestation in the horse. Removal of fetal gonads results in an immediate fall in maternal plasma concentrations of conjugated and unconjugated estrogens whereas progestogens levels remain unchanged [18].

4. Androgen signaling and placenta function

To exert a cellular response, steroid hormones need to bind to either a membrane receptor or an intracellular, nuclear or cytoplasmic receptor. T and DHT can bind to either type of receptor, AR (encoded by *AR*, in the human Xq11-12), or a membrane-bound receptor, such as G protein-coupled receptor family C group 6 member A (GPRC6A) [19]. DHEA and A4 require conversion to T or DHT to exert their androgenic effects.

AR is expressed at all levels of the female hypothalamic-pituitary-gonadal axis, including the brain, ovarian stroma, ovarian follicles and corpus luteum. Furthermore, AR is present in first trimester and term placenta, and localizes to the cytosol of placental villi, and in cytotrophoblast, differentiated syncytiotrophoblast, and placental stroma [20]. In ruminant placentomes, nuclear signals are predominantly observed in invasive TGC and uninucleate trophoblast cells, stromal cells of the chorionic villi, caruncular epithelial, and stromal cells during late gestation [21, 22].

AR belongs to the steroid hormone intracellular receptor family. Exon 1 of the *AR* gene encodes the N-terminal domain, which contains an activation function 1 (AF1) region that interacts with coregulatory proteins to enhance transcriptional regulation of AR target genes. Exons 2 and 3 encode two distinct zinc-fingers (DNA-binding domain) required for interaction with a palindromic androgen response elements (ARE) of the core sequence, 5′-TGTTCT-3′, separated by 3 nucleotides located within the promoter regions of AR target genes. The remaining exons encode a hinge region which contains the nuclear localization signal, and the ligand binding domain [23].

When localized to the cytoplasm, AR is bound by a number of chaperone proteins including heat shock protein 90 (Hsp90) as well as immunophilins. When ligands, T or DHT, bind to AR, there is a conformational change which exposes the nuclear localization signal, allowing the interaction with importin-α, which facilitates nuclear translocation. Once inside the nucleus, two subunits of the AR dimerize and bind the ARE on promoter regions of AR-target genes, resulting in transcriptional regulation, leading to either activation or suppression of expression. Co-regulatory proteins, such as histone lysine demethylases (KDMs), modulate transcriptional activity of AR-target genes. In sheep for example, KDMs have been found to act as co-regulators in trophoblast cells [22, 24]. This interaction with regulator factors is critical for signaling processes in the placenta.

Androgens are known to stimulate proliferation of human umbilical vein endothelial cells, indicating a key role for androgens during pregnancy. During establishment of pregnancy, androgens play a role in embryo implantation. Early in pregnancy, before implantation, T is converted to DHT which regulates transcription of factors necessary for initiation of decidualization and early endometrial receptivity. Near the time of implantation, T itself promotes endometrial remodeling, and soon after implantation it serves as an important precursor for E2 which regulates vascular remodeling [25]. Studies in mice reveal that insufficient androgens may delay embryo implantation, whereas excess androgens lead to aberrant gene expression at implantation sites.

Studies on ovine placentas revealed vascular endothelial growth factor A (VEGFA) expression to be androgen responsive, and androgens are thought to regulate the expression of VEGFA and play a key role in placental angiogenesis [21, 23]. More specifically, AR and the KDM1A coregulator are recruited to an ARE in the ovine VEGFA promoter. On gestational day 90, placenta VEGFA mRNA and VEGFA and AR protein levels increased in testosterone-treated ewes compared to control placentas [22].

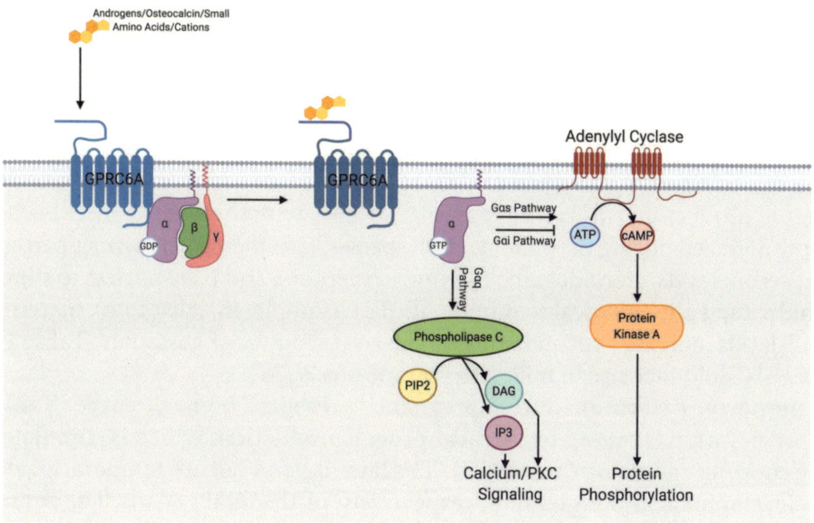

Figure 3.
Androgen signaling through GPRC6A in target tissue. Image created with BioRender.com.

In addition to the classical genomic intracellular AR mediated signaling pathways, androgens also act through membrane receptors. GPRC6A is a G protein-coupled receptor (GPCR) that functions as a membrane receptor for small amino acids, cations, osteocalcin, and androgens [26]. GPRC6A is known to have a long extracellular domain to allow for the binding of these different ligands [26]. GPRC6A mediates the effects of osteocalcin, a protein hormone released by osteoblasts, and results in the activation of the cAMP pathway and subsequently, testosterone synthesis by the Leydig cells of the testis. GPRC6A ligand binding can result in the activation of the Gαs, Gαi, and Gαq pathways (**Figure 3**). The presence of GPRC6A has been identified in placental trophoblast cell membranes, indicating the possibility of androgens eliciting a non-genomic effect on cells of the placenta.

Another membrane receptor that androgens elicit a non-genomic effect through is Zrt- and Irt-like protein 9 (ZIP9) [27]. ZIP9 is a zinc transporter that also acts as a receptor for androgens via G-protein coupling. Studies have revealed the presence of ZIP9 in ovarian tissue of Atlantic croakers, and act as a receptor for androgens inducing apoptosis in follicular cells, as well as promoting zinc uptake. Studies also show a similar action in breast and prostate tissue [28]. Ultimately, these two studies reveal that androgens binding to ZIP9 results in the activation of pro-apoptotic genes and the regulation of zinc homeostasis within target tissues [28].

Similarly, Transient receptor potential cation channel subfamily M (melastatin) member 8 (TRPM8) and Oxoeicosanoid receptor 1 (OXER1) bind a variety of ligands including androgens [29]. However, their expression during pregnancy or in placental cells is currently unknown.

5. Androgens and pregnancy

Androgens play a fundamental role in female physiology, particularly during pregnancy. In women, androgens are synthesized by cells within the ovaries, the adrenal glands, fat, and also in placenta, acting in an endocrine or paracrine fashion [30]. DHEA, mainly from the adrenal glands, acts as a crucial precursor for E2 and T in the ovary and other target tissues such as fat [31]. Depending on the intracellular availability of steroidogenic enzymes in target tissues, DHEA is converted to A4 which is a precursor for T, both of which can be aromatized to estrogens [32]. Some studies have reported an elevated level of T during pregnancy. An increase in T levels occurs from the first trimester of pregnancy, becoming more pronounced towards the third trimester, being three-folds higher than observed in non-pregnant women (**Table 1**) [36]. In contrast, maternal circulating DHEA levels decrease in pregnant women due to it being converted to T and E2 [37].

Steroid production varies widely among species, with these differences becoming more pronounced during pregnancy. Each species have their own distinct pattern of steroid serum levels, steroidogenic enzymes, receptors, and transporters to support their individual physiological requirements. For example, in dairy cows, maternal serum T levels increase ~100-fold during the last trimester of gestation (**Table 1**), as well as a ~50-fold increase in milk testosterone levels [38].

In the horse, T elevation during pregnancy presents a biphasic curve (**Table 1**). The first elevation is caused by luteal androgen production, which is stimulated by equine chorionic gonadotropin (eCG). The late rise and fall are temporally related to the development and regression, respectively, of the fetal gonads. The equine placenta has little capacity to synthesize androgens, as it lacks CYP17A1. Hence, androgens in the form of DHEA are substrates for E2 synthesis, and must be supplied mostly by fetal gonads, forming a true feto-placental unit [39].

As androgen levels increase during pregnancy, the mother and developing fetuses usually are protected from excess bioactive androgens by increased secretion of sex hormone-binding and placental aromatase, which converts T into E2. Hyperandrogenism can result from a number of conditions, the most common being luteomas and theca-lutein cysts within the ovary. Luteomas are benign tumors that occur during pregnancy with excess androgen production in 25-35% of the cases [33, 40, 41]. These often go unnoticed and in most cases are non-virilizing.

Humans	**Testosterone (ng/ml)**	
	Pimiparous	**Multiparous**
1st trimester	1.34	0.66
2nd trimester	1.98	0.73
3rd trimester	2.56	0.71
7-20 wks	0.69	
21-40 wks	1.095	
Horse		
Days from ovulation		
0-35	0.04	
35-120	0.14	
180–240	2.5	
240-300	3.5	
>300	1.5	
Cow		
Days from ovulation		
0-90	0.020-0.050	
90-270	0.22	

Table 1.
Testosterone serum levels during pregnancy in human [33], horses [34], and cows [35].

Additional causes of excess androgen production during pregnancy are conditions such as polycystic ovarian syndrome (PCOS), one of the most common endocrine disorders in women of reproductive age, and congenital adrenal hyperplasia (CAH). Both conditions result in pregnancy complications, including pregnancy induced hypertension and pre-eclampsia, a human pregnancy syndrome characterized by the onset of hypertension and proteinuria after 20 weeks of gestation, and can lead to maternal or fetal mortality [42]. In humans, clinical observations have established that women with PCOS exhibit similar features as seen in classical 21-hydroxylase deficiency in CAH, such as anovulation, ovarian hyperandrogenism, LH hypersecretion, polycystic appearing ovaries, and insulin resistance, despite normalization of adrenal androgen excess after birth [43]. Furthermore, animal studies have demonstrated that intrauterine exposure to excessive amounts of androgens can lead to development of PCOS after birth (reviewed in [44, 45]). In fact, prenatal androgenization in pregnant ewes has revealed reproductive and metabolic phenotypes in female offspring that closely resemble PCOS in women. These observations suggest that androgen excess during early life, whether derived from fetal or maternal sources, may provide one possible mechanism to explain the occurrence of PCOS in adulthood.

Less common causes leading to androgen excess during pregnancy include placental aromatase deficiency. Aromatase is encoded by the CYP19A1 gene, and is responsible for converting T to E2. At least 10 different promoters have been identified in its regulatory region, enabling regulation in a tissue-specific manner [46]. Mutations in CYP19A1 prevent aromatization of testosterone, leading to hyperandrogenism and phenotypes similar to androgen excess, including maternal and fetal virilization and development of ambiguous genitalia at birth [47]. Of particular interest is the observation that placental aromatase deficiency is associated with pre-eclampsia [48, 49]. Women with pre-eclampsia have significantly lower levels of placental aromatase, and significantly lower levels of both 17β-estradiol:testosterone and estrone:androstenedione ratios, as well as higher levels of T. In fact, this placental defect in steroidogenesis appears before clinical symptoms of pre-eclampsia and thus may serve as a diagnostic marker.

6. Conclusions

The focus of this chapter was on androgens and their potential role in pregnancy and placental development and function. Normal pregnancy in women is associated with increased maternal serum levels of androgens, which are derived from the adrenal glands, adipose tissue, ovaries, and placenta. Species differences in androgen production exist reflecting species-specific needs for pregnancy maintenance and/or placental function. Furthermore, the placenta contains classical androgen receptors as well as non-classical membrane receptors, indicating the placenta is a target of androgen signaling. Preliminary and ongoing studies suggest a role for androgen signaling in trophoblast cell differentiation and placental angiogenesis.

Acknowledgements

The authors would like to thank Ms. Coni Hoerndli, Science Design (chsciencedesign.com), for help with **Figures 1** and **2**. Funding for this work was provided and supported by Agriculture and Food Research Initiative Competitive Grant 2019-67015-29000 from the U.S. Department of Agriculture (USDA) National Institute of Food and Agriculture.

Author details

Agata M. Parsons Aubone, River Evans and Gerrit J. Bouma*
Colorado State University, Fort Collins, USA

*Address all correspondence to: gerrit.bouma@colostate.edu

References

[1] Itskovitz J, Hodgen GD. Endocrine basis for the initiation, maintenance and termination of pregnancy in humans. Psychoneuroendocrinology 1988;13:155-70. DOI: 10.1016/0306-4530(88)90012-1

[2] Astle S, Slater DM, Thornton S. The involvement of progesterone in the onset of human labour. Eur J Obstet Gynecol Reprod Biol 2003;108:177-81. DOI: 10.1016/s0301-2115(02)00422-0.

[3] Rosenfeld CR, Chen C, Roy T, Liu X. Estrogen selectively up-regulates eNOS and nNOS in reproductive arteries by transcriptional mechanisms. J Soc Gynecol Investig 2003;10: 205 – 15. DOI: 10.1016/s1071-5576(03)00049-2

[4] Pepe GJ, Albrecht ED. Actions of placental and fetal adrenal steroid hormones in primate pregnancy. Endocr Rev 1995;16:608-48. DOI: 10.1210/edrv-16-5-608

[5] Makieva, Sofia et al. Androgens in pregnancy: roles in parturition. Human reproduction update vol. 20,4 (2014): 542-59. doi:10.1093/humupd/dmu008

[6] Furukawa, Satoshi et al. A comparison of the histological structure of the placenta in experimental animals. Journal of toxicologic pathology vol. 27,1 (2014): 11-8. doi:10.1293/tox.2013-0060

[7] Leiser R, Kaufmann P. Placental structure: in a comparative aspect. Exp Clin Endocrinol. 1994; 102(3):122-134. doi:10.1055/s-0029-1211275

[8] Seo, Heewon; Bazer, Fuller W.; Burghardt, Robert C.; Johnson, Greg A. 2019. "Immunohistochemical Examination of Trophoblast Syncytialization during Early Placentation in Sheep." *Int. J. Mol. Sci.* 20, no. 18: 4530. DOI:org/10.3390/ijms20184530

[9] Ghayee HK, Auchus RJ. Basic concepts and recent developments in human steroid hormone biosynthesis. Rev Endocr Metab Disord. 2007; 8(4): 289-300. doi:10.1007/s11154-007-9052-2

[10] Penning TM. New frontiers in androgen biosynthesis and metabolism. Curr Opin Endocrinol Diabetes Obes. 2010; 17(3): 233-239. doi:10.1097/MED.0b013e3283381a31

[11] Abraham G., Ovarian and Adrenal Contribution to Peripheral Androgens During the Menstrual Cycle, The Journal of Clinical Endocrinology and Metabolism, Volume 39, Issue 2, 1 August 1974, Pages 340-346, doi:10.1210/jcem-39-2-340

[12] Longcope C. Adrenal and gonadal androgen secretion in normal females. Clin Endocrinol Metab. 1986; 15(2): 213-228. doi:10.1016/s0300-595x(86)80021-4

[13] Kazuyoshi Taya, Gilbert S. Greenwald, In vivo and in vitro Ovarian Steroidogenesis in the Pregnant Rat, *Biology of Reproduction*, Volume 25, Issue 4, 1 November 1981, Pages 683-691, doi:10.1095/biolreprod25.4.683

[14] Thorburn GD, Challis JR. Endocrine control of parturition. Physiol Rev. 1979; 59(4): 863-918. doi:10.1152/physrev.1979.59.4.863

[15] Legacki EL, Corbin CJ, Ball BA, Scoggin KE, Stanley SD, Conley AJ. Steroidogenic enzyme activities in the pre- and post-parturient equine placenta. Reproduction. 2018; 155(1): 51-59. doi:10.1530/REP-17-0472

[16] J. C. Escobar, S. S. Patel, V. E. Beshay, T. Suzuki, B. R. Carr, The Human Placenta Expresses CYP17 and Generates Androgens *De Novo, The Journal of Clinical Endocrinology and Metabolism*, Volume 96, Issue 5, 1 May

2011, Pages 1385-1392, doi:10.1210/jc.2010-2504

[17] Vu TT, Hirst JJ, Stark M, et al. Changes in human placental 5alpha-reductase isoenzyme expression with advancing gestation: effects of fetal sex and glucocorticoid exposure. Reprod Fertil Dev. 2009; 21(4): 599-607. doi:10.1071/RD08224

[18] Pashen RL, Allen WR. The role of the fetal gonads and placenta in steroid production, maintenance of pregnancy and parturition in the mare. J Reprod Fertil Suppl. 1979;(27):499-509. PMID: 289829.

[19] Grigorova M, Punab M, Kahre T, et al. The number of CAG and GGN triplet repeats in the Androgen Receptor gene exert combinatorial effect on hormonal and sperm parameters in young men. Andrology. 2017;5(3):495-504. doi:10.1111/andr.12344

[20] McWhorter, E.S., Russ, J.E., Winger, Q.A. *et al.* Androgen and estrogen receptors in placental physiology and dysfunction. *Front. Biol.* **13,** 315-326 (2018). https://doi.org/10.1007/s11515-018-1517-z

[21] P.Khatri, B.Hoffmann, G.Schuler. 2013. Androgen receptor is widely expressed in bovine placentomes and up-regulated during differentiation of bovine trophoblast giant cells. Placenta. DOI.org/10.1016/j.placenta.2013.01.018

[22] Cleys ER, Halleran JL, Enriquez VA, da Silveira JC, West RC, Winger QA, et al. (2015) Androgen Receptor and Histone Lysine Demethylases in Ovine Placenta. PLoS ONE 10(2): e0117472. https://doi.org/10.1371/journal.pone.0117472

[23] Davey RA, Grossmann M. Androgen Receptor Structure, Function and Biology: From Bench to Bedside. Clin Biochem *Rev*. 2016;37(1):3-15. PMID: 27057074, PMCID: PMC4810760

[24] Hord, Taylor Kimberly, et al. "Placenta Specific Gene Targeting to Study Histone Lysine Demethylase and Androgen Signaling in Ruminant Placenta." *Animal Reproduction*, vol. 17, no. 3, 2020, doi:10.1590/1984-3143-ar2020-0069.

[25] Gibson DA, Simitsidellis I, Saunders PT. Regulation of androgen action during establishment of pregnancy. *J Mol Endocrinol*. 2016;57(1):R35-R47. doi:10.1530/JME-16-0027

[26] Pi, Min, et al. "GPRC6A: Jack of All Metabolism (or Master of None)". *Molecular Metabolism*, vol. 6, no. 2, 2017, pp. 185-193., doi:10.1016/j.molmet.2016.12.006.

[27] Thomas, Peter, et al. "ZIP9, a Novel Membrane Androgen Receptor and Zinc Transporter Protein." *General and Comparative Endocrinology*, vol. 257, 2018, pp. 130-136., doi:10.1016/j.ygcen.2017.04.016.

[28] Pascal, Laura E., and Zhou Wang. "Unzipping Androgen Action Through ZIP9: A Novel Membrane Androgen Receptor." *Endocrinology*, vol. 155, no. 11, 2014, pp. 4120-4123., doi:10.1210/en.2014-1749.

[29] Thomas, Peter. "Membrane Androgen Receptors Unrelated to Nuclear Steroid Receptors." *Endocrinology*, vol. 160, no. 4, 2019, pp. 772-781., doi:10.1210/en.2018-00987.

[30] Lebbe M, Woodruff TK. Involvement of androgens in ovarian health and disease. Mol Hum Reprod. 2013 Dec;19(12):828-37. doi: 10.1093/molehr/gat065. Epub 2013 Sep 10. PMID: 24026057; PMCID: PMC3843026

[31] Labrie, 2010. Chapter 4 - DHEA, Important Source of Sex Steroids in Men and Even More in Women. doi.org/10.1016/S0079-6123(10)82004-7

[32] Buster JE, Chang RJ, Preston DL, et al. Interrelationships of circulating maternal steroid concentrations in third trimester pregnancies. II. C18 and C19 steroids: estradiol, estriol, dehydroepiandrosterone, dehydroepiandrosterone sulfate, delta 5-androstenediol, delta 4-androstenedione, testosterone, and dihydrotestosterone. J Clin Endocrinol Metab. 1979;48(1):139-142. doi:10.1210/jcem-48-1-139

[33] Hakim C, Padmanabhan V, Vyas AK. Gestational Hyperandrogenism in Developmental Programming. *Endocrinology*. 2017;158(2):199-212. doi:10.1210/en.2016-1801

[34] Esteller-Vico A, Ball BA, Troedsson MHT, Squires EL. Endocrine changes, fetal growth, and uterine artery hemodynamics after chronic estrogen suppression during the last trimester of equine pregnancy. *Biol Reprod*. 2017;96(2):414-423. doi:10.1095/biolreprod.116.140533

[35] Gaiani R, Chiesa F, Mattioli M, Nannetti G, Galeati G. Androstenedione and testosterone concentrations in plasma and milk of the cow throughout pregnancy. *J Reprod Fertil*. 1984;70(1):55-59. doi:10.1530/jrf.0.0700055

[36] Dawood MY, Saxena BB. Testosterone and dihydrotestosterone in maternal and cord blood and in amniotic fluid. Am J Obstet Gynecol. 1977;129(1):37-42. doi:10.1016/0002-9378(77)90815-8

[37] Bird CE, Cook SJ, DresselDE, Clark AF. Plasma C_{19}-$^{\Delta 5}$-steroid levels during normal human pregnancy. https://doi.org/10.1016/S0009-9120(80)90795-X

[38] Mattioli M et al., Androstendione and testosterone concentrations in plasma and milk of the cow throughout pregnancy, J Reprod Fertil. 1984. DOI: 10.1530/jrf.0.0700055

[39] Ginther O.J. Reproductive Biology of the Mare: Basic and Applied Aspects, Volumen2. Equiservices, 1992. ISBN: 9780964007215

[40] McClamrock HD, Adashi EY. Gestational hyperandrogenism. *Fertil Steril*. 1992;57(2):257-274. doi:10.1016/s0015-0282(16)54828-6

[41] Kaňová N, Bičíková M. Hyperandrogenic states in pregnancy. *Physiol Res*. 2011;60(2):243-252. doi:10.33549/physiolres.932078

[42] Palomba S, de Wilde MA, Falbo A, Koster MP, La Sala GB, Fauser BC. Pregnancy complications in women with polycystic ovary syndrome. Hum Reprod Update. 2015;21(5):575-592. doi:10.1093/humupd/dmv029

[43] Barnes, R B et al. "Ovarian hyperandrogynism as a result of congenital adrenal virilizing disorders: evidence for perinatal masculinization of neuroendocrine function in women. The Journal of clinical endocrinology and metabolism vol. 79,5 (1994): 1328-33. doi:10.1210/jcem.79.5.7962325

[44] Cardoso RC, Padmanabhan V. Developmental Programming of PCOS Traits: Insights from the Sheep. *Med Sci (Basel)*. 2019;7(7):79. Published 2019 Jul 11. doi:10.3390/medsci7070079

[45] Dumesic DA, Hoyos LR, Chazenbalk GD, Naik R, PadmanabhanV, AbbottDH. Mechanisms of intergenerational transmission of polycystic ovary syndrome. *Reproduction*. 2020;159(1):R1-R13. doi:10.1530/REP-19-0197

[46] Belgorosky A, Guercio G, Pepe C, Saraco N, Rivarola MA. Genetic and clinical spectrum of aromatase deficiency in infancy, childhood and adolescence.

Horm Res. 2009;72(6):321-330. doi:10.1159/000249159

[47] Lin L, Ercan O, Raza J, et al. Variable phenotypes associated with aromatase (CYP19) insufficiency in humans. *J Clin Endocrinol Metab*. 2007;92(3):982-990. doi:10.1210/jc.2006-1181

[48] Perez-Sepulveda A, Monteiro LJ, Dobierzewska A, et al. Placental Aromatase Is Deficient in Placental Ischemia and Preeclampsia. *PLoS One*. 2015;10(10):e0139682. Published 2015 Oct 7. doi:10.1371/journal.pone.0139682

[49] Berkane N, Liere P, Lefevre G, et al. Abnormal steroidogenesis and aromatase activity in preeclampsia. *Placenta*. 2018;69:40-49. doi:10.1016/j.placenta.2018.07.004

Chapter 5

Testosterone

Kizito Omona

Abstract

Testosterone is a hormone produced majorly by the testicles in adult human _ men. The hormone affects a man's appearance and sexual development, stimulates sperm production and regulates a man's sex drive. It also helps build muscles and bone mass. Testosterone production decreases with age. Its production is at its highest in a man's early adulthood and drops slowly each year afterwards. The normal range of testosterone in the body is typically 300 to 1000 ng/dL for men and 15 to 70 ng/dL for women. A range of symptoms can occur if its production drastically drops below normal. Men with low T can experience a range of symptoms if its decrease becomes significant. Low testosterone, or low T, is diagnosed when levels fall below 300 ng/dL. A blood test, called 'a serum testosterone test', is used to determine the level of circulating testosterone. When the body does not produce the right amount of testosterone, the condition is called hypogonadism. This is sometimes called "low T". Men diagnosed with hypogonadism can benefit from testosterone therapy. However, therapy is not usually recommended, unless testosterone level falls quite below the normal range for age. This is because there are some natural remedies which can help.

Keywords: low T, Hypogonadism, sex drive, erection, semen volume, mood

1. Introduction

The term Hormones refer to substances or molecules that are produced by the endocrine system. This system sends messages to various parts of the body and hormones are the messengers used to do so. Hormones help to regulate body processes, like hunger, blood pressure and sexual desire, among others. Whereas hormones are key molecules in reproduction in human, they are fundamental to *all* the body systems [1]. Chemically, hormones may be classified as either proteins or steroids. All of the hormones in the human body, except the sex hormones and those from the adrenal cortex, are proteins or protein derivatives [2].

Hormones flow through the whole body by blood but only affect certain cells designed to receive their messages _ target cells. These specific cells that respond to a given hormone have receptor sites for the said hormone [1, 2]. This is a sort of lock-and-key mechanism, in that if the hormone fits the receptor site then there will be an effect. It is synonymous with lock and key, where if the key fits, then the lock opens. If a hormone and a receptor do not match, there will be no reaction. In some cases, target cells are localized in a single gland or organ whereas in other instances, they are diffuse and scattered throughout the whole body in which case many areas will be affected. Through modifying activities of the cells, hormones are able to bring about their associated effects on those target cells.

When certain types of hormones called protein hormones react with receptors on the surface of the target cell, the sequence of events that results in hormone action is relatively fast. On the other hand, steroid hormones basically react with receptor sites inside a target cell. Since this method of action involves synthesis of proteins, the actions of these hormones are relatively slow [2].

2. The male reproductive hormones

2.1 General male reproductive hormones

Male reproductive functions are mediated by different hormones [3]. The 'master' regulator hormonal axis is the hypothalamo-pituitary-gonadal/testicular axis which is led by the pulsatile release of hypothalamic gonadotropin-releasing hormone (GnRH). This, in turn, stimulates anterior pituitary trophic hormones _ luteinizing hormone (LH) and follicle-stimulating hormone (FSH). Luteinizing hormone acts upon the testicular cells, the Leydig cells for steroidogenesis while follicle stimulating hormone acts on the Sertoli cells to aid spermatogenesis. This primary axis is influenced by an array of other testicular hormones, metabolic hormones and different regulatory factors. These hormonal cross-talks influence the intricate testicular functions, sexual behavior and semen quality in men, including semen volume [3]. See **Figure 1** for the illustration.

Testes secrete steroids known as androgens. These androgens, in turn, are responsible for maintenance of male characteristics as well as male behaviors. Follicle stimulating hormones (FSH) released from pituitary gland stimulates the growth of the seminiferous tubules. Seminiferous tubules constitute much of the

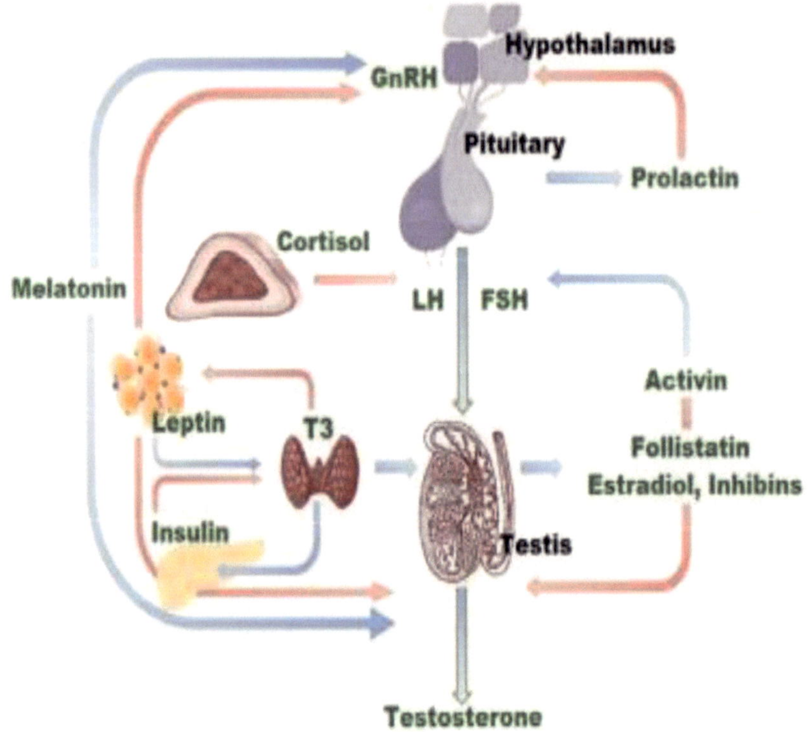

Figure 1.
Hypothalamo-pituitary-testicular Axis and its crosstalk with other hormones in the regulation of male reproductive functions [3].

structure of the testes. The hormone, FSH, promotes within seminiferous tubules cell divisions which will result in the production of mature sperm [4].

The luteinizing hormones (LH), also released from pituitary gland, promotes the development of certain endocrine tissues within the testes. These tissues are composed of groups of cells (interstitial tissue) between the seminiferous tubules.

Under the influence of LH, the interstitial tissues secrete the steroid hormone testosterone. Even though testosterone may be secreted by the adrenal cortex, the amount of secretion is usually insignificant [4]. Testosterone is also produced in ovary in females [5].

Testosterone, in the presence of normal amounts of growth hormone, promotes growth of the bony skeleton. This is in addition to promoting male characteristics, male behaviors and the maintenance of the spermatic tubules [4, 6, 9]. The secretion of androgen markedly increases at puberty accounting for rapid growth at that stage of life [4, 7].

Illustration is shown in **Figure 1**.

2.2 Testosterone

Testosterone is the primary male sex hormone and anabolic steroid [6]. It is the main anabolic steroid hormone produced by the body but serving two main effects on the body:

- Anabolic effects, which promote muscle building
- Androgenic effects, which are responsible for male traits, such as facial hair and a deeper voice, among others.

Some athletes take testosterone to boost their performance because of its anabolic effects [6].

Testosterone is produced majorly by the testicles in adult human _ men [7]. In women, the ovaries produce the hormone [8]. The hormone affects a man's appearance and sexual development, stimulates sperm production and regulates a man's sex drive, including semen volume. It also helps build muscles and bone masses [7, 8, 11].

Testosterone production decreases with age. Its production is at its highest in a man's early adulthood and drops slowly each year afterwards [9]. The normal range of testosterone in the body is typically 300 to 1000 ng/dL (nanogram per deciliter). A range of symptoms can occur if its production drastically drops below normal. Men with low testosterone level, also known as 'low T', can experience a range of symptoms if its decrease becomes significant. Low testosterone, or low T, is diagnosed when levels fall severely below 300 ng/dL in male or 15 ng/dL in female. A blood test, called 'a serum testosterone test', is usually used to determine the level of circulating testosterone [7, 9]. When the body does not produce the right amount of testosterone, the condition is called hypogonadism. This is sometimes called "low T". Men diagnosed with hypogonadism can benefit from testosterone therapy. However, therapy is not usually recommended, unless testosterone level falls quite below the normal range for a given age. This is because there are some natural remedies which can help [9].

2.2.1 Normal and abnormal levels of testosterone

A normal testosterone level range for men is 300 to 1000 nanograms per deciliter (ng/dL) [7]. For women, its normal level is between 15 and 70 ng/dL. However, it's also considered normal to have changes in the level of testosterone throughout life [8].

Testosterone levels can decrease naturally due to age or other health conditions. After the age of 40, men's testosterone levels decrease. The decrease, on average, is about one percent (1%) every year. When men reach above 40 years of age, some symptoms of low testosterone become commonly seen. The commonest symptom to appear is erectile dysfunction. Irrespective of age, low testosterone levels have often been observed in people with obesity [8].

Hypogonadism, also called low testosterone, is the most common problem related to testosterone, in men.

As discussed earlier (Section 2.2), Testosterone is responsible for traits such as body hair, muscle mass and strength. Therefore, men with low levels of testosterone might notice a reduction in these traits whereas women with too much testosterone might notice an increase in these traits [8].

2.2.2 Chemical properties of testosterone

The molecular formula is $\mathbf{C_{19}H_{28}O_2}$ [10]. The molecular weight is 288.42 g/mol [11]. In medical treatment, the therapeutic testosterone is a synthetic form of endogenous androgenic steroid testosterone [12].

Generally speaking, in vivo, testosterone is converted into dihydrotestosterone (DHT) in the target tissues irreversibly by the enzyme 5-alpha reductase. The testosterone or DHT ligand-androgen receptor complexes then act as transcription factor complexes. In this way, it stimulates the expression of various responsive genes. In comparison, DHT binds with higher affinity to androgen receptors than testosterone, thus activating gene expression more efficiently. Testosterone, in addition, is irreversibly converted to estradiol by the enzyme complex aromatase. This occurs particularly in the liver and adipose tissue. Both testosterone and DHT promote the development and maintenance of male sex traits related to the internal and external genitalia, skeletal muscle and hair follicles. On the other hand, estradiol promotes epiphyseal maturation and bone mineralization. However, because of rapid metabolism by the liver, therapeutic testosterone is generally administered as an ester derivative (**Figure 2**) [11].

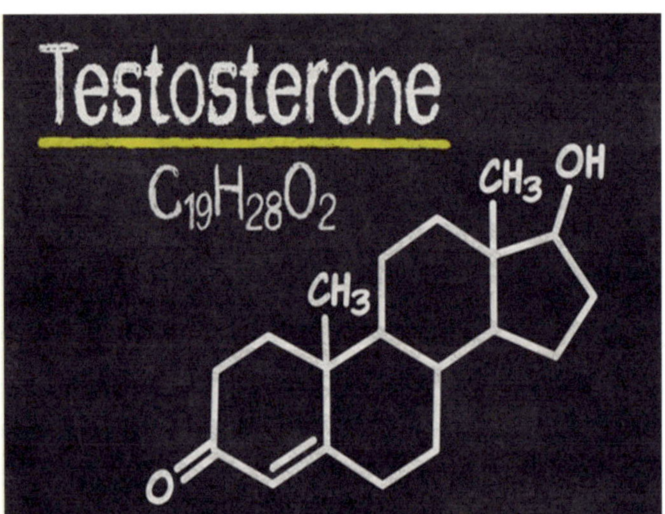

Figure 2.
Chemical structure of testosterone [5].

2.2.3 The role of testosterone

In males, testosterone is the predominant sex hormone [6, 9]. It plays a number of important roles. These roles include;

a. Development of penis and testes

b. Deepening of voice at puberty

c. Appearance of facial and pubic hair at puberty. It starts at puberty but later in life, it may play a role in balding

d. Building muscle mass and strength

e. Bone growth and strength

f. Sex drive (libido)

g. Sperm production, including semen volume

Therefore, males in adolescent stages of life, who have too little testosterone may not experience normal masculinization. The genitals of such males may not enlarge, as well as their facial and body hair may be scanty. The voice may also not deepen as normally expected [5].

Notably, testosterone also helps in the maintenance of normal mood [7]. Scholars have argued that there may be other important functions of this hormone, testosterone, that have not yet been discovered [5].

To control the production of testosterone in men, signals have to be sent from the hypothalamus in the brain to the pituitary gland at the base of the brain. In turn, the pituitary gland then relays signals to the testes to produce testosterone [4]. Thus, a "feedback loop" closely regulates the amount of this hormone in the blood. Notably, when the level of testosterone rise too high, the brain (hypothalamus) then sends signals to the pituitary to reduce the production [5]. See **Figure 1** about the 'Hypothalamo-pituitary-testicular Axis'.

For normal working of the ovaries in females, there must be proper balance between testosterone and estrogen. It is a known fact that androgens also play an important role in normal brain functions, including mood, sex drive and cognitive functions, although these areas may still require more studies [1–5].

2.2.4 Too little testosterone

A range of symptoms can occur if testosterone production drastically drops below normal [7]. In past few years, scholars have focused on the effects of testosterone deficiency among men. As already known, that as men grow older, their levels of testosterone drop gradually, about 1–2% each year. The rate of this drop is slower compared to the relatively rapid drop in estrogen in females that culminates in menopause [5]. Majority of men, more than a third, who are above 45 years of age, have reduced levels of testosterone [5].

The following symptoms of deficiency of testosterone in adult males occur: they are but not limited to;

a. Reduced body and facial hair

b. Loss of muscle mass

c. Low libido, impotence, small testicles, reduced sperm count and infertility

d. Increased breast size

e. Hot flashes

f. Irritability, poor concentration and depression

g. Loss of body hair

h. Brittle bones and an increased risk of fracture

Indeed some men who have testosterone deficiency have related symptoms or conditions. These symptoms or conditions appear to improve when testosterone replacement is done [4, 5, 9].

Therefore, in a nutshell, men with low levels of testosterone might notice a reduction in body hair, muscle mass and strength, while women with too much testosterone might notice an increase in these traits [8].

2.2.5 Too much testosterone

Having too much naturally-occurring testosterone is not a common problem among men [5]. Too much testosterone is common only in male athletes who inject themselves with the hormone in order to make use of its anabolic effects. This is because anabolic steroids, testosterone or related hormones, increase muscle mass and athletic performance [5].

Thus, problems associated with abnormally high testosterone levels in men include but not limited to;

a. Low sperm counts, shrinking of the testicles and impotence

b. Heart muscle damage and increased risk of heart attack

c. Prostate enlargement with difficulty urinating

d. Liver disease

e. Acne

f. Fluid retention with swelling of the legs and feet

g. Weight gain, perhaps related in part to increased appetite

h. High blood pressure and cholesterol

i. Insomnia

j. Headaches

k. Increased muscle mass

l. Increased risk of blood clots

m. Stunted growth in adolescents

n. Uncharacteristically aggressive behavior

o. Mood swings, euphoria, irritability, impaired judgment and delusions

On another hand, women with too much testosterone may grow facial hair, develop a deeper voice or experience decreased breast size. Too much testosterone in women can also cause acne [8].

Among women, perhaps the most common cause of a high testosterone level is polycystic ovary syndrome (PCOS). It affects 6–10% of premenopausal women [5, 7].

Therefore, women with too much testosterone might notice an increase in these traits; body hair, muscle mass and strength [8].

2.2.6 Misuse of testosterone in athletes

As already discussed, the effects of testosterone in the body are two; (1) anabolic effects and (2) Virilizing or androgenic effects. Anabolic effects are related to protein synthesis and growth [13]. Male athletes who inject themselves with the hormone in order to make use of its anabolic effects tend to do so to make use of this advantage. This is because anabolic steroids, testosterone or related hormones, increase muscle mass and athletic performance [5]. Anabolic effects involve growth of muscle mass, increased bone density, as well as stimulation of linear growth and bone maturation [13].

Meanwhile, the Virilizing effects, also called androgenic effects, are related to the biological development of male sexual traits. This includes maturation of sex organs, specifically growth of penis and formation of scrotum in male fetus. However, at puberty, testosterone also coordinates development of masculine characteristics such as deepening of the voice and growth of facial hair [13].

2.2.7 Diseases and conditions affecting testosterone

As shown in **Figure 1** about the 'Hypothalamo-pituitary-testicular Axis', men will experience drop in testosterone when a disease or condition affects the axis. Thus, conditions or diseases affecting the testes, pituitary and hypothalamus glands also affect testosterone levels in the body.

- Testes – Conditions or disease of testes affecting testosterone include direct injury, castration, infection, radiation treatment, chemotherapy and tumors

- Pituitary and hypothalamus glands – Conditions or disease of pituitary and hypothalamus affecting testosterone include tumors, HIV/AIDS, certain infections and autoimmune conditions and lastly medications. These medications include steroids, morphine or related drugs and major tranquilizers, such as haloperidol, among others.

Klinefelter syndrome and hemochromatosis also affect testosterone levels. Klinefelter syndrome is a genetic disease in which a man has an extra x-chromosome whereas hemochromatosis is a genetic disease in which an abnormal gene causes excessive iron to accumulate throughout the body. These two conditions can also affect testosterone.

On the other hand, women may have a testosterone deficiency due to diseases of the pituitary, hypothalamus or adrenal glands, in addition to removal of the ovaries [5].

Therefore, high T levels can indicate ovarian or testicular cancer. Low T levels can indicate chronic illness or a problem with the pituitary gland, which releases hormones [8].

2.2.8 Testosterone therapy

Therapy Option: Currently, testosterone therapy is approved primarily for the treatment of delayed male puberty, low production of testosterone and certain inoperable female breast cancers [5].

Testosterone treatment can improve symptoms in men with significantly low levels of active testosterone, such as:

- Generalized weakness
- Low energy
- Disabling frailty
- Depression
- Problems with sexual function
- Problems with cognition.

The most common treatment for low testosterone is testosterone replacement therapy (TRT). TRT is given as an injection, a skin patch, or a topical gel containing testosterone that replaces the testosterone missing from the body [8].

Currently, there is no serious risk from acute poisoning with testosterone replacement therapy but chronic use can cause harm. Major risks of using the hormone are those of excessive androgens [12]. These are menstrual irregularities and virilization in women and impotence, premature cardiovascular disease and prostatic hypertrophy in men. It must be noted that both men and women can suffer liver damage with oral anabolic steroids containing a substituted product, 17-alpha-carbon. Again, psychiatric changes can occur during use or after cessation [12]. TRT falls against the recommendations by American College of Obstetricians and Gynecologists (ACOG) [14].

No Therapy Option: There's no magic solution for boosting testosterone but some natural remedies [9] may help;

a. Get eight hours night's sleep daily

b. Lose that excess weight _ weight reduction

c. Eat food rich with enough Zinc _ Zinc supplements

d. Reduce dietary sugary intake

e. Do regular physical exercise

These five remedies can be of help [9].

Eight (8) hours of sleep in every 24 hour is sufficient [9]. However, reduced hours of sleep have tremendous effects on testosterone level [15].

Low levels of testosterone have been discovered in overweight individuals. For this matter, weight reduction is paramount the no therapy option for treating testosterone related problems.

Scholars [9] have coined that men with hypogonadism often have zinc deficiencies. In other literature [16], it is coined that testosterone deficiency is associated with late-onset hypogonadism. Micronutrients [16], such as copper and zinc influence testosterone synthesis. These coupled with reduced dietary sugary intake and regular physical exercise can treat most of your testosterone related problems [9].

2.2.9 Performing testosterone test

A normal testosterone level for men is a range of 300 to 1000 nanograms per deciliter (ng/dL) [7]. For women, its normal level is between 15 and 70 ng/dL. However, it is considered normal to have changes in the level of testosterone throughout life [8].

To have testosterone levels checked requires a simple blood test. The test is usually performed in the morning, when T levels are highest. Sometimes, the test needs to be re-taken to confirm the measurements [8].

Some medications affect testosterone levels and so, the clinician or doctor may require one to stop taking such medication before testosterone test is performed. The medications below can artificially increase testosterone levels. They are;

- Steroids (T levels fall rapidly after one has stopped using steroids)
- Anticonvulsants
- Barbiturates
- Androgen or estrogen therapies

Opiates, in particular, are known to artificially decrease the levels of testosterone [8].

Studies, have confirmed that saliva offers a relatively accurate measurement of testosterone levels. This is especially true when diagnosing male hypogonadism [17]. In an earlier study, it was shown that salivary testosterone, dropped by 47% in 1454 males aged 20-89 years during their life time. However, in a later study (second), it was found that salivary testosterone was strongly correlated with bioavailable testosterone ($p < 0.000001$). It was also strongly correlated with calculated free testosterone ($p < 0.00001$) and total testosterone ($p < 0.002$). Hence forth, salivary testosterone was significantly related to hypogonadal symptoms [17].

However, American College of Obstetricians and Gynecologists Committee (ACOG) and other scholars, recommend against salivary testing for hormone replacement in females [14].

3. Conclusion

Men and women need the proper amount of testosterone to develop and function normally. Checking testosterone levels is quite important. The levels usually vary and for that matter, single low level may not be meaningful, except in the presence of symptoms related to low T. It is even more meaningless if the level of testosterone was normal at one time. To know when to measure level of testosterone, how best to respond to the results of measurement and when it is necessary to accept the risks of treatment are all areas of more research. Anything less of research might not be helpful.

Acknowledgements

I do acknowledge the technical guidance of my colleagues in the Faculty of Health Sciences of Uganda Martyrs' University. In a special way I appreciate Ms. Scovia Mbabazi, the former Associate Dean and Mr. Mathias Lwenge, the current Associate Dean at the faculty.

Conflict of interest

The author declares no conflict of interest.

Author details

Kizito Omona
Faculty of Health Sciences, Uganda Martyrs' University, Kampala, Uganda

*Address all correspondence to: komona@umu.ac.ug; kizitoomona@gmail.com

References

[1] Toler, S. What you should know about hormones. *Clue.* [Online] 2019. https://helloclue.com/articles/cycle-a-z/what-you-should-know-about-hormones.

[2] National Institute of Health. Characteristics of Hormones. *NIH.* [Online] 2020. https://training.seer.cancer.gov/.

[3] Sulagna, D., Pallav, S. and Suriyani, M. Male Reproductive Hormones and Semen Quality. 2019. Vol. 8, 5, pp. 189-194.

[4] Ernest, J. W. B. *Hormones.* Britannica: Encyclopædia Britannica, inc, 2019.

[5] Harvard Medical School. *Testosterone — What It Does And Doesn't Do.* New York: Harvard Health Publishing, 2019.

[6] Mayo Clinic. *Performance-enhancing Drugs: Know the risks.* 2019.

[7] Ryan, W. and Kathleen, Y. 12 Signs of Low Testosterone. *Healthline.* [Online] 2019. https://www.healthline.com/health/low-testosterone/warning-signs.

[8] Heitz, D. *When to Consider a Testosterone Test.* 2017.

[9] Pietrangelo, A. 5 Natural Testosterone Boosters. *Healthline.* [Online] 2015. https://www.healthline.com/health/low-testosterone/natural-boosters.

[10] ChemSpider. Testosterone. *ChemSpider.com.* s.l.: ChemSpider, 2020.

[11] National Center for Biotechnology Information. *PubChem Compound Summary for CID 6013, Testosterone.* 2020.

[12] Sylvana, V. C., et al. Testosterone. s.l.: InChem.org, 1994.

[13] New World Encyclopaedia. Testoterone. *New World Encyclopaedia.* [Online] 2020. https://www.newworldencyclopedia.org/entry/Testosterone.

[14] ACOG, ASRM. Compounded bioidentical menopausal hormone therapy. 2012. Vol. 98, 2, pp. 308-312.

[15] Leproult, R. and Van-Cauter, E. Effect of 1 Week of Sleep Restriction on Testosterone Levels in Young Healthy Men. 2011. Vol. 305, 21, pp. 2173-2174.

[16] Chang, C. S., et al. Correlation between serum testosterone level and concentrations of copper and zinc in hair tissue. 2011. Vol. 144, 1-3, pp. 264-271.

[17] John, E. M., et al. Validation of Salivary Testosterone as a Screening Test for Male Hypogonadism. 2009. Vol. 9, 3, pp. 165-169.

Chapter 6

Androgens and Cardiovascular Risk Factors in Polycystic Ovary Syndrome

Licy L. Yanes Cardozo, Alexandra M. Huffman, Jacob E. Pruett and Damian G. Romero

Abstract

Polycystic Ovary Syndrome (PCOS) is the most common endocrine disorder in reproductive-aged women. Clinical or biochemical signs of androgen excess is a cardinal feature of the syndrome and are present in approximately 80% of women with PCOS. Increased blood pressure and insulin resistance, two major cardiovascular risk factors, are frequently present in women with PCOS. This chapter aims to highlight the fundamental role of androgens in mediating the increased blood pressure and insulin resistance in women with PCOS. This chapter is also a call for action to develop new pharmacological therapies that target the androgen synthesis and androgen receptor activation dysregulation present in women with PCOS. These novel therapies will allow to prevent or mitigate the excess androgen-mediated cardiovascular risk factors that affect women with PCOS.

Keywords: polycystic ovary syndrome, androgens, androgen receptor, blood pressure, insulin resistance

1. Introduction

Polycystic Ovary Syndrome (PCOS) is the most common endocrine disorder and cause of androgen excess in reproductive-age women [1, 2]. The etiology of the syndrome is unknown, and the pathophysiological characteristics are complex. There are three different sets of diagnostic criteria available to diagnose PCOS; the Rotterdam criteria is the most commonly used. The key difference among those three criteria is that hyperandrogenism is considered an essential component of the syndrome for the Androgen Excess Society guidelines [3] and National Institutes of Health (NIH) [4], but not for the Rotterdam criteria [5]. More recently, the Rotterdam criteria for PCOS diagnosis were endorsed by the NIH at an NIH-sponsored workshop [6] as well as by the International evidence-based guideline for the assessment and management of PCOS [7]. Insulin resistance (IR) is frequently present in lean and obese women with PCOS, but it is not included in the diagnostic criteria. Women with PCOS may seek medical care due to a broad range of clinical manifestations such as infertility, menstrual dysfunction, excessive hair growth or hirsutism, alopecia, or acne. More recently, it became clear that the cardiometabolic risk factors, such as IR, increases in blood pressure (BP), and obesity affect a high percentage of women with PCOS compared to normal cycling women [8–11].

Importantly, in women with PCOS, plasma levels of androgens positively correlate with BP and IR. Whether and how androgen excess causes increased BP and IR in women with PCOS is unknown. Unfortunately, limited effective evidence-based therapeutic agents are available to treat those cardiovascular risk factors in PCOS patients. Furthermore, the use of antiandrogens in PCOS is often only recommended to manage the dermatological manifestations of the syndrome, but neither the IR nor increases in BP [12]. This chapter aims to highlight the fundamental role of androgens in mediating increases in BP and IR in women with PCOS and the lack of therapeutic options to ameliorate the hyperandrogenism and cardiometabolic complications in these patients.

2. Androgen synthesis in PCOS

In women, the concentration of plasmatic androgens is higher than of estrogens [13]. Excess androgens are secreted by the ovaries in most women with PCOS, but in 20–30% of them, excess androgens are also secreted by the adrenal gland. Plasma levels of total and free testosterone (T), dihydrotestosterone (DHT), dehydroepiandrosterone (DHEA), DHEA sulfate (DHEAS), and androstenedione are significantly elevated in PCOS [2, 14]. Androstenedione, DHEA, and DHEAS are pro-hormones synthesized by the adrenal gland, they circulate at a higher concentration than T. Those pro-hormones could be converted into more potent T and DHT in the adipose tissue, liver, and the skin [3, 15]. Depending on the type of androgens measured, hyperandrogenemia is present in ~80% of PCOS diagnosed cases [16]. Recently, a study showed that the 11-oxygenated androgens, 11β-hydroxyandrostenedione, 11-ketoandrostenedione, and 11-ketotestosterone, represent the majority of circulating androgens in women with PCOS [17]. Moreover, 11β-hydroxyandrostenedione, 11-ketoandrostenedione circulating levels positively correlate with circulating insulin and IR assessed by the Homeostatic Model Assessment of Insulin Resistance (HOMA-IR) in women with PCOS [17]. The HOMA-IR is an index of IR calculated according to the formula: fasting insulin (microU/L) x fasting glucose (nmol/L)/22.5 [18]. The HOMA-IR is extensively used in epidemiological studies, but rarely in the clinical setting. On the other hand, the hyperinsulinemic eulgycemic clamp is considered the gold standard to determine IR; but, unfortunately, it is impractical for routine use in the clinic [19]. Local production or activation of androgens at the tissular level have been reported, and they may constitute a key factor in the cardiometabolic abnormality in these patients. For example, the subcutaneous adipose tissue in women with PCOS has a higher concentration of androgens than in control subjects [20, 21]. Testosterone can be converted to its more biologically active form, DHT, by the 5α-reductase, and to estradiol by the aromatase. DHT is more biologically active than testosterone, binding to the androgen receptor (AR) with a 2-fold higher affinity and a 5-fold decreased dissociation rate compared to testosterone [22]. The synthesis of androgens in women is complex. The local activation of androgens is not well understood during normal physiology or diseases such as PCOS.

3. Androgen receptor in PCOS

AR is a member of the steroid hormone receptor superfamily, a class of receptors that function through their ability to regulate the transcription of specific genes. It contains an N-terminal transactivation domain, a central DNA-binding domain, and a C-terminal ligand-binding domain [23]. Androgens act by binding to the

AR and subsequently translocate to the nucleus to act as a transcription factor and promote gene expression. The unbound AR is inactive in the cytoplasm as a large dynamic heterocomplex, together with heat shock proteins (Hsp70 and Hsp90) and their co-chaperones [24]. Ligand binding dissociates the AR from heat shock proteins, causing its activation and translocation to the nuclei to exert its transcription regulatory role.

Androgen actions in the cardiovascular system could be genomic or non-genomic [25], although most of the basic research data available derived from experiments performed in male rats. The activity of AR is modulated by a polyglutamine tract of variable size in its N-terminal transactivation domain. This polyglutamine tract is encoded by a highly polymorphic CAG repeat sequence in exon 1 of the AR gene located on the X-chromosome. Shorter CAG repeats lengths in exon 1 of the AR gene are associated with a stronger transcriptional activity of the AR. The shorter CAG repeats have been associated with the androgen actions in male conditions such as prostate cancer [24] and benign prostatic hyperplasia [26]. Moreover, abnormal expansion of the CAG repeat length leads to Kennedy's disease, which is associated with hypogonadism and impaired spermatogenesis in men [27, 28]. However, studies in women with PCOS did not find significant differences in the mean values of CAG repeat sizes compared to controls [29, 30]. The fundamental role of AR in the development of metabolic and reproductive features of PCOS was demonstrated by the lack of effect of DHT in AR knockout (ARKO) mice, supporting the fundamental concept that androgen excess, via AR activation, is a key factor in PCOS [31]. More recent studies further demonstrated that AR signaling pathways within the brain and adipocytes are key in the physiopathology of metabolic PCOS characteristics [32]. Pharmacological strategies safely targeting the brain and adipocyte AR-could constitute a novel and effective way to ameliorate the cardiometabolic complications in PCOS.

4. Cardiovascular disease in PCOS

Several studies have shown that the odds ratio for cardiovascular disease (CVD) is significantly higher in women with PCOS compared to the control women [33–35]. Whether women with PCOS suffer from higher mortality from CVD is still unclear, pending high-quality data. Obesity is frequently observed in women with PCOS, but, even after BMI adjustment, the increased risk for cardiovascular events in PCOS persists, suggesting that additional factors play a role in mediating the higher prevalence of CVD in women with PCOS [35]. Hypertension, the most important modifiable cardiovascular risk factor for cardiovascular disease, is commonly diagnosed in women with PCOS. Moreover, insulin resistance, another risk factor for CVD, is also frequently present in women with PCOS, and independent of those subjects' BMI. Data from clinical and basic research suggest that hyperandrogenism may underlie these cardinal cardiovascular risk factors in patients with PCOS. Below we describe whether and how androgens mediate the increases in BP and IR in women with PCOS.

5. Hyperandrogenism is a key factor mediating increases in blood pressure in women with PCOS

Increased BP remains the leading risk factor for death globally, accounting for 10.4 million deaths per year [36]. There is a sexual dimorphic relationship between androgens and BP in women compared to men. Free androgen index

(FAI), a measure of bioavailable androgens, is positively correlated with systolic and diastolic blood pressure [37]. A recent meta-analysis reported a greater risk of developing hypertension in reproductive age women with PCOS [38]. In contrast, epidemiological studies have shown an inverse relationship between androgens and BP in men, and this association persisted after adjusting for age and body mass index [39]. The mechanisms behind the elevated BP in response to hyperandrogenism in women remain unclear. Some of the possible mechanisms involved in androgen-mediated regulation of BP are discussed below.

6. Potential mechanisms that could mediate increases in blood pressure in PCOS

The kidneys are a key regulator of long-term BP control and body fluid homeostasis in the body. The renin-angiotensin-aldosterone system (RAAS) plays a major role in several forms of hypertension, and it is composed of the classical and non-classical arms with opposite physiological effects [40, 41]. The classical RAS pathway starts with angiotensinogen (AGTN) which is enzymatically cleaved to Angiotensin I (ANG I) by renin. ANG I is then cleaved by angiotensin I converting enzyme (ACE) to Angiotensin II (ANG II), which binds to the ANG II receptor type 1 (AT1R) and ANG II type 2 receptor (AT2R). High levels of ANG II had been related to metabolic disorders. The non-classical pathway, the angiotensin I converting enzyme 2 (ACE2) reduces Ang II levels by transforming it in Angiotensin (1–7) (ANG (1–7)), which also can be generated from ANG I passing through Angiotensin (1–9) (ANG (1–9)) by the action of the endopeptidases: prolyl-endopeptidase and neutral endopeptidase. The main known biological effects of ANG (1–7) are associated with Mas receptor activation, causing an improvement in metabolic syndrome, obesity, and hypertension.

The rate-limiting step of the RAS is the conversion of AGTN to ANG I by renin [42]. Women with PCOS have hyperreninemia [43], and blockade of the AT1R is effective in decreasing their BP [44]. We and others have shown that androgens stimulate the synthesis of intrarenal AGTN in male and female rats [45–48]. In the kidney, the AR is highly expressed in proximal tubule cells [49], glomerular endothelial cells [50], and podocytes [51]. Moreover, the enzymes involved in androgen biosynthesis are expressed and active in the kidney [52]. In experimental models of hypertension, androgens can shift the pressure-natriuresis curve to the right, promoting sodium reabsorption [53, 54]. Androgens could also directly increase sodium reabsorption via upregulation of epithelial sodium channel (ENaC) α, β, and γ subunits expression [55]. Renal medullary blood flow and the sensitivity of the pressure-natriuresis response are regulated by various paracrine and humoral factors known to play an important role in the control of renal function and BP. Those regulatory factors include ANG II, kinins, prostaglandins, atrial natriuretic peptide (ANP), and nitric oxide (NO). Whether changes in the renal medulla microcirculation play a role in mediating the increases in BP under excess of androgens in women with PCOS remains unclear.

Plasma ACE2 activity is low in healthy subjects but elevated in patients with cardiovascular risk factors or cardiovascular disease. Hypertensive men have a high higher level of plasma ACE2 compared to women [56]. The role of increased levels of plasmatic ACE2 in men remains unknown. It has been reported that male mice have higher renal ACE2 mRNA and protein expression, as well as higher ACE2 activity, than their female counterparts [57, 58]. However, the effect of androgen excess in the non-classical RAS pathway is still not well understood. Androgens downregulate AT2R expression levels in the aorta, *in vivo*, and *ex vivo* [59]. ACE2 is the receptor for SARS-CoV and SARS-CoV-2 [60, 61]. SARS-CoV and probably SARS-CoV-2, Spike protein binding to the ACE2 receptor causes its downregulation through internalization [62]. SARS-CoV causes an imbalance in ACE/ACE2 and consequently ANG II/ANG (1–7) that leads to lung injury [62]. Men have suffered a higher rate of severity and mortality from COVID-19 [63]. Whether such sex difference in COVID-19 outcomes is due to ACE2 expression modulation by androgens remains unknown. Further research is needed to elucidate whether and how androgens modulate the non-classical RAS pathway in PCOS and how its regulation could impact COVID-19 outcomes in this population.

Our research teams' studies focus on the cardiometabolic complications associated with androgen excess in female rats. The hyperandrogenic female (HAF) rat, an animal experimental model of PCOS, is generated by the chronic administration of the non-aromatizable androgen DHT. This model exhibits upregulation of intrarenal angiotensinogen and ACE mRNA expression, which are associated with a ~ 10 mmHg increase in BP compared to control female rats [46]. When HAF rats are treated with enalapril, an ACE inhibitor, their BP is lowered to values comparable to that of control rats, suggesting that the RAAS activation has a role in mediating androgens' effect on BP [64]. The stimulatory effect of androgens upon the intrarenal RAAS persisted after discontinuation of androgen exposure in female rats, suggesting a cardiometabolic androgenic memory in female rats. Interestingly, in the kidney medulla, AGTN and AT1R were still elevated after six months of DHT withdrawal [65]. AT1R blockers or ACE inhibitors are widely used as antihypertensive drugs. Women should be advised about the potential teratogenic and fetotoxic risks of ACE inhibitors or AT1R blockers if they become pregnant. ACE inhibitors and AT1R blockers use in the first trimester of pregnancy may not present significant risks for malformations in live births but a high risk of miscarriage [66]. Novel and tissue-selective RAAS inhibitors that do not cross the placental barrier are warranted to ameliorate the increases in BP in women with PCOS in the future.

In the US, a frequent finding in PCOS patients is an increase in body mass index (BMI), with up to 80% being either overweight or obese [67]. There is a strong link between adiposity and hypertension, with multiple mechanisms being suggested [68]. Hypertrophy of adipocytes is associated with local hypoxia, leading to increased oxidative stress and inflammatory cytokines, followed by capillary rarefaction [69, 70]. These processes can lead to a positive feedback loop, ultimately releasing more inflammatory cytokines and reactive oxidative species into the systemic circulation. Chronic inflammation can ultimately lead to increased BP. In HAF rats, there is increased fat mass and BP coupled with increased plasma tumor necrosis factor alpha and renal mRNA expression of NADPH oxidase 4 [46, 71]. Increased adiposity is also associated with increased circulating adipokines, such as leptin [69]. Chronic hyperleptinemia is known to stimulate the sympathetic nervous system [72], which could lead to vasoconstriction. It has been reported that in women with PCOS, leptin levels can be elevated [73]. Furthermore, using heart rate variability as a measure of autonomic dysfunction, women with PCOS have increased sympathetic activity compared to control women matched for body mass index, systolic and diastolic BP [74]. Additionally, leptin is linked to activation of the RAAS via the renal sympathetic nervous system [72]. All the findings mentioned above suggest that BP control is complex and depends on multiples pathways in women with PCOS.

Endothelial dysfunction refers to the impaired function in the endothelium, the inner lining of blood vessels, which could lead to inappropriate vasoconstriction and atherosclerosis [75]. Endothelial dysfunction frequently occurs under chronic inflammation conditions or high oxidative stress, which interfere with the nitric oxide production needed for vasodilation [76]. Interestingly, this occurs not just in obese females but also in lean females with PCOS. A recent study found that normotensive lean females with PCOS, even without insulin resistance, had increased endothelial dysfunction compared to controls [77]. One of the major vascular oxygen-derived free radicals is superoxide anion. Superoxide is routinely scavenged by superoxide dismutase (SOD). Superoxide can also combine with nitric oxide (NO), which results in quenching of NO and, theoretically, can induce vasoconstriction. There is an interaction between NO and oxidative stress to maintain endothelial function. We previously showed that an intact NO system is necessary for antioxidants to elicit a BP-lowering effect [78]. Furthermore, Huirliman and colleagues demonstrated that the presence of endothelial dysfunction and IR develops in pair-fed DHT-treated female rats, suggesting an obesity-independent mechanism [79]. Increased endothelial dysfunction has also been found in transgender men compared to cisgender women matched for body mass index [80], suggesting a broader link between endothelial dysfunction and female androgen excess in addition to women with PCOS. Another study with lean females with PCOS also found that they had decreased plasma total antioxidant status [81]. This reduced ability to handle oxidative stress can contribute to the endothelial dysfunction in hyperandrogenic females.

Cardiovascular diseases are the leading cause of death in women. Furthermore, there have been an overall decline in CVD mortality over the past 40 years; however, the mortality in younger women has plateaued since 2000 [82]. Increases in BP is a primary cardiovascular risk factor. The carotid artery intima-media thickness (cIMT) has emerged as an important surrogate marker of target organ damage in hypertensive heart disease. A recent prospective cross-sectional study in PCOS women showed that cIMT was significantly increased in women with PCOS compared to controls, and this increase was independent of BMI, age, and smoking status [83]. Consequenly, the cIMT could be used to determine the cardiovascular risk profile in women with PCOS.

In summary, hyperandrogenemia in females has multiple mechanisms of causing increased BP and impaired vascular function. Pharmacological agents that target multiple pathways could constitute effective therapeutic agents to be used in women with PCOS.

7. Hyperandrogenism is a key factor mediating insulin resistance in PCOS

IR is recognized as a significant contributor to metabolic homeostasis disturbances in women with PCOS, especially in obese individuals, due to increased lipid accumulation in muscle and liver from impaired insulin signaling. Decreased insulin sensitivity and glucose tolerance have been reported in women with PCOS versus healthy individuals in several studies [84]. Additionally, both metabolic syndrome and hyperinsulinemia have a characteristic increase in low-grade inflammation markers [85], which has also been observed in women with PCOS [86]. IR prevalence among women with PCOS is varied between different measurement methods but is reported to be between 40% and 70%, approximately [87]. Women with insulin receptor mutations, and thus high levels of insulin, develop severe hyperandrogenemia [88].

Hyperandrogenism and or hyperandrogenemia is present in about 80% of women with PCOS [89]. Both circulating testosterone and its precursor androstenedione have been shown in positive association with the severity of metabolic dysfunction in women with PCOS [90]. The prevalence of type 2 Diabetes Mellitus (T2DM) in the US is 10-times higher among young women with PCOS compared to age-matched, normal-cycling women [91]. Insulin and insulin signaling can influence androgens in women with PCOS. Insulin can stimulate the ovaries of theca cells to produce androgens. This dysfunctional androgen stimulation is suggested to induce hyperandrogenism in women with PCOS in a positive feedback mechanism with hyperinsulinemia. Specifically, the P450c17 (CYP17A1) enzyme in the theca cells has been addressed as having modulated activity in response to insulin and IGF. This is specifically relevant to PCOS because the enzyme is necessary for the production of androgens [92]. Additionally, high circulating plasma insulin may itself influence androgen availability due to its suppression of sex hormone-binding globulin (SHBG) synthesis, a steroid transport protein, and subsequent increase in the bioavailability of unbound testosterone [93]. PCOS patients have been shown to have reduced SHBG level [94], that could lead to increases in free T. In addition to its role in glucose homeostasis and metabolism, in the central nervous system insulin can effectively modulate food intake and signal satiety. Insulin has also been shown to influence gonadotropin-releasing hormone (GnRH) in the hypothalamic neurons by increasing its expression and activity [95]. In PCOS, GnRH pulse frequency modifications and subsequent LH timing alterations have been suggested as another potential trigger to prevent inhibition of androgens and lead to their increased biosynthesis [96, 97]. This relationship illustrates the importance of the interplay between the neuroendocrine system, insulin, and androgen production in women with PCOS. Clinically, in a randomized controlled trial, women with PCOS treated for three months with Resveratrol, a natural polyphenol able to reduce androgen production via CYP17A1, showed a 30% reduction in fasting insulin and increased insulin sensitivity [98]. Together, these findings suggest the potential therapeutic importance of androgen targeted drugs to treat IR in PCOS patients.

The main target tissues of insulin action and subsequent insulin resistance and dysfunction include white adipose tissue, skeletal muscle, and the liver. Androgens play a significant role in each of these insulin-responsive target tissues in women.

7.1 Androgen actions on the adipose tissue

Androgens regulate several different aspects of adipose cell function and lipid accumulation and are themselves synthesized by the adipose tissue. Adipose tissue is known to play a role in whole-body insulin sensitivity, inflammation, and intracellular stress. The adipose tissue is crucial for the storage of lipids, and adipocytes are the primary storage cells to serve this purpose. The adipose tissue can also release adipokines, like leptin and adiponectin, which may directly influence insulin sensitivity, inflammatory response, fatty acid oxidation, sex steroids, and even energy expenditure. Several adipokines are dysregulated in PCOS [99]. Women with high androgens have been shown to display a fat distribution pattern more similar to men, with increased abdominal visceral adipose accumulation [100]. Although the expansion of the subcutaneous adipose depot is also associated with PCOS [101]. Additionally, after administration of androgen antagonists, women with PCOS were shown to lose visceral adiposity, which suggests that androgens have a role in fat distribution [102]. This increased adiposity is considered to be due to a hypertrophic adipocyte expansion compared to a hyperplasic response, which is more highly indicative of metabolic syndrome. Hypertrophy of adipocytes is influenced by androgens directly by increasing visceral adipocyte mass. Women with PCOS have an increase in adipocyte size [103]. Androgens influence adipogenesis by limiting the differentiation of preadipocytes. In preadipocytes taken from the subcutaneous adipose depots of healthy women were shown to have impaired insulin-induced glucose uptake in response to testosterone [104]. This study suggests that androgens, via the androgen receptor, mediate insulin resistance in adipocytes. Interestingly, the relationship between circulating testosterone and elevated fasting insulin in PCOS is independent of adiposity [105], supporting that insulin resistance is intrinsic to PCOS and may be mediated by hyperandrogenemia independently of obesity.

7.2 Androgens actions on the skeletal muscle

Glucose can be used as a primary fuel source in the skeletal muscle when insulin is high, instead of fatty acids, or can be stored in the form of glycogen for future periods of exercise. Glucose may enter the skeletal muscle in response to insulin by the specific cell surface transporter GLUT4. Skeletal muscle alone may show insulin resistance, which is defined as a reduced ability for glucose uptake and glycogen storage in response to insulin. Skeletal muscle serves as a primary organ for glucose disposal [87].

Several studies suggest that adiponectin and lower AMPK phosphorylation may be important in skeletal muscle-specific insulin resistance in PCOS [106], even in non-obese hyperandrogenic women. Adiponectin is an adipokine that has an inverse relationship with a degree of adiposity. Adiponectin has both insulin-sensitizing properties, including skeletal muscle, and is decreased by androgens [107].

Androgens have been shown to alter lean muscle mass. Both healthy and women with PCOS who exercised using resistance strength training, which focuses on skeletal muscle contractions, along with aerobic training showed reduced fasting glucose concentration and serum testosterone profiles [108]. Together, this suggests the potential to target the skeletal muscle to improve insulin-sensitive tissue sensitivity and improve hyperandrogenemia.

7.3 Androgens actions on the liver

Of crucial importance following a meal, glucose is allowed entry into the liver and stored as glycogen in the liver due to the effects of insulin. In a healthy adult, storage is especially important to help varying energy levels in the body to prevent blood glucose from changing rapidly between meals and allow it to be released when energy is needed.

Hyperandrogenemia in PCOS has been associated with several different disturbances of the liver. Alanine aminotransferase (ALT), often used as a clinical biomarker of liver injury, has been shown in positive association to androgen levels in young women with PCOS [109]. Women with PCOS with high androgens display a distinct metabolic phenotype different than women with normal levels of androgens. There is evidence that women with PCOS are at an increased risk of developing a spectrum of nonalcoholic fatty liver disease, the most common liver disease. Women with PCOS and obesity have an increased risk for NAFLD [110]. Interestingly, even after adjusting for BMI, other PCOS cohorts have shown that hyperandrogenemic women with PCOS have a significantly higher liver fat than women with normal levels of androgens [111]. Those findings suggest that androgens may be an independent risk factor for steatosis and the development of NAFLD.

8. Pharmacological management of cardiometabolic complications in women with PCOS

Recent studies have shown that women with PCOS frequently report long delays in the syndrome's diagnosis, dissatisfaction with information and care provided, and distrust in primary care providers' opinions [112, 113]. Those patients' concerns with their diagnosis and health care providers are shocking, considering that PCOS is the most common endocrine disorder in reproductive-age women. We described below the current therapeutic options for the management of cardiometabolic complications in women with PCOS.

8.1 Oral contraceptives

Oral contraceptives (OCPs) are the first-line therapy in women with PCOS to improve their irregular menstrual cycles. OCPs reduce circulating androgens by suppression of Luteinizing Hormone and stimulation of sex hormone-binding globulin (SHBG), leading to a decrease in free testosterone plasma levels. In some women, OCPs can exacerbate hypertension and are associated with a 2-fold increase in the risk of cardiovascular diseases in the general female population [114]. Exogenous estrogens can stimulate the production of AGTN by the liver in female rats [115, 116], which theoretically could lead to higher levels of ANG II. OCPs are contraindicated for smokers due to the higher risk of cardiovascular diseases in this population [117]. OCPs do not seem to affect glucose and insulin homeostasis in healthy individuals [118]. However, the effect of OCPs on women with PCOS remains controversial, mainly due to the heterogeneity of the studies, as shown in a recent meta-analysis [119]. Furthermore, several clinical studies have suggested that the use of oral contraceptives may aggravate insulin resistance and worsen hyperglycemia in obese women with PCOS [120–123]. The long-term impact of OCPs in IR and cardiovascular diseases in women with PCOS remains unknown. Interestingly, previous use of OCPs was associated with an increased risk of development of CVD in PCOS in a Danish study [33]. Prospective randomized long-term clinical trials analyzing the effect of OCPs on cardiovascular morbidity and mortality in women with PCOS, obese and lean, are lacking and desperately needed.

8.2 Androgen receptor blockers

Recommendations from the International evidence-based guideline for the assessment and management of Polycystic Ovary Syndrome [7] recommend that AR blockers be used mostly towards the dermatological manifestations of the syndrome, not the metabolic ones. AR blockers can be used in addition to OCPs and insulin sensitizers to ameliorate excessive hair growth or hirsutism. Antiandrogen monotherapy is not recommended because of its teratogenic potential [124]. In the US, the AR blocker most commonly used in the clinic is spironolactone [124]. Spironolactone is also a progesterone and mineralocorticoid receptor blocker. Blockade of the mineralocorticoid receptor causes a diuretic effect that potentially can cause serious side effects such as hyperkalemia and hypotension [124]. Other potent antiandrogens are flutamide and cyproterone acetate. Cyproterone acetate is not currently available in the US and recently has been linked to an increased risk of meningioma among high dose users [125]. Flutamide use has been associated with severe hepatoxicity, and it is not FDA-approved for use in women with PCOS. Bicalutamide, an androgen receptor blocker, has been used in combination with OCPs in a study where hirsutism was the primary endpoint [126]. Safe, effective, and specific AR blockers are necessary to positively impact the management of the cardiometabolic risk factors in women with PCOS.

8.3 Insulin sensitizers

Metformin is the most frequent insulin sensitizer agent used in women with PCOS [124, 127]. Obesity exacerbates the IR in women with PCOS, and weight loss in women with PCOS ameliorates it. However, weight loss is very difficult to achieve and sustain. Since insulin resistance is present in obese and lean women with PCOS, it has been proposed to be the key factor in mediating the adverse cardiovascular risk profile observed in PCOS subjects. Metformin has been used for years to treat insulin resistance in women with PCOS. The effectiveness of metformin to improve IR and prevent T2DM in women with PCOS is unclear. Metformin reduces the risk of progression from insulin resistance to T2DM in only 30% of patients in the Diabetes Prevention Trial [128]. Metformin can lower testosterone levels; thereby, some of the beneficial effects in women with PCOS may be due to lowering their androgen levels [129]. A recent metanalysis showed no effect of metformin on indexes of fasting insulin, homeostasis model assessment of insulin resistance, sex hormone-binding globulin, high-density lipoprotein cholesterol, total cholesterol, triglycerides, fasting blood glucose, and androstenedione in overweight women with PCOS [130]. Long-term prospective randomized controlled trials assessing the effect of metformin on cardiovascular morbidity and mortality in women with PCOS are not available at present.

8.4 Incretins

Glucagon-like peptide-1 (GLP-1) is an incretin that potentiates the food-mediated release of insulin leading to a decrease in plasma glucose levels and delaying gastric emptying, and exerting satiety effects. Several short-term clinical trials showed that administration of GLP-1 receptor agonists caused significant improvement in metabolic abnormalities and also cause weight loss in women with PCOS [131]. Similar beneficial effects of GLP-1 were observed in hyperandrogenic female rats [132]. In contrast, we recently reported that administration of the GLP-1 receptor agonist (GLP-1 RA) liraglutide to a model of postmenopausal PCOS, elicits several beneficial metabolic effects but the BP-lowering effect of GLP-1 RA was blunted compared with control rats [64]. These results suggest that GLP-1 RA treatment could improve DHT-induced metabolic and BP abnormalities in reproductive-aged PCOS. It is possible to hypothesize that GLP-1 RA's BP-lowering effect in PCOS animals could be mediated by estrogens, which are significantly decreased in postmenopausal PCOS rodents, leading to the lack of effect in those aging animals. This concept of a role for estrogens in the age-differential effect of GLP-1 RA in BP regulation in PCOS is an exciting hypothesis that needs to be tested.

8.5 SGLT2 inhibitors

Among therapies in clinical trials for women with PCOS are the sodium-glucose cotransporter-2 inhibitors (SGLT2i), which are antidiabetic agents. SGLT2i has recently been shown to be superior to metformin for weight loss in women with PCOS [133]. Additionally, SGLT2i is cardioprotective in patients with T2DM or with heart failure [134]. For example, in the EMPA-REG trial, SGLT2i reduced the relative risk of cardiovascular death by 38% in patients with T2DM on the background of the blockade of the renin-angiotensin system (RAS) [135]. A possible mechanism to explain why SGLT2i has dramatic cardiovascular protection includes its interactions with the RAS, which is affected by sex steroids and is a major regulator of BP [45, 136].

9. Conclusions

PCOS, the most common endocrine disorder in reproductive-aged women, is associated with increases in BP and IR. Excess of androgens, a cardinal feature of the syndrome, may underlie those cardiovascular risk factors in PCOS. Effective and safe pharmacological agents that target the androgen excess and the androgen receptor are desperately needed to treat the cardiometabolic abnormalities found in women with PCOS.

Acknowledgements

This work was supported by the National Institute of General Medical Sciences of the National Institutes of Health under Award Number P20GM121334 (L.L.Y.C. and D.G.R.), and National Institute of Diabetes and Digestive and Kidney Diseases under Award Number R21DK113500 (D.G.R.). The content is solely the responsibility of the authors and does not necessarily represent the official views of the National Institutes of Health.

Conflict of interest

The authors declare no conflict of interest.

Author details

Licy L. Yanes Cardozo[1,2,3,4,5*], Alexandra M. Huffman[2,3,4,5], Jacob E. Pruett[2,3,4,5] and Damian G. Romero[2,3,4,5*]

1 Department of Medicine, University of Mississippi Medical Center, Jackson, MS, United States

2 Department of Cell and Molecular Biology, University of Mississippi Medical Center, Jackson, MS, United States

3 Mississippi Center of Excellence in Perinatal Research, University of Mississippi Medical Center, Jackson, MS, United States

4 Women's Health Research Center, University of Mississippi Medical Center, Jackson, MS, United States

5 Cardio Renal Research Center, University of Mississippi Medical Center, Jackson, MS, United States

*Address all correspondence to: lyanes@umc.edu and dromero@umc.edu

References

[1] Bozdag G, Mumusoglu S, Zengin D, Karabulut E, Yildiz BO. The prevalence and phenotypic features of polycystic ovary syndrome: a systematic review and meta-analysis. Hum Reprod. 2016;31(12):2841-2855.

[2] Azziz R, Sanchez LA, Knochenhauer ES, Moran C, Lazenby J, Stephens KC, et al. Androgen excess in women: experience with over 1000 consecutive patients. J Clin Endocrinol Metab. 2004;89(2):453-462.

[3] Azziz R, Carmina E, Dewailly D, Diamanti-Kandarakis E, Escobar-Morreale HF, Futterweit W, et al. Positions statement: criteria for defining polycystic ovary syndrome as a predominantly hyperandrogenic syndrome: an Androgen Excess Society guideline. J Clin Endocrinol Metab. 2006;91(11):4237-4245.

[4] Zawadski JK, Dunaif A. Diagnostic criteria for polycystic ovary syndrome: towards a rational approach. In: Dunaif A, Givens JR, Haseltine FP, Merrian GR, editors. Polycystic Ovary Syndrome. Boston: Blackwell Scientific Publications; 1992. p. 377-384.

[5] Rotterdam EA-SPCWG. Revised 2003 consensus on diagnostic criteria and long-term health risks related to polycystic ovary syndrome. Fertil Steril. 2004;81(1):19-25.

[6] National Institutes of Health. Evidence-based Methodology Workshop on Polycystic Ovary Syndrome. Bethesda, MD2012.

[7] Teede HJ, Misso ML, Costello MF, Dokras A, Laven J, Moran L, et al. Recommendations from the international evidence-based guideline for the assessment and management of polycystic ovary syndrome. Fertil Steril. 2018;110(3):364-379.

[8] Paradisi G, Steinberg HO, Hempfling A, Cronin J, Hook G, Shepard MK, et al. Polycystic ovary syndrome is associated with endothelial dysfunction. Circulation. 2001;103(10):1410-1415.

[9] Rizzo M, Berneis K, Spinas G, Rini GB, Carmina E. Long-term consequences of polycystic ovary syndrome on cardiovascular risk. Fertil Steril. 2009;91(4 Suppl):1563-1567.

[10] Tock L, Carneiro G, Togeiro SM, Hachul H, Pereira AZ, Tufik S, et al. Obstructive sleep apnea predisposes to nonalcoholic Fatty liver disease in patients with polycystic ovary syndrome. Endocr Pract. 2014;20(3):244-251.

[11] Kargili A, Karakurt F, Kasapoglu B, Derbent A, Koca C, Selcoki Y. Association of polycystic ovary syndrome and a non-dipping blood pressure pattern in young women. Clinics (Sao Paulo). 2010;65(5):475-479.

[12] Moghetti P, Tosi F, Tosti A, Negri C, Misciali C, Perrone F, et al. Comparison of spironolactone, flutamide, and finasteride efficacy in the treatment of hirsutism: a randomized, double blind, placebo-controlled trial. J Clin Endocrinol Metab. 2000;85(1):89-94.

[13] Burger HG. Androgen production in women. Fertil Steril. 2002;77 Suppl 4:S3–S5.

[14] Huang A, Brennan K, Azziz R. Prevalence of hyperandrogenemia in the polycystic ovary syndrome diagnosed by the National Institutes of Health 1990 criteria. Fertil Steril. 2010;93(6):1938-1941.

[15] Kirschner MA, Bardin CW. Androgen production and metabolism in normal and virilized women. Metabolism. 1972;21(7):667-688.

[16] Lizneva D, Suturina L, Walker W, Brakta S, Gavrilova-Jordan L, Azziz R. Criteria, prevalence, and phenotypes of polycystic ovary syndrome. Fertil Steril. 2016;106(1):6-15.

[17] O'Reilly MW, Kempegowda P, Jenkinson C, Taylor AE, Quanson JL, Storbeck KH, et al. 11-Oxygenated C19 Steroids Are the Predominant Androgens in Polycystic Ovary Syndrome. J Clin Endocrinol Metab. 2017;102(3):840-848.

[18] Matthews DR, Hosker JP, Rudenski AS, Naylor BA, Treacher DF, Turner RC. Homeostasis model assessment: insulin resistance and beta-cell function from fasting plasma glucose and insulin concentrations in man. Diabetologia. 1985;28(7):412-419.

[19] DeFronzo RA, Tobin JD, Andres R. Glucose clamp technique: a method for quantifying insulin secretion and resistance. Am J Physiol. 1979;237(3):E214–E223.

[20] Quinkler M, Sinha B, Tomlinson JW, Bujalska IJ, Stewart PM, Arlt W. Androgen generation in adipose tissue in women with simple obesity--a site-specific role for 17beta-hydroxysteroid dehydrogenase type 5. J Endocrinol. 2004;183(2):331-342.

[21] O'Reilly M, Gathercole L, Capper F, Arlt W, Tomlinson J. Effect of insulin on AKR1C3 expression in female adipose tissue: in-vivo and in-vitro study of adipose androgen generation in polycystic ovary syndrome. Lancet. 2015;385 Suppl 1:S16.

[22] Grino PB, Griffin JE, Wilson JD. Testosterone at high concentrations interacts with the human androgen receptor similarly to dihydrotestosterone. Endocrinology. 1990;126(2):1165-1172.

[23] Tan MH, Li J, Xu HE, Melcher K, Yong EL. Androgen receptor: structure, role in prostate cancer and drug discovery. Acta Pharmacol Sin. 2015;36(1):3-23.

[24] Pratt WB, Toft DO. Steroid receptor interactions with heat shock protein and immunophilin chaperones. Endocr Rev. 1997;18(3):306-360.

[25] Lucas-Herald AK, Alves-Lopes R, Montezano AC, Ahmed SF, Touyz RM. Genomic and non-genomic effects of androgens in the cardiovascular system: clinical implications. Clin Sci (Lond). 2017;131(13):1405-1418.

[26] Giovannucci E, Platz EA, Stampfer MJ, Chan A, Krithivas K, Kawachi I, et al. The CAG repeat within the androgen receptor gene and benign prostatic hyperplasia. Urology. 1999;53(1):121-125.

[27] Belsham DD, Yee WC, Greenberg CR, Wrogemann K. Analysis of the CAG repeat region of the androgen receptor gene in a kindred with X-linked spinal and bulbar muscular atrophy. J Neurol Sci. 1992;112(1-2):133-138.

[28] Yoshida KI, Yano M, Chiba K, Honda M, Kitahara S. CAG repeat length in the androgen receptor gene is enhanced in patients with idiopathic azoospermia. Urology. 1999;54(6):1078-1081.

[29] Jaaskelainen J, Korhonen S, VoutilainenR,HippelainenM,HeinonenS. Androgen receptor gene CAG length polymorphism in women with polycystic ovary syndrome. Fertil Steril. 2005;83(6):1724-1728.

[30] Dasgupta S, Sirisha PV, Neelaveni K, Anuradha K, Reddy AG, Thangaraj K, et al. Androgen receptor CAG repeat polymorphism and epigenetic influence among the south Indian women with Polycystic Ovary Syndrome. PLoS One. 2010;5(8):e12401.

[31] Caldwell ASL, Edwards MC, Desai R, Jimenez M, Gilchrist RB, Handelsman DJ, et al. Neuroendocrine androgen action is a key extraovarian mediator in the development of polycystic ovary syndrome. Proc Natl Acad Sci U S A. 2017;114(16):E3334-E3E43.

[32] Cox MJ, Edwards MC, Rodriguez Paris V, Aflatounian A, Ledger WL, Gilchrist RB, et al. Androgen Action in Adipose Tissue and the Brain are Key Mediators in the Development of PCOS Traits in a Mouse Model. Endocrinology. 2020;161(7).

[33] Glintborg D, Rubin KH, Nybo M, Abrahamsen B, Andersen M. Cardiovascular disease in a nationwide population of Danish women with polycystic ovary syndrome. Cardiovasc Diabetol. 2018;17(1):37.

[34] Zhou Y, Wang X, Jiang Y, Ma H, Chen L, Lai C, et al. Association between polycystic ovary syndrome and the risk of stroke and all-cause mortality: insights from a meta-analysis. Gynecol Endocrinol. 2017;33(12):904-910.

[35] de Groot PC, Dekkers OM, Romijn JA, Dieben SW, Helmerhorst FM. PCOS, coronary heart disease, stroke and the influence of obesity: a systematic review and meta-analysis. Hum Reprod Update. 2011;17(4):495-500.

[36] Collaborators GBDRF. Global, regional, and national comparative risk assessment of 84 behavioural, environmental and occupational, and metabolic risks or clusters of risks for 195 countries and territories, 1990-2017: a systematic analysis for the Global Burden of Disease Study 2017. Lancet. 2018;392(10159):1923-1994.

[37] Chen MJ, Yang WS, Yang JH, Chen CL, Ho HN, Yang YS. Relationship between androgen levels and blood pressure in young women with polycystic ovary syndrome. Hypertension. 2007;49(6):1442-1447.

[38] Amiri M, Ramezani Tehrani F, Behboudi-Gandevani S, Bidhendi-Yarandi R, Carmina E. Risk of hypertension in women with polycystic ovary syndrome: a systematic review, meta-analysis and meta-regression. Reprod Biol Endocrinol. 2020;18(1):23.

[39] Khaw KT, Barrett-Connor E. Blood pressure and endogenous testosterone in men: an inverse relationship. J Hypertens. 1988;6(4):329-332.

[40] Santos RAS, Oudit GY, Verano-Braga T, Canta G, Steckelings UM, Bader M. The renin-angiotensin system: going beyond the classical paradigms. Am J Physiol Heart Circ Physiol. 2019;316(5):H958-HH70.

[41] Li XC, Zhang J, Zhuo JL. The vasoprotective axes of the renin-angiotensin system: Physiological relevance and therapeutic implications in cardiovascular, hypertensive and kidney diseases. Pharmacol Res. 2017;125(Pt A):21-38.

[42] Alreja G, Joseph J. Renin and cardiovascular disease: Worn-out path, or new direction. World J Cardiol. 2011;3(3):72-83.

[43] Diamanti-Kandarakis E, Economou FN, Livadas S, Tantalaki E, Piperi C, Papavassiliou AG, et al. Hyperreninemia characterizing women with polycystic ovary syndrome improves after metformin therapy. Kidney Blood Press Res. 2009;32(1):24-31.

[44] Jensterle M, Janez A, Vrtovec B, Meden-Vrtovec H, Pfeifer M, Prezelj J, et al. Decreased androgen levels and improved menstrual pattern after angiotensin II receptor antagonist telmisartan treatment in four hypertensive patients with polycystic

ovary syndrome: case series. Croat Med J. 2007;48(6):864-870.

[45] Yanes LL, Sartori-Valinotti JC, Iliescu R, Romero DG, Racusen LC, Zhang H, et al. Testosterone-dependent hypertension and upregulation of intrarenal angiotensinogen in Dahl salt-sensitive rats. Am J Physiol Renal Physiol. 2009;296(4):F771–F779.

[46] Yanes LL, Romero DG, Moulana M, Lima R, Davis DD, Zhang H, et al. Cardiovascular-renal and metabolic characterization of a rat model of polycystic ovary syndrome. Gend Med. 2011;8(2):103-115.

[47] Ellison KE, Ingelfinger JR, Pivor M, Dzau VJ. Androgen regulation of rat renal angiotensinogen messenger RNA expression. J Clin Invest. 1989;83(6):1941-1945.

[48] Chen YF, Naftilan AJ, Oparil S. Androgen-dependent angiotensinogen and renin messenger RNA expression in hypertensive rats. Hypertension. 1992;19(5):456-463.

[49] Quinkler M, Bujalska IJ, Kaur K, Onyimba CU, Buhner S, Allolio B, et al. Androgen receptor-mediated regulation of the alpha-subunit of the epithelial sodium channel in human kidney. Hypertension. 2005;46(4):787-798.

[50] Torres-Estay V, Carreno DV, San Francisco IF, Sotomayor P, Godoy AS, Smith GJ. Androgen receptor in human endothelial cells. J Endocrinol. 2015;224(3):R131–R137.

[51] Doublier S, Lupia E, Catanuto P, Periera-Simon S, Xia X, Korach K, et al. Testosterone and 17beta-estradiol have opposite effects on podocyte apoptosis that precedes glomerulosclerosis in female estrogen receptor knockout mice. Kidney Int. 2011;79(4):404-413.

[52] Quinkler M, Bumke-Vogt C, Meyer B, Bahr V, Oelkers W, Diederich S. The human kidney is a progesterone-metabolizing and androgen-producing organ. J Clin Endocrinol Metab. 2003;88(6):2803-2809.

[53] Ivy JR, Bailey MA. Pressure natriuresis and the renal control of arterial blood pressure. J Physiol. 2014;592(18):3955-3967.

[54] Reckelhoff JF, Zhang H, Granger JP. Testosterone exacerbates hypertension and reduces pressure-natriuresis in male spontaneously hypertensive rats. Hypertension. 1998;31(1 Pt 2):435-439.

[55] Loh SY, Giribabu N, Salleh N. Sub-chronic testosterone treatment increases the levels of epithelial sodium channel (ENaC)-alpha, beta and gamma in the kidney of orchidectomized adult male Sprague-Dawley rats. PeerJ. 2016;4:e2145.

[56] SantosRAS,SampaioWO,AlzamoraAC, Motta-Santos D, Alenina N, Bader M, et al. The ACE2/Angiotensin-(1-7)/MAS Axis of the Renin-Angiotensin System: Focus on Angiotensin-(1-7). Physiol Rev. 2018;98(1):505-553.

[57] Ji H, de Souza AM, Bajaj B, Zheng W, Wu X, Speth RC, et al. Sex-specific modulation of blood pressure and the renin-angiotensin system by ACE (Angiotensin-Converting Enzyme) 2. Hypertension. 2020;76(2):478-487.

[58] Liu J, Ji H, Zheng W, Wu X, Zhu JJ, Arnold AP, et al. Sex differences in renal angiotensin converting enzyme 2 (ACE2) activity are 17β-oestradiol-dependent and sex chromosome-independent. Biology of sex differences. 2010;1(1):6.

[59] Mishra JS, Hankins GD, Kumar S. Testosterone downregulates angiotensin II type-2 receptor via androgen receptor-mediated ERK1/2 MAP kinase pathway in rat aorta. J Renin Angiotensin Aldosterone Syst. 2016;17(4).

[60] Zhou P, Yang XL, Wang XG, Hu B, Zhang L, Zhang W, et al. A pneumonia outbreak associated with a new coronavirus of probable bat origin. Nature. 2020;579(7798):270-273.

[61] Li W, Moore MJ, Vasilieva N, Sui J, Wong SK, Berne MA, et al. Angiotensin-converting enzyme 2 is a functional receptor for the SARS coronavirus. Nature. 2003;426(6965):450-454.

[62] Kuba K, Imai Y, Rao S, Gao H, Guo F, Guan B, et al. A crucial role of angiotensin converting enzyme 2 (ACE2) in SARS coronavirus-induced lung injury. Nat Med. 2005;11(8):875-879.

[63] Brandi ML, Giustina A. Sexual Dimorphism of Coronavirus 19 Morbidity and Lethality. Trends Endocrinol Metab. 2020;31(12):918-927.

[64] Torres Fernandez ED, Huffman AM, Syed M, Romero DG, Yanes Cardozo LL. Effect of GLP-1 Receptor Agonists in the Cardiometabolic Complications in a Rat Model of Postmenopausal PCOS. Endocrinology. 2019;160(12):2787-2799.

[65] Torres Fernandez ED, Adams KV, Syed M, Maranon RO, Romero DG, Yanes Cardozo LL. Long-Lasting Androgen-Induced Cardiometabolic Effects in Polycystic Ovary Syndrome. J Endocr Soc. 2018;2(8):949-964.

[66] Moretti ME, Caprara D, Drehuta I, Yeung E, Cheung S, Federico L, et al. The Fetal Safety of Angiotensin Converting Enzyme Inhibitors and Angiotensin II Receptor Blockers. Obstet Gynecol Int. 2012;2012:658310.

[67] Dumesic DA, Oberfield SE, Stener-Victorin E, Marshall JC, Laven JS, Legro RS. Scientific Statement on the Diagnostic Criteria, Epidemiology, Pathophysiology, and Molecular Genetics of Polycystic Ovary Syndrome. Endocr Rev. 2015;36(5):487-525.

[68] Mendoza MF, Kachur SM, Lavie CJ. Hypertension in obesity. Curr Opin Cardiol. 2020;35(4):389-396.

[69] Choe SS, Huh JY, Hwang IJ, Kim JI, Kim JB. Adipose Tissue Remodeling: Its Role in Energy Metabolism and Metabolic Disorders. Front Endocrinol (Lausanne). 2016;7:30.

[70] Okuno Y, Fukuhara A, Hashimoto E, Kobayashi H, Kobayashi S, Otsuki M, et al. Oxidative Stress Inhibits Healthy Adipose Expansion Through Suppression of SREBF1-Mediated Lipogenic Pathway. Diabetes. 2018;67(6):1113-1127.

[71] Manneras L, Cajander S, Holmang A, Seleskovic Z, Lystig T, Lonn M, et al. A new rat model exhibiting both ovarian and metabolic characteristics of polycystic ovary syndrome. Endocrinology. 2007;148(8):3781-3791.

[72] Hall JE, do Carmo JM, da Silva AA, Wang Z, Hall ME. Obesity, kidney dysfunction and hypertension: mechanistic links. Nat Rev Nephrol. 2019;15(6):367-385.

[73] Rojas J, Chavez M, Olivar L, Rojas M, Morillo J, Mejias J, et al. Polycystic ovary syndrome, insulin resistance, and obesity: navigating the pathophysiologic labyrinth. Int J Reprod Med. 2014;2014:719050.

[74] Yildirir A, Aybar F, Kabakci G, Yarali H, Oto A. Heart rate variability in young women with polycystic ovary syndrome. Ann Noninvasive Electrocardiol. 2006;11(4):306-312.

[75] Hadi HA, Carr CS, Al Suwaidi J. Endothelial dysfunction: cardiovascular risk factors, therapy, and outcome. Vasc Health Risk Manag. 2005;1(3):183-198.

[76] Schulz E, Gori T, Munzel T. Oxidative stress and endothelial dysfunction in

hypertension. Hypertens Res. 2011;34(6):665-673.

[77] Usselman CW, Yarovinsky TO, Steele FE, Leone CA, Taylor HS, Bender JR, et al. Androgens drive microvascular endothelial dysfunction in women with polycystic ovary syndrome: role of the endothelin B receptor. J Physiol. 2019;597(11):2853-2865.

[78] Yanes L, Romero D, Iliescu R, Cucchiarelli VE, Fortepiani LA, Santacruz F, et al. Systemic arterial pressure response to two weeks of Tempol therapy in SHR: involvement of NO, the RAS, and oxidative stress. Am J Physiol Regul Integr Comp Physiol. 2005;288(4):R903–R908.

[79] Hurliman A, Keller Brown J, Maille N, Mandala M, Casson P, Osol G. Hyperandrogenism and Insulin Resistance, Not Changes in Body Weight, Mediate the Development of Endothelial Dysfunction in a Female Rat Model of Polycystic Ovary Syndrome (PCOS). Endocrinology. 2015;156(11):4071-4080.

[80] Gulanski BI, Flannery CA, Peter PR, Leone CA, Stachenfeld NS. Compromised endothelial function in transgender men taking testosterone. Clin Endocrinol (Oxf). 2020;92(2):138-144.

[81] Yilmaz M, Bukan N, Ayvaz G, Karakoc A, Toruner F, Cakir N, et al. The effects of rosiglitazone and metformin on oxidative stress and homocysteine levels in lean patients with polycystic ovary syndrome. Hum Reprod. 2005;20(12):3333-3340.

[82] Wilmot KA, O'Flaherty M, Capewell S, Ford ES, Vaccarino V. Coronary Heart Disease Mortality Declines in the United States From 1979 Through 2011: Evidence for Stagnation in Young Adults, Especially Women. Circulation. 2015;132(11):997-1002.

[83] Jabbour R, Ott J, Eppel W, Frigo P. Carotid intima-media thickness in polycystic ovary syndrome and its association with hormone and lipid profiles. PLoS One. 2020;15(4):e0232299.

[84] Gilbert EW, Tay CT, Hiam DS, Teede HJ, Moran LJ. Comorbidities and complications of polycystic ovary syndrome: An overview of systematic reviews. Clin Endocrinol (Oxf). 2018;89(6):683-699.

[85] Shanik MH, Xu Y, Skrha J, Dankner R, Zick Y, Roth J. Insulin resistance and hyperinsulinemia: is hyperinsulinemia the cart or the horse? Diabetes Care. 2008;31 Suppl 2:S262–S268.

[86] Peng Z, Sun Y, Lv X, Zhang H, Liu C, Dai S. Interleukin-6 Levels in Women with Polycystic Ovary Syndrome: A Systematic Review and Meta-Analysis. PLoS One. 2016;11(2):e0148531.

[87] Diamanti-Kandarakis E, Dunaif A. Insulin resistance and the polycystic ovary syndrome revisited: an update on mechanisms and implications. Endocr Rev. 2012;33(6):981-1030.

[88] Moller DE, Cohen O, Yamaguchi Y, Assiz R, Grigorescu F, Eberle A, et al. Prevalence of mutations in the insulin receptor gene in subjects with features of the type A syndrome of insulin resistance. Diabetes. 1994;43(2):247-255.

[89] Sanchez-Garrido MA, Tena-Sempere M. Metabolic dysfunction in polycystic ovary syndrome: Pathogenic role of androgen excess and potential therapeutic strategies. Mol Metab. 2020;35:100937.

[90] O'Reilly MW, Taylor AE, Crabtree NJ, Hughes BA, Capper F, Crowley RK, et al. Hyperandrogenemia predicts metabolic phenotype in

polycystic ovary syndrome: the utility of serum androstenedione. J Clin Endocrinol Metab. 2014;99(3):1027-1036.

[91] Ehrmann DA, Barnes RB, Rosenfield RL, Cavaghan MK, Imperial J. Prevalence of impaired glucose tolerance and diabetes in women with polycystic ovary syndrome. Diabetes Care. 1999;22(1):141-146.

[92] Rosenfield RL, Ehrmann DA. The Pathogenesis of Polycystic Ovary Syndrome (PCOS): The Hypothesis of PCOS as Functional Ovarian Hyperandrogenism Revisited. Endocr Rev. 2016;37(5):467-520.

[93] Nestler JE, Powers LP, Matt DW, Steingold KA, Plymate SR, Rittmaster RS, et al. A direct effect of hyperinsulinemia on serum sex hormone-binding globulin levels in obese women with the polycystic ovary syndrome. J Clin Endocrinol Metab. 1991;72(1):83-89.

[94] Deswal R, Yadav A, Dang AS. Sex hormone binding globulin - an important biomarker for predicting PCOS risk: A systematic review and meta-analysis. Syst Biol Reprod Med. 2018;64(1):12-24.

[95] Gamba M, Pralong FP. Control of GnRH neuronal activity by metabolic factors: the role of leptin and insulin. Mol Cell Endocrinol. 2006;254-255:133-9.

[96] Chaudhari N, Dawalbhakta M, Nampoothiri L. GnRH dysregulation in polycystic ovarian syndrome (PCOS) is a manifestation of an altered neurotransmitter profile. Reprod Biol Endocrinol. 2018;16(1):37.

[97] Coutinho EA, Kauffman AS. The Role of the Brain in the Pathogenesis and Physiology of Polycystic Ovary Syndrome (PCOS). Med Sci (Basel). 2019;7(8).

[98] Banaszewska B, Wrotynska-Barczynska J, Spaczynski RZ, Pawelczyk L, Duleba AJ. Effects of Resveratrol on Polycystic Ovary Syndrome: A Double-blind, Randomized, Placebo-controlled Trial. J Clin Endocrinol Metab. 2016;101(11):4322-4328.

[99] Spritzer PM, Lecke SB, Satler F, Morsch DM. Adipose tissue dysfunction, adipokines, and low-grade chronic inflammation in polycystic ovary syndrome. Reproduction. 2015;149(5):R219–R227.

[100] Lovejoy JC, Bray GA, Bourgeois MO, Macchiavelli R, Rood JC, Greeson C, et al. Exogenous androgens influence body composition and regional body fat distribution in obese postmenopausal women--a clinical research center study. J Clin Endocrinol Metab. 1996;81(6):2198-2203.

[101] Wehr E, Moller R, Horejsi R, Giuliani A, Kopera D, Schweighofer N, et al. Subcutaneous adipose tissue topography and metabolic disturbances in polycystic ovary syndrome. Wien Klin Wochenschr. 2009;121(7-8):262-269.

[102] Gambineri A, Patton L, Vaccina A, Cacciari M, Morselli-Labate AM, Cavazza C, et al. Treatment with flutamide, metformin, and their combination added to a hypocaloric diet in overweight-obese women with polycystic ovary syndrome: a randomized, 12-month, placebo-controlled study. J Clin Endocrinol Metab. 2006;91(10):3970-3980.

[103] Manneras-Holm L, Leonhardt H, Kullberg J, Jennische E, Oden A, Holm G, et al. Adipose tissue has aberrant morphology and function in PCOS: enlarged adipocytes and low serum adiponectin, but not circulating sex steroids, are strongly associated with insulin resistance. J Clin Endocrinol Metab. 2011;96(2):E304–E311.

[104] Corbould A. Chronic testosterone treatment induces selective insulin resistance in subcutaneous adipocytes of women. J Endocrinol. 2007;192(3):585-594.

[105] Luotola K, Piltonen TT, Puurunen J, Morin-Papunen LC, Tapanainen JS. Testosterone is associated with insulin resistance index independently of adiposity in women with polycystic ovary syndrome. Gynecol Endocrinol. 2018;34(1):40-44.

[106] Hansen SL, Svendsen PF, Jeppesen JF, Hoeg LD, Andersen NR, Kristensen JM, et al. Molecular Mechanisms in Skeletal Muscle Underlying Insulin Resistance in Women Who Are Lean With Polycystic Ovary Syndrome. J Clin Endocrinol Metab. 2019;104(5):1841-1854.

[107] Nishizawa H, Shimomura I, Kishida K, Maeda N, Kuriyama H, Nagaretani H, et al. Androgens decrease plasma adiponectin, an insulin-sensitizing adipocyte-derived protein. Diabetes. 2002;51(9):2734-2741.

[108] Kogure GS, Miranda-Furtado CL, Silva RC, Melo AS, Ferriani RA, De Sa MF, et al. Resistance Exercise Impacts Lean Muscle Mass in Women with Polycystic Ovary Syndrome. Med Sci Sports Exerc. 2016;48(4):589-598.

[109] Chen MJ, Chiu HM, Chen CL, Yang WS, Yang YS, Ho HN. Hyperandrogenemia is independently associated with elevated alanine aminotransferase activity in young women with polycystic ovary syndrome. J Clin Endocrinol Metab. 2010;95(7):3332-3341.

[110] Gambarin-Gelwan M, Kinkhabwala SV, Schiano TD, Bodian C, Yeh HC, Futterweit W. Prevalence of nonalcoholic fatty liver disease in women with polycystic ovary syndrome. Clin Gastroenterol Hepatol. 2007;5(4):496-501.

[111] Jones H, Sprung VS, Pugh CJ, Daousi C, Irwin A, Aziz N, et al. Polycystic ovary syndrome with hyperandrogenism is characterized by an increased risk of hepatic steatosis compared to nonhyperandrogenic PCOS phenotypes and healthy controls, independent of obesity and insulin resistance. J Clin Endocrinol Metab. 2012;97(10):3709-3716.

[112] Gibson-Helm M, Teede H, Dunaif A, Dokras A. Delayed Diagnosis and a Lack of Information Associated With Dissatisfaction in Women With Polycystic Ovary Syndrome. J Clin Endocrinol Metab. 2017;102(2):604-612.

[113] Lin AW, Bergomi EJ, Dollahite JS, Sobal J, Hoeger KM, Lujan ME. Trust in Physicians and Medical Experience Beliefs Differ Between Women With and Without Polycystic Ovary Syndrome. J Endocr Soc. 2018;2(9):1001-1009.

[114] Araujo LF, de Matos Soeiro A, Fernandes JL, Pesaro AE, Serrano CV, Jr. Coronary artery disease in women: a review on prevention, pathophysiology, diagnosis, and treatment. Vasc Health Risk Manag. 2006;2(4):465-475.

[115] Klett C, Hellmann W, Hackenthal E, Ganten D. Modulation of tissue angiotensinogen gene expression by glucocorticoids, estrogens, and androgens in SHR and WKY rats. Clin Exp Hypertens. 1993;15(4):683-708.

[116] Klett C, Ganten D, Hellmann W, Kaling M, Ryffel GU, Weimar-Ehl T, et al. Regulation of hepatic angiotensinogen synthesis and secretion by steroid hormones. Endocrinology. 1992;130(6):3660-3668.

[117] Tanis BC, van den Bosch MA, Kemmeren JM, Cats VM, Helmerhorst FM, Algra A, et al. Oral contraceptives and the risk of myocardial infarction. N Engl J Med. 2001;345(25):1787-1793.

[118] Troisi RJ, Cowie CC, Harris MI. Oral contraceptive use and glucose metabolism in a national sample of women in the united states. Am J Obstet Gynecol. 2000;183(2):389-395.

[119] Halperin IJ, Kumar SS, Stroup DF, Laredo SE. The association between the combined oral contraceptive pill and insulin resistance, dysglycemia and dyslipidemia in women with polycystic ovary syndrome: a systematic review and meta-analysis of observational studies. Hum Reprod. 2011;26(1):191-201.

[120] Meyer C, McGrath BP, Teede HJ. Effects of medical therapy on insulin resistance and the cardiovascular system in polycystic ovary syndrome. Diabetes Care. 2007;30(3):471-478.

[121] Nader S, Riad-Gabriel MG, Saad MF. The effect of a desogestrel-containing oral contraceptive on glucose tolerance and leptin concentrations in hyperandrogenic women. J Clin Endocrinol Metab. 1997;82(9):3074-3077.

[122] Adeniji AA, Essah PA, Nestler JE, Cheang KI. Metabolic Effects of a Commonly Used Combined Hormonal Oral Contraceptive in Women With and Without Polycystic Ovary Syndrome. J Womens Health (Larchmt). 2016;25(6):638-645.

[123] Morin-Papunen LC, VauhkonenI, KoivunenRM, RuokonenA, MartikainenHK,TapanainenJS.Endocrine and metabolic effects of metformin versus ethinyl estradiol-cyproterone acetate in obese women with polycystic ovary syndrome: a randomized study. J Clin Endocrinol Metab. 2000;85(9):3161-3168.

[124] Goodman NF, Cobin RH, Futterweit W, Glueck JS, Legro RS, Carmina E, et al. American Association of Clinical Endocrinologists, American College of Endocrinology, and Androgen Excess and Pcos Society Disease State Clinical Review: Guide to the Best Practices in the Evaluation and Treatment of Polycystic Ovary Syndrome--Part 1. Endocr Pract. 2015;21(11):1291-1300.

[125] Gil M, Oliva B, Timoner J, Macia MA, Bryant V, de Abajo FJ. Risk of meningioma among users of high doses of cyproterone acetate as compared with the general population: evidence from a population-based cohort study. Br J Clin Pharmacol. 2011;72(6):965-968.

[126] Moretti C, Guccione L, Di Giacinto P, Simonelli I, Exacoustos C, Toscano V, et al. Combined Oral Contraception and Bicalutamide in Polycystic Ovary Syndrome and Severe Hirsutism: A Double-Blind Randomized Controlled Trial. J Clin Endocrinol Metab. 2018;103(3):824-838.

[127] Goodman NF, Cobin RH, Futterweit W, Glueck JS, Legro RS, Carmina E, et al. American Association of Clinical Endocrinologists, American College of Endocrinology, and Androgen Excess and Pcos Society Disease State Clinical Review: Guide to the Best Practices in the Evaluation and Treatment of Polycystic Ovary Syndrome - Part 2. Endocr Pract. 2015;21(12):1415-1426.

[128] Knowler WC, Barrett-Connor E, Fowler SE, Hamman RF, Lachin JM, Walker EA, et al. Reduction in the incidence of type 2 diabetes with lifestyle intervention or metformin. N Engl J Med. 2002;346(6):393-403.

[129] Nestler JE, Jakubowicz DJ. Decreases in ovarian cytochrome P450c17 alpha activity and serum free testosterone after reduction of insulin secretion in polycystic ovary syndrome. N Engl J Med. 1996;335(9):617-623.

[130] Guan Y, Wang D, Bu H, Zhao T, Wang H. The Effect of Metformin on

Polycystic Ovary Syndrome in Overweight Women: A Systematic Review and Meta-Analysis of Randomized Controlled Trials. Int J Endocrinol. 2020;2020:5150684.

[131] Jensterle Sever M, Kocjan T, Pfeifer M, Kravos NA, Janez A. Short-term combined treatment with liraglutide and metformin leads to significant weight loss in obese women with polycystic ovary syndrome and previous poor response to metformin. Eur J Endocrinol. 2014;170(3):451-459.

[132] Hoang V, Bi J, Mohankumar SM, Vyas AK. Liraglutide improves hypertension and metabolic perturbation in a rat model of polycystic ovarian syndrome. PLoS One. 2015;10(5):e0126119.

[133] Javed Z, Papageorgiou M, Deshmukh H, Rigby AS, Qamar U, Abbas J, et al. Effects of empagliflozin on metabolic parameters in polycystic ovary syndrome: a randomized controlled study. Clinical endocrinology. 2019;90(6):805-813.

[134] Butler J, Handelsman Y, Bakris G, Verma S. Use of sodium–glucose co-transporter-2 inhibitors in patients with and without type 2 diabetes: implications for incident and prevalent heart failure. European Journal of Heart Failure. 2020.

[135] Zinman B, Wanner C, Lachin JM, Fitchett D, Bluhmki E, Hantel S, et al. Empagliflozin, cardiovascular outcomes, and mortality in type 2 diabetes. New England Journal of Medicine. 2015;373(22):2117-2128.

[136] Mompeón A, Lázaro-Franco M, Bueno-Betí C, Pérez-Cremades D, Vidal-Gómez X, Monsalve E, et al. Estradiol, acting through ERα, induces endothelial non-classic renin-angiotensin system increasing angiotensin 1-7 production. Mol Cell Endocrinol. 2016;422:1-8.

Section 3

Estrogens

Chapter 7

Serum Sex Hormone Profiles in Potentially Resectable Esophageal Cancer

Waleed Al-Khyatt and Syed Yusuf Iftikhar

Abstract

Esophageal cancer (EC) affects men far more commonly than women. Numerous epidemiological studies have suggested that the hormonal milieu may play a role in this gender bias. However, there is little known about circulating sex hormone levels in relation to the risk of EC development. In this chapter, the correlation between circulating sex hormone levels and mRNA expression of estrogen receptors (ER) in normal esophageal mucosal samples and EC biopsies from patients with potentially resectable EC is studied. Moreover, the association of serum sex hormones levels with and clinico-pathological features of EC is analysed.

Keywords: esophageal, cancer, squamous, adenocarcinoma, sex hormones, estrogen, testosterone, estradiol

1. Introduction

Sex steroid hormones are essential for normal reproductive health in both sexes. Estrogens in women and androgens in men are crucial for development of sexual organs and regulation of gametogenesis. They also play vital roles in regulating physiological functions of other non-target tissues and organs. For instance, estrogens are involved in the maintenance of bone mass, regulation of lipoprotein synthesis, prevention of urogenital atrophy, regulation of insulin responsiveness, and maintenance of cognitive function.

Sex steroids hormones are also linked with development, progression, or treatment of several cancers that include breast, uterine, prostate, and testicular cancer [1].

Indeed, the correlation between endogenous sex steroid hormones and the risk of developing breast cancer is well described in the literature. Besides, the use of anti-estrogenic therapy is associated with better local control and survival outcome in patients with breast cancer [2].

Esophageal cancer (EC) is the eighth most common cancer and the sixth most common cause of cancer mortality worldwide [3]. Despite developments in treatment modalities, estimated overall five-year survival rate for patients with EC is still poor, one of the characteristic features of EC, especially esophageal adenocarcinoma (EAC) is a persistence gender bias over several decades, in all races and across the world [3–5]. Although EC is not a hormone-dependant tumour, several epidemiological studies suggested that female sex hormones may have a protective role against

IntechOpen

the development of this aggressive malignancy [6, 7]. There is mounting evidence that the male predominance associated with oesophageal cancer is age dependent. The gender ratio is at its highest at a younger age, whereas the incidence difference between older men and women is smaller afterwards [8, 9]. This gender ratio seems to have been consistent during the last decades, despite the increasing incidence in EAC.

Several epidemiological studies investigated the possible association between the endogenous and exogenous sex hormonal exposure and EC. Lindblad et al. suggested that the use of HRT was not associated with a reduced risk of EC of any histological type [10]. Similarly, two recent studies examined the association between the use of HRT and the risk of EAC and squamous cell carcinoma (ESCC) in postmenopausal women [11, 12]. Freedman et al. found that the use of HRT was significantly associated with lower risk of ESCC and with a non-significant lower risk of EAC. Moreover, older age at menopause was inversely associated with ESCC. This risk reduction was more evident in women with intact uteri and who received estrogen and progestin containing HRT. Therefore, it was suggested that higher estrogen and progesterone levels may be related inversely to EC and in this way help explain the lower incidence rates in women compared to men [11]. In contrast, another study of 161,086 postmenopausal women involved in the Women's Health Initiative (WHI), showed that the risk of ESCC was only lower among HRT users with a decreased risk mainly among current users of estrogen and progestin containing HRT. No association was observed between the use of HRT and the risk of EAC. Also, no other reproductive or hormonal factors were significantly associated with the risk of either ESCC or EAC [12].

A nested case–control study within a prospective UK cohort and meta-analysis found that women prescribed HRT had a reduced risk of OC (adjusted RR for HRT versus no HRT prescriptions, 0.68, 95% CI 0.53–0.88; $p < 0.004$) [13]. There were no significant differences in cancer risk by HRT type, estimated duration of HRT use or between past and current users [13]. Recently, the Million Women Study (MWS) by Green et al examined risk of esophageal and gastric cancers in relation to reproductive factors in a large UK cohort [14]. They have shown that risks of both esophageal and gastric cancers were higher in postmenopausal than in pre- or peri-menopausal women, and, among postmenopausal women, risks were higher the younger the women were at menopause [14]. In contrast to some studies where no association of childbearing on the risk of AEC was identified [15], the MWS demonstrated that the association between parity and risk of EC was more significant for ESCC than for EAC and age at menarche was significantly associated with EAC but not ESCC [14]. Green et al therefore suggested that the reduced risks associated with menopausal status and with hormone therapy use are consistent with a hypothesis that exposure to estrogens reduces the risk of EC [14].

On the other hand, in a large population-based cohort of 87, 323 postmenopausal women with breast cancer, the potential effects of tamoxifen (Selective ER modulator mostly acts as an anti-estrogen) used for breast cancer treatment was evaluated. In this study, there was no increase in the risk of developing EC in breast cancer patients who received adjuvant tamoxifen treatment in comparison to the control group [16, 17]. However, a different large population-based study of 138,885 women (by Chandanos et al.) suggested a 60% risk increase of EAC among the exposed group but did not achieve statistical significance. In contrast, there was an increased risk of ESCC and lung cancer observed only in the unexposed cohort, indicating that the confounding factor of smoking might explain the increased incidence during the unexposed period [18].

Interestingly, a dose-dependent risk reduction in EC by breastfeeding was suggested [19]. In a recent study, based on pooled data from several large case–control studies, endogenous reproductive factors and exogenous factors were evaluated in women. Breastfeeding was associated dose-dependently with a reduced risk of

EAC, while parity, menstruation, history of pregnancy, use of oral contraceptives or of HRT were not associated with the risk of developing this tumour [20, 21].

In a cohort of patients with prostate cancer, a reduced risk of EAC but not of ESCC was noted. Hence, it was suggested that a diagnosis of prostate cancer may be linked with aetiological factors that are negatively associated with EAC, or anti-androgen therapy may influence the development of EAC [22]. In contrast, estrogen exposure in a national cohort of men with prostate cancer did not show any reduced risk of a second AEC [23]. Despite these efforts to explain the relation between female reproductive factors and risk of development of EC, the results are rather unclear and contradict each other. This could be partially explained by the fact that the number of women with EC included in those studies was relatively small, which could have the affected potential significance of the results [24].

Recently, it has suggested that the ER system is involved in EC progression and thus may provide a novel target for the treatment of EC [25]. However, there is little known about sex hormones levels in relation to the risk of EC development. In this study we aimed to:

1. Describe sex hormones profiles in a cohort of patients with established OC.

2. Identify whether there is any correlation between circulating sex hormone levels and mRNA expression of estrogen receptors (ER) in normal esophageal mucosal samples and EC biopsies.

3. Analyse the correlation between circulating sex hormone levels and clinic-pathological features of EC.

2. Material and methods

2.1 Patient cohort

Joint ethical approval for the research protocol was acquired from the Derbyshire Research Ethics Committee and Derbyshire Hospitals Research and Development office. Written, informed consent was obtained from all patients included in this study. EC samples and matched normal tissue taken from adjacent macroscopic mucosa from the same patient were collected from resected EC specimens of 34 patients [EAC: n = 28; ESCC: n= 6] who underwent esophagectomy. Normal samples were microscopically examined by a consultant pathologist to confirm normal features.

2.2 mRNA analysis by qRT-PCR

Total RNA was extracted from tissue samples (30 mg), ground in liquid N_2 with a pestle and mortar and from cell lines (10^4 cells) using the RNeasy Mini kit method (QIAGEN, UK) as per manufacturer's protocol. 300 ng of total RNA was reverse transcribed with (+RT) or without (-RT) reverse transcriptase (RT) using the high-capacity cDNA reverse transcription kit (Life Technologies, Paisley, UK). 2 µl of cDNA were amplified by real time PCR with commercially available TaqMan assays (Life Technologies, Paisley, UK) for *ESR1* (Hs00174860_m1), *ESR2* (Hs01100353_m1), and the reference genes *GAPDH* (Hs02758991_g1), *PGK1* (Hs00943178_g1), and *ACTB* (Hs01060665_g1) in a Chromo 4 thermal cycler (Bio-Rad Laboratories LTD, Hemel Hempstead, UK). Expression of *ESR1* and *ESR2* was quantified relative to the geometric mean of three reference genes and reported as relative to max using the GenEX software Version 5 (MultiD, DE) in accordance with MIQE guidelines [26].

2.3 Immunohistochemistry

Immunohistochemistry (IHC) slides were prepared in the Histopathology Department at the Royal Derby Hospital. Normal mucosa and EC samples were stained using ERα and ERβ antibodies (NCL-L-ER-6F11 and 6007907, respectively, Novacastra, Newcastle, UK). ERα and ERβ positive breast cancer samples were used as positive controls. The 'H-score method was used to measure the strength of ER-staining in normal esophageal mucosa and matched tumour samples [27]. Positive staining was defined as an H-score ≥ 10 in this study.

2.4 Blood samples

Blood samples were collected from 34 patients with histologically proven EC. Once the patient was anaesthetised, 10 ml of central venous blood was taken using gold-top Vacutainer Serum Separation Tubes (BD Vacutainer® SST™). Blood samples were immediately transported to the Clinical Chemistry laboratory in Royal Derby Hospital for analysis. Fasting serum level of testosterone, luteinizing hormone (LH), follicle stimulating hormone (FSH), sex hormone binding globulin (SHBG), 17-β oestradiol (E2) were measured using *ElectroChemiLuminescence ImmunoAssay* (ECLIA, Roche) and as per manufacturer's protocols. *Elecsys and Cobas e immunoassay 411 analyzer* was used for running of ECLIA (Roche-diagnostic, USA). The free androgen index (FAI) was calculated as the total testosterone to SHBG ratio [28].

2.5 Statistical analysis

For qRT-PCR on primary tissues, the two-tailed Wilcoxon signed rank test was used for matched cases while the two-tailed Mann-Whitney *U* test was used for non-matched variables. Either the two-tailed Mann-Whitney *U* test or Kruskal-Wallis test, as appropriate, was used to establish relationships between hormone levels, ER mRNA and clinico-pathological features. Correlation coefficient (r) was calculated using two-tail Spearman correlation. Statistical differences were calculated using SPSS Statistics® for Windows™ v21 software from IBM SPSS Statistics (Feltham, UK) and GraphPad Prism® v6 (La Jolla, CA, USA). A value of $p \leq 0.05$ was considered as statistically significant.

3. Results

3.1 Clinico-pathological characteristics of recruited patients

The clinico-pathological characteristics of EC patients included in the analysis are summarised in **Table 1**. Median age was 65 years (range, 30 – 79 years). There were 28 males and 6 females with male-to-female ratio of 5.7:1. Of those 34 patients, 28 patients had EAC and 6 patients had ESCC. One-year disease specific survival was approximately 73.5%. Twenty-five (74%) patients received neoadjuvant therapy.

3.2 Sex hormones profiles

The median (Inter quartile range) (IQR) of the serum sex hormones levels (34 patients) against their corresponding laboratory reference ranges (Derby Hospital biochemistry department) is summarised in **Table 2**. Median serum levels of FSH and LH hormone were higher than normal. However, the median of serum levels of E2, progesterone, testosterone, and SHBG were within the normal ranges **Table 2**.

Patients recruited		**34**
Median age (years)		65 (range, 30-79)
One-year disease-specific survival		73.5%
Gender	Male	28 (83%)
	Female	6 (17%)
Histology	EAC	28 (76%)
	ESCC	6 (24%)
Tumour depth (T-stage)	T1	8 (24%)
	T2	3 (9%)
	T3	23 (67%)
Nodal involvement	No (N0)	15 (44%)
	Yes (N1)	19 (56%)
Tumor differentiation	Moderate	25 (74%)
	Poor	9 (26%)
Vascular invasion	No	21(62%)
	Yes	13 (38%)
Barrett's Metaplasia	No	13 (46%)
	Yes	15 (54%)
Circumferential resection margin	Not involved	23 (68%)
	Involved	11 (32%)
Preoperative chemotherapy	No	9 (26%)
	Yes	25 (74%)

Table 1.
Patient Characteristics.

In a gender-based analysis, there were significant higher median (IQR) levels of LH and FSH in female patients compared to LH and FSH levels in male patients. In contrast, women had significantly lower median levels E2, testosterone compared to men. There was no significant difference in serum levels of progesterone and SHBG between men and women (**Table 3**).

3.3 Correlation between serum sex hormones level and estrogen receptor expression

The results of correlation between serum sex hormones and ERα and ERβ expression at mRNA are summarised in **Tables 4** and **5**. There was no significant correlation between the expression of ERα or ERβ mRNA in normal mucosa or tumour samples and serum level of LH, FSH, E2, Testosterone, FAI, or SHBG. In analysis of the correlation of hormones levels with estrogen receptors expression in both genders, we found that there was significant inverse correlation between testosterone level and ERβ mRNA expression in normal mucosa from male patients ($r = -0.41, p = 0.03$) (**Table 6**). In female patients, there was significant inverse correlation between progesterone level and ERα mRNA expression in EC samples ($r = -0.87, p = 0.04$) level (**Table 7**). No correlation was demonstrated between the levels of rest of sex hormones and ERs expression in either gender (**Tables 6** and **7**).

Hormone (reference range)	Median (IQR) of serum level
LH (1.7 – 8.6 IU/L)	9.9 (7, 17) IU/L
FSH (1.5 – 12.4 IU/L)	17 (9.6, 28) IU/L
E2 (28 – 167 pmol/L)	73 (50, 95) pmol/L
Progesterone (0.7 – 4.3 nmol/L)	1.1 (0.5, 1.15) nmol/L
Testosterone (8.3 – 27.8 nmol/L)	12 (6.5, 16.5) nmol/L
SHBG (14.5 – 48.4 nmol/L)	52 (32, 68) nmol/L
FAI (34 – 106 %)	20.5% (12%, 31%)

LH, luteinizing hormone; FSH, follicular stimulating hormone; E2, 17β-Oestradiol; SHBG, serum hormone binding globulin; FHI, free androgen index.

Table 2.
The median (IQR) of serum sex hormones levels of patients with EC (n = 34).

Hormone (reference range)	Median (IQR) of serum level		
	Male (n = 28)	Female (n = 6)	*p* value*
LH (1.7 – 8.6 IU/L)	9.5 (6.5 – 12) IU/L	33.5 (21 – 45.5) IU/L	0.004
FSH (1.5 – 12.4 IU/L)	13 (7.8 - 23) IU/L	62 (40 – 90) IU/L	0.001
E2 (28 – 167 pmol/L)	78 (59 – 98) pmol/L	50 (35 – 50) pmol/L	0.002
Progesterone (0.7 – 4.3 nmol/L)	1.2 (0.8 – 2.4) nmol/L	0.9 (0.8 – 1.5) nmol/L	0.51
Testosterone (8.3 – 27.8 nmol/L)	14 (8 – 20) nmol/L	0.5 (0.3 – 1.1) nmol/L	0.0001
SHBG (14.5 – 48.4 nmol/L)	54 (32 – 65) nmol/L	40 (28.5 – 89) nmol/L	0.84
FAI (34 – 106 %)	21.5% (16% – 35%)	1% (0.5% – 3%)	0.001

LH, luteinizing hormone; FSH, follicular stimulating hormone; E2, 17β-Oestradiol; SHBG, serum hormone binding globulin; FHI, free androgen index.
**Calculated using two-tail Mann Whitney U test.*

Table 3.
Gender-based comparison of serum sex hormones levels in patients with EC.

Hormone	ESR1 (ERα) mRNA expression			
	Normal mucosa		Tumour	
	r	p-value*	r	p-value*
LH	0.08	0.69	0.16	0.41
FSH	- 0.16	0.38	0.04	0.83
E2	0.11	0.55	0.03	0.99
Progesterone	0.2	0.26	0.22	0.2
Testosterone	0.10	0.56	0.10	0.57
SHBG	- 0.2	0.32	0.08	0.68
FAI	0.31	0.11	- 0.08	0.7

LH, luteinizing hormone; FSH, follicle stimulating hormone; E2, 17β-Oestradiol; SHBG, serum hormone binding globulin; FHI, free androgen index; r, the correlation coefficient.
**Calculated using two-tail Spearman correlation.*

Table 4.
Correlation between serum sex hormones levels and ERα mRNA expression.

Hormone	ESR2 (ERβ) mRNA expression			
	Normal mucosa		Tumour	
	r	p-value*	r	p-value*
LH	- 0.22	0.24	- 0.01	0.94
FSH	0.08	0.67	- 0.03	0.85
E2	0.02	0.92	- 0.16	0.38
Progesterone	0.08	0.66	- 0.18	0.33
Testosterone	- 0.03	0.08	- 0.14	0.43
SHBG	0.07	0.7	0	1
FAI	- 0.14	0.49	- 0.25	0.21

LH, luteinizing hormone; FSH, follicle stimulating hormone; E2, 17β-Oestradiol; SHBG, serum hormone binding globulin; FHI, free androgen index; r, the correlation coefficient.
**Calculated using two-tail Spearman correlation.*

Table 5.
Correlation between serum sex hormones levels and ERβ mRNA expression.

Hormone	ESR1 (ERα) mRNA expression				ESR1 (ERβ) mRNA expression			
	Normal mucosa		Tumour		Normal mucosa		Tumour	
	r	p-value*	r	p-value*	r	p-value*	r	p-value*
LH	0.13	0.53	0.19	0.36	- 0.26	0.21	- 0.06	0.77
FSH	- 0.13	0.52	- 0.04	0.85	0.07	0.72	- 0.17	0.41
E2	0.07	0.73	0.08	0.69	0.05	0.80	- 0.07	0.73
Progesterone	- 0.13	0.54	0.08	0.71	- 0.27	0.19	0.10	0.62
Testosterone	0.09	0.64	0.26	0.19	- 0.41	0.03	- 0.03	0.88
SHBG	0.13	0.52	0.08	0.69	- 0.01	0.99	- 0.07	0.74
FAI	0.35	0.11	0.09	0.68	- 0.22	0.36	- 0.14	0.53

LH, luteinizing hormone; FSH, follicle stimulating hormone; E2, 17β-Oestradiol; SHBG, serum hormone binding globulin; FHI, free androgen index; r, the correlation coefficient.
**Calculated using two-tail Spearman correlation.*

Table 6.
Correlation between serum sex hormones levels and estrogen receptors mRNA expression in male patients (n = 28).

Hormone	ESR1 (ERα) mRNA expression				ESR1 (ERβ) mRNA expression			
	Normal mucosa		Tumour		Normal mucosa		Tumour	
	r	p-value*	r	p-value*	r	p-value*	r	p-value*
LH	- 0.80	0.20	- 0.80	0.20	- 0.40	0.60	0.40	0.60
FSH	- 0.36	0.55	-0.22	0.74	0.10	0.87	0.31	0.61
E2	0.71	0.18	0.71	0.18	- 0.35	0.56	0.35	0.56
Progesterone	- 0.62	0.27	- 0.87	0.04	- 0.21	0.74	0.36	0.55
Testosterone	0	1.0	- 0.20	0.75	0.60	0.29	- 0.70	0.19
SHBG	- 0.56	0.32	- 0.15	0.81	0.46	0.43	- 0.21	0.74
FAI	0.37	0.54	0	1.00	0	1.00	- 0.16	0.80

LH, luteinizing hormone; FSH, follicle stimulating hormone; E2, 17β-Oestradiol; SHBG, serum hormone binding globulin; FHI, free androgen index; r, the correlation coefficient.
**Calculated using two-tail Spearman correlation.*

Table 7.
Correlation between serum sex hormones levels and estrogen receptors mRNA expression in female patients (n = 6).

Hormone	Disease specific one-year survival			
	Males		Females	
LH	R	- 0.33	R	0.26
	*p-value**	0.10	*p-value**	0.74
FSH	R	0.12	r	0.36
	*p-value**	0.56	*p-value**	0.55
E2	R	0.32	r	1.000**
	*p-value**	0.10	*p-value**	< 0.0001
Progesterone	R	0.16	R	0.36
	*p-value**	0.46	*p-value**	0.55
Testosterone	R	0.19	R	0.35
	*p-value**	0.37	*p-value**	0.56
SHBG	R	0.21	R	0.36
	*p-value**	0.29	*p-value**	0.55
FAI	r	0.21	r	0.19
	*p-value**	0.35	*p-value**	0.76

LH, luteinizing hormone; FSH, follicle stimulating hormone; E2, 17β-Oestradiol; SHBG, serum hormone binding globulin; FHI, free androgen index; r, the correlation coefficient.
**Calculated using two-tail Spearman correlation.*

Table 8.
Correlation of serum sex hormones level & 1-year disease specific survival.

Hormone		Histology (EAC vs ESSC)	T-Stage	LN-stage	Grade	VI	BM	CRM
LH	r	0.04	- 0.08	0.21	0.18	0.04	- 0.01	- 0.06
	*p-value**	0.87	0.71	0.30	0.39	0.83	0.98	0.78
FSH	r	- 0.03	- 0.18	0.25	- 0.13	- 0.28	- 0.02	- 0.16
	*p-value**	0.88	0.36	0.21	0.61	0.16	0.943	0.50
E2	r	- 0.27	- 0.125	0.12	0	0.10	-.018	0.02
	*p-value**	0.17	0.53	0.54	1.00	0.61	0.93	0.92
Progesterone	r	- 0.25	- 0.21	0.39	0.27	- 0.16	- 0.06	- 0.25
	*p-value**	0.28	0.32	0.05	0.19	0.46	0.77	0.23
Testosterone	r	0.21	0.18	0.15	0.12	0.06	- 0.04	0.05
	*p-value**	0.28	0.35	0.44	0.53	0.78	0.86	0.81
SHBG	r	0.24	0.13	0.08	0.13	- 0.09	- 0.17	- 0.01
	*p-value**	0.24	0.51	0.69	0.53	0.65	0.39	0.96
FAI	r	- 0.17	- 0.08	- 0.24	- 0.22	- 0.15	0.20	- 0.50
	*p-value**	0.61	0.72	0.29	0.33	0.61	0.37	0.02

LH, luteinizing hormone; FSH, follicle stimulating hormone; E2, 17β-Oestradiol; SHBG, serum hormone binding globulin; FHI, free androgen index; T-stage, tumour depth; LN-stage, lymph node involvement; VI, vascular invasion; BM, barrett's metaplasia; CRM, circumferential resection margin; r, the correlation coefficient.
**Calculated using two-tail Spearman correlation.*

Table 9.
Correlation between serum sex hormones levels and pathological features in male patients (n = 28).

Hormone		Histology (AEC vs ESSC)	T-Stage	LN-stage	Grade	VI	BM	CRM
LH	r	- 0.78	- 0.78	0.78	- 0.26	0.78	- 0.78	0
	*p-value**	0.23	0.23	0.23	0.74	0.23	0.23	1.00
FSH	r	- 0.18	- 0.74	0.74	0.18	0	-.725	- 0.15
	*p-value**	0.77	0.15	0.15	0.77	1.00	0.17	0.81
E2	r	- 0.25	- 0.41	0.41	0.25	- 0.41	0.25	- 0.61
	*p-value**	0.69	0.50	0.50	0.69	0.50	0.69	0.27
Progesterone	r	- 0.73	- 0.44	0.44	- 0.18	0.74	- 0.73	0.15
	*p-value**	0.17	0.45	0.45	0.77	0.15	0.17	0.81
Testosterone	r	0	0.58	- 0.58	0.71	0.87	- 0.35	0.87
	*p-value**	1.00	0.31	0.31	0.18	0.06	0.56	0.06
SHBG	r	0.73	0	0	- 0.18	- 0.44	- 0.18	0.15
	*p-value**	0.17	1.00	1.00	0.77	0.45	0.77	0.81
FAI	R	0.56	0.15	- 0.15	0.56	0.76	- 0.19	0.30
	*p-value**	0.33	0.81	0.81	0.33	0.14	0.76	0.62

LH, luteinizing hormone; FSH, follicle stimulating hormone; E2, 17β-Oestradiol; SHBG, serum hormone binding globulin; FHI, free androgen index; T-stage, tumour depth; LN-stage, lymph node involvement; VI, vascular invasion; BM, barrett's metaplasia; CRM, circumferential resection margin; r, the correlation coefficient.
**Calculated using two-tail Spearman correlation.*

Table 10.
Correlation between serum sex hormones levels and pathological features in female patients (n = 6).

3.4 Correlation between serum sex hormones levels and clinico-pathological features

Gender-based analysis of correlation between serum hormones levels and survival outcome at one year and pathological features after intended curative resection was performed using two-tail Spearman test. There was highly significant positive correlation between 1-year disease survival outcome and serum E2 level in female patients ($r = 1$, $p < 0.0001$) (**Table 8**). However, no significant association was determined between sex hormones levels and 1-year disease specific survival in male patients (**Table 7**).

No correlation was demonstrated between serum hormonal levels and pathological features of EC from either male or female patients (**Tables 9** and **10**).

4. Discussion

In this study, we investigated sex steroid hormones profiles in patients with established EC. Our results demonstrated that there was no correlation between serum level of LH, FHS, E2, SHBG, or FAI and ER expression in normal esophageal mucosa or EC from both genders. Whilst 1-year disease survival is significantly correlated with high E2 level in female patients, no significant correlation is identified between survival outcome and sex hormones level in male patients.

The disparity in the incidence of EC between males and females has always raised the question regarding the role of sex hormones and sex EC in esophageal carcinogenesis. In an *in vitro* study, Matsuoka et al. were first to investigate the effect of E2 and testosterone on the growth of newly established cancer cell lines of ESCC origin, which expressed both ER and androgen receptor (AR). They found that the growth rate of the cell lines was inhibited by estrogen and enhanced by testosterone [29]. In a similar way, Utsumi et al. suggested that the presence of ER arbitrates the inhibitory effect of estrogen when it was noted that the growth of ER positive transplanted tumour was significantly greater in male than it was in female nude mice. Such a difference was not observed for ER negative tumour. Also, the growth rate of ER positive tumours was enhanced in oophorectomised female mice and significantly suppressed with a physiological dose of E2 compared to ER negative cancer [30, 31]. Likewise, Ueo et al studied sex hormone dependency and hormone responsiveness on both ER positive (KSE-1) and ER negative (KSE-2) ESCC cell lines transplanted in male and female nude mice. They found that the administration of E2 significantly inhibited the growth of KSE-1 tumours in both males and females in conjunction with an increase in E2 levels. No similar influence on KSE-2 growth was identified. Therefore, they suggested that the growth of human EC cells with sex hormone receptor is influenced by circulating hormone levels and can be manipulated by systemic E2 administration [32].

EAC often expresses ER, which suggests a possible biological involvement of steroid hormones. Wang et al. suggested that ER and their signalling could have a role in EC development when he found that 43.75% (21/48) and 20.83% (10/48) of EC cases were positive for ER and progesterone receptor (PR) respectively, while these receptors were negative in esophageal tissues taken from normal subjects [33]. Similarly, Tiffin et al suggested that the role of ER may warrant further investigation when they identified mild to moderate ER staining in most of their esophageal tissue samples. However, the author did not discriminate between the ER subtypes detected [34]. Interestingly, Nozoe et al found that ERα expression was significantly higher in male patients with ESCC in comparison to females. Also, a positive expression of ERα plus negative expression of ERβ was found to be an unfavourable independent prognostic indicator in patients with ESCC. Therefore, they suggested that hormonal therapy using estrogen may have a role in improving the outcome in this type of cancer and its possible anti-tumour effect requires more in depth both laboratory and clinical based investigations [35]. Akgun et al. studied the expression of ERβ in Barrett's metaplasia and associated EAC. They concluded that all EAC and most precursor lesions, Barrett's metaplasia with or without dysplasia, express ERβ in a significantly high percentage of the cells. These findings raise the possibility that EAC may benefit from treatment and/or chemoprevention by SERM [36]. Likewise, Liu et al. found that ERβ1, ERβ2, ERβ3 and ERβ5 are overexpressed in EAC compared to its precursor lesion Barrett's metaplasia negative for dysplasia, suggesting a significant biological role [37]. In contrast, Kalayarasan et al. studied the expression of ERα and ERβ as well as Progesterone Receptors (PR) in both tumour tissue and adjacent normal mucosa samples of 45 cases of EC (ESCC = 30 cases, EAC= 15 cases). They found neither tumours nor normal mucosa expressed ERα or PR. However, all cases of EAC, irrespective of their stage/grade, were strongly positive for ERβ and the intensity of staining in tumours was significantly higher than in normal adjacent mucosa. Therefore, they suggested that estrogen may have an effect on the growth of EAC and this effect may be mediated by ERβ [38]. Despite numerous studies assessing the role of sex hormones in AEC development, the findings are still featured by some inconsistency. It seems therefore important that the molecular mechanisms of ER in esophageal carcinogenesis are further clarified.

Recently, Zuguchi et al found that there is increased nuclear ERβ reactivity in human ESCC in comparison to matched normal mucosa [39]. Moreover, increased ERβ expression seems to have unfavourable correlation to the histo-pathological stage of the disease [39]. Therefore, they concluded that EC is an estrogen dependant malignancy and ERβ might provide an additional therapeutic target for treatment of ESCC [39]. Another study by Sukocheva et al demonstrated that tamoxifen and raloxifen inhibited the growth of esophageal AC cell lines proliferation by inducing apoptosis and cell cycle arrest [40]. However, the study did not differentiate between the role of each receptor, especially when we know for fact that SERMs have different agonist and antagonist function of ER in different body tissues.

Several studies demonstrated that women undergoing curative EC resection have better long term survival outcome compared to men [6, 7]. In a case control study, Wang et al, found that there was a low serum E2 level from healthy controls from an area with a high incidence of ESCC compared to counterparts from a low incidence area in China [41]. Hence, they suggested that the discrepancy in incidence of ESCC may be explained by the lack of a protective E2 effect [41]. In another study, Petrick JL et al identified a high ratio of androgens to estrogens – particularly testosterone:estradiol ratio – was more common in EAC patients than controls, including after restriction to cases without weight loss in the previous 5 years [42]. The lack of association between circulating E2 and ER expression in this study may reflect the theoretical possibility that ER expression is influenced more by intra-tumor E2 rather than circulating hormone concentrations [43, 44]. For instance, Recchione et el found that E2 level in breast cancer samples is significantly higher compared to serum level of E2. Similarly, in a comparison of blood and breast cancer tissue concentrations sex steroids by Secreto et al showed that there was significantly higher level of E2 in the tumours than in the blood [45].

Recently, Xie, S-H et al found that an increased disease-specific mortality with lower SHBG levels and higher FSH levels in male EAC patients without surgical treatment. No clear associations were observed for dehydroepiandrosterone sulphate, LH, prolactin, testosterone, 17-OH-progesterone, progesterone, E2, androstenedione, testosterone:estradiol ratio or free testosterone index [46]. In our study, there was no correlation between sex hormones level and pathological features. However, we found higher serum E2 level had significant positive correlation with 1-year disease specific survival in women. This may indicate that E2 may play antiproliferative effect and in turn reduce the risk of developing distant micro metastases. For example, high dose estrogens, like diethylstilbestrol found to paradoxically inhibit breast cancer growth by activation of Fas/FasL apoptotic pathway [47]. In another in vitro study, Al-Khyatt et al found that ERs antagonists induced apoptosis in EC cell lines proliferation. Thus, they concluded that their findings may indicate that the ER system is involved in OC progression and thus may provide a novel target for the treatment of OC [25].

In a study by Awan et al [48], a raised testosterone level had a positive correlation with the presence of EC compared to control group. Furthermore, serum testosterone levels decreased after surgical resection of the tumour [48]. In this study it was demonstrated that testosterone had an inverse correlation with ERβ mRNA expression in normal mucosa from male patients. Several studies investigated the role of androgens in the pathogenesis of estrogen-dependant cancers like breast cancer [49]. Nevertheless, the significance of cross-talk between androgens and ER in EC is not clear and warrants further investigation [50].

The number of patients used in this study is relatively small, especially female patients. This could be the reason behind the lack of any association between serum sex hormones and ER expression or pathological features. Another limitation is there was no matched healthy control. The serum sex hormones levels of healthy controls could have been used for comparison as well as studying the correlation between hormones levels and risk factors profiles for EC.

In summary, in this study, there was no association between sex hormones profiles and the expression of ER or pathological features of EC in both genders.

Interestingly, survival outcome was better in women with increased serum level of E2. Current published evidence supports that sex hormones may play a role in esophageal carcinogenesis. Hence, future research work may include a population-based study looking into the correlation of sex hormones and risk factors profiles for EC in healthy volunteers and patients is required. Likewise, a well-designed *in vivo* study to address the potential therapeutic role of ERα and ERβ in treatment of EC is warranted.

Author details

Waleed Al-Khyatt* and Syed Yusuf Iftikhar
Department of Upper GI Surgery, Royal Derby Hospital, Derby, UK

*Address all correspondence to: waleed.al-khyatt@nhs.net

References

[1] Chen, C., et al., *The roles of estrogen and estrogen receptors in gastrointestinal disease.* Oncol Lett, 2019. **18**(6): p. 5673-5680.

[2] Syed, B.M., et al., *Long-term clinical outcome of oestrogen receptor-positive operable primary breast cancer in older women: a large series from a single centre.* Br J Cancer, 2011. **104**(9): p. 1393-400.

[3] Arnold, M., et al., *Global incidence of oesophageal cancer by histological subtype in 2012.* Gut, 2015. **64**(3): p. 381-7.

[4] Vial, M., L. Grande, and M. Pera, *Epidemiology of adenocarcinoma of the esophagus, gastric cardia, and upper gastric third.* Recent Results Cancer Res. **182**: p. 1-17.

[5] Vizcaino, A.P., et al., *Time trends incidence of both major histologic types of esophageal carcinomas in selected countries, 1973-1995.* Int J Cancer, 2002. **99**(6): p. 860-8.

[6] Badwe, R.A., et al., *Impact of age and sex on survival after curative resection for carcinoma of the esophagus.* Cancer, 1994. **74**(9): p. 2425-9.

[7] Hidaka, H., et al., *Sex difference in survival of patients treated by surgical resection for esophageal cancer.* World J Surg, 2007. **31**(10): p. 1982-7.

[8] Rutegard, M., et al., *Oesophageal adenocarcinoma: the new epidemic in men?* Maturitas, 2011. **69**(3): p. 244-8.

[9] Derakhshan, M.H., et al., *Oesophageal and gastric intestinal-type adenocarcinomas show the same male predominance due to a 17 year delayed development in females.* Gut, 2009. **58**(1): p. 16-23.

[10] Lindblad, M., et al., *Hormone replacement therapy and risks of oesophageal and gastric adenocarcinomas.* Br J Cancer, 2006. **94**(1): p. 136-41.

[11] Freedman, N.D., et al., *The association of menstrual and reproductive factors with upper gastrointestinal tract cancers in the NIH-AARP cohort.* Cancer, 2010. **116**(6): p. 1572-81.

[12] Bodelon, C., et al., *Hormonal factors and risks of esophageal squamous cell carcinoma and adenocarcinoma in postmenopausal women.* Cancer Prev Res (Phila), 2011. **4**(6): p. 840-50.

[13] Green, J., et al., *Menopausal hormone therapy and risk of gastrointestinal cancer: nested case-control study within a prospective cohort, and meta-analysis.* Int J Cancer, 2012. **130**(10): p. 2387-96.

[14] Green, J., et al., *Reproductive factors and risk of oesophageal and gastric cancer in the Million Women Study cohort.* Br J Cancer, 2012. **106**(1): p. 210-6.

[15] Lagergren, J. and C. Jansson, *Sex hormones and oesophageal adenocarcinoma: influence of childbearing?* Br J Cancer, 2005. **93**(8): p. 859-61.

[16] Andersson, M., H.H. Storm, and H.T. Mouridsen, *Incidence of new primary cancers after adjuvant tamoxifen therapy and radiotherapy for early breast cancer.* J Natl Cancer Inst, 1991. **83**(14): p. 1013-7.

[17] Curtis, R.E., et al., *Second cancers after adjuvant tamoxifen therapy for breast cancer.* J Natl Cancer Inst, 1996. **88**(12): p. 832-4.

[18] Chandanos, E., et al., *Tamoxifen exposure and risk of oesophageal and gastric adenocarcinoma: a population-based cohort study of breast cancer patients in Sweden.* Br J Cancer, 2006. **95**(1): p. 118-22.

[19] Cheng, K.K., et al., *A case-control study of oesophageal adenocarcinoma*

in women: a preventable disease. Br J Cancer, 2000. **83**(1): p. 127-32.

[20] Cronin-Fenton, D.P., et al., *Reproductive and sex hormonal factors and oesophageal and gastric junction adenocarcinoma: a pooled analysis.* Eur J Cancer, 2010. **46**(11): p. 2067-76.

[21] Gallus, S., et al., *Oesophageal cancer in women: tobacco, alcohol, nutritional and hormonal factors.* Br J Cancer, 2001. **85**(3): p. 341-5.

[22] Cooper, S.C., et al., *Patients with prostate cancer are less likely to develop oesophageal adenocarcinoma: could androgens have a role in the aetiology of oesophageal adenocarcinoma?* Cancer Causes Control, 2009. **20**(8): p. 1363-8.

[23] Lagergren, J. and O. Nyren, *Do sex hormones play a role in the etiology of esophageal adenocarcinoma? A new hypothesis tested in a population-based cohort of prostate cancer patients.* Cancer Epidemiol Biomarkers Prev, 1998. **7**(10): p. 913-5.

[24] Rashid, F., R.N. Khan, and S.Y. Iftikhar, *Probing the link between oestrogen receptors and oesophageal cancer.* World J Surg Oncol, 2010. **8**: p. 9.

[25] Al-Khyatt, W., et al., *Selective oestrogen receptor antagonists inhibit oesophageal cancer cell proliferation in vitro.* BMC Cancer, 2018. **18**(1): p. 121.

[26] Bustin, S.A., et al., *The MIQE guidelines: minimum information for publication of quantitative real-time PCR experiments.* Clin Chem, 2009. **55**(4): p. 611-22.

[27] McClelland, R.A., et al., *Automated quantitation of immunocytochemically localized estrogen receptors in human breast cancer.* Cancer Res, 1990. **50**(12): p. 3545-50.

[28] Szulc, P., et al., *Osteoprotegerin serum levels in men: correlation with age, estrogen, and testosterone status.* J Clin Endocrinol Metab, 2001. **86**(7): p. 3162-5.

[29] Matsuoka, H., et al., *Sex hormone response of a newly established squamous cell line derived from clinical esophageal carcinoma.* Cancer Res, 1987. **47**(15): p. 4134-40.

[30] Utsumi, Y., et al., *Role of estrogen receptors in the growth of human esophageal carcinoma.* Cancer, 1989. **64**(1): p. 88-93.

[31] Utsumi, Y., et al., *Effect of 17 beta-estradiol on the growth of an estrogen receptor-positive human esophageal carcinoma cell line.* Cancer, 1991. **67**(9): p. 2284-9.

[32] Ueo, H., et al., *Inhibitory effects of estrogen on the growth of a human esophageal carcinoma cell line.* Cancer Res, 1990. **50**(22): p. 7212-5.

[33] Wang, L.Y., *[Estrogen and progesterone receptors in esophageal carcinoma cells].* Zhonghua Zhong Liu Za Zhi, 1991. **13**(1): p. 23-5.

[34] Tiffin, N., et al., *Sex hormone receptor immunohistochemistry staining in Barrett's oesophagus and adenocarcinoma.* Histopathology, 2003. **42**(1): p. 95-6.

[35] Nozoe, T., et al., *Significance of immunohistochemical expression of estrogen receptors alpha and beta in squamous cell carcinoma of the esophagus.* Clin Cancer Res, 2007. **13**(14): p. 4046-50.

[36] Akgun, H., J. Lechago, and M. Younes, *Estrogen receptor-beta is expressed in Barrett's metaplasia and associated adenocarcinoma of the esophagus.* Anticancer Res, 2002. **22**(3): p. 1459-61.

[37] Liu, L., M. Chirala, and M. Younes, *Expression of estrogen receptor-beta isoforms in Barrett's metaplasia, dysplasia*

and esophageal adenocarcinoma. Anticancer Res, 2004. **24**(5A): p. 2919-24.

[38] Kalayarasan, R., et al., *Estrogen and progesterone receptors in esophageal carcinoma.* Dis Esophagus, 2008. **21**(4): p. 298-303.

[39] Zuguchi, M., et al., *Estrogen receptor alpha and beta in esophageal squamous cell carcinoma.* Cancer Sci, 2012. **103**(7): p. 1348-55.

[40] Sukocheva, O.A., et al., *Effect of estrogen on growth and apoptosis in esophageal adenocarcinoma cells.* Dis Esophagus, 2013. **26**(6): p. 628-35.

[41] Wang, Q.M., et al., *Estrogen analogues: promising target for prevention and treatment of esophageal squamous cell carcinoma in high risk areas.* Med Sci Monit, 2010. **16**(7): p. HY19-22.

[42] Petrick, J.L., et al., *Association between circulating levels of sex steroid hormones and esophageal adenocarcinoma in the FINBAR Study.* PloS one, 2018. **13**(1): p. e0190325-e0190325.

[43] Lukanova, A., et al., *Circulating levels of sex steroid hormones and risk of ovarian cancer.* Int J Cancer, 2003. **104**(5): p. 636-42.

[44] Recchione, C., et al., *Testosterone, dihydrotestosterone and oestradiol levels in postmenopausal breast cancer tissues.* The Journal of Steroid Biochemistry and Molecular Biology, 1995. **52**(6): p. 541-546.

[45] Secreto, G., et al., *Intratumour amount of sex steroids in elderly breast cancer patients. An approach to the biological characterization of mammary tumours in the elderly.* J Steroid Biochem Mol Biol, 1996. **58**(5-6): p. 557-61.

[46] Xie, S.-H., et al., *Prediagnostic circulating levels of sex hormones and survival in esophageal adenocarcinoma.* International Journal of Cancer. **n/a**(n/a).

[47] Lewis-Wambi, J.S. and V.C. Jordan, *Estrogen regulation of apoptosis: how can one hormone stimulate and inhibit?* Breast Cancer Res, 2009. **11**(3): p. 206.

[48] Awan, A.K., et al., *Androgen receptors may act in a paracrine manner to regulate oesophageal adenocarcinoma growth.* Eur J Surg Oncol, 2007. **33**(5): p. 561-8.

[49] Higa, G.M. and R.G. Fell, *Sex hormone receptor repertoire in breast cancer.* Int J Breast Cancer, 2013. **2013**: p. 284036.

[50] Campagnoli, C., et al., *Postmenopausal breast cancer, androgens, and aromatase inhibitors.* Breast Cancer Res Treat, 2013. **139**(1): p. 1-11.

Chapter 8

Small Molecules Inhibit Extranuclear Signaling by Estrogen: A Promising Strategy to Halt Breast Cancer Progression and Metastasis

Imaobong Etti, Chukwuemeka Nwafor and Grace Essien

Abstract

The sex hormone estrogen plays critical roles in reproductive and sexual development. It regulates the expression and activity of key signaling molecules critical in various cellular signaling pathways. These signals are mediated by its binding to estrogen receptors alpha (ERα) and beta (ERβ). ERα has been shown to greatly participate in extranuclear signaling, inducing tumorogenesis and breast cancer metastasis. Small molecules from plants are reported with better selectivity toward tumorigenic cells with negligible toxicity when compared to their synthetic counterpart. The molecules used in this study were first probed for their drug-likeness and their pharmacokinetic profile was elucidated before docking them to the ligand binding domain of the human ERα followed by a post docking prime analysis. All tested molecules had good drug-like and pharmacokinetic properties when compared to about 95% of orally available drugs as predicted by qikprop. The docking results revealed a strong binding interaction with ERα, influenced mostly by the vicinal diol groups of the studied molecules. These resulted in a conformational change, inducing receptor dimerization and altering the interactions of the sex hormone with other proteins. The studied ligands are promising in strongly inhibiting the binding of estrogen to ERα, thus limiting its extranuclear signaling.

Keywords: sex hormones, human estrogen receptor alpha (hERα), molecular docking, pharmacokinetics, extracellular signaling, breast cancer

1. Introduction

Estrogen plays an important role in mammary gland development and has been implicated in the initiation and progression of breast cancer [1]. There are two major receptors with which this sex hormone binds to mediate its biological activities. These receptors are estrogen receptors, alpha and beta (ERα and ERβ). ERα is present mainly in mammary gland, uterus, ovary (thecal cells), bone, male reproductive organs (testes and epididymis), prostate (stroma), liver, and adipose tissue. By contrast, ERβ is found mainly in the prostate (epithelium), bladder, ovary (granulosa cells), colon, adipose tissue, and immune system. Both subtypes are markedly expressed in the cardiovascular and central nervous systems. The alpha subtype has a more prominent role on the mammary gland and uterus, as well as on the preservation of skeletal homeostasis and the regulation of metabolism. The beta subtype seems to have a more profound effect on the central nervous and immune systems [2]. In terms of sequence homology, the ER_{β} shows a high homology to ER_{α} in the DBD (more than 95% amino acid identity) and in the LBD (~55% amino acid identity) [3, 4]. However, the NTD of ER_{β} is shorter than that of ER_{α} with a very poor sequence homology of only ~15% compared to that of ER_{α} (**Figure 1A** and **B**).

The major ER subtype is the ERα which has been reported in about 70% of breast cancer cases [7]. In addition to the well-studied nuclear functions of ERα, it also participates in extranuclear signaling which involve growth factor signaling components, adaptor molecules and the stimulation of cytosolic kinases [8]. ERα extranuclear pathways have the potential to activate gene transcription, modulate cytoskeleton, and promote tumor cell proliferation, survival, and metastasis. Inhibition of ERα extranuclear actions is, thus, a promising strategy to curb breast tumor progression and may be useful in preventing ERα positive metastasis.

Commonly used endocrine therapies include: selective estrogen receptor modulators (such as tamoxifen, raloxifene, toremifene), aromatase inhibitors (such as anastrozole, letrozole and exemstane) and selective estrogen receptor downregulators (such as fulvestrant). Unfortunately, tumor cells readily develop resistance to these therapies in a progressive manner, a major obstacle limiting the success of breast cancer treatment. Resiatance may be de novo or acquired and has been shown to be influenced by complicated crosstalks. These resistance to available therapies combined with their undue toxicities provoke the search into small molecules from plant, deemed

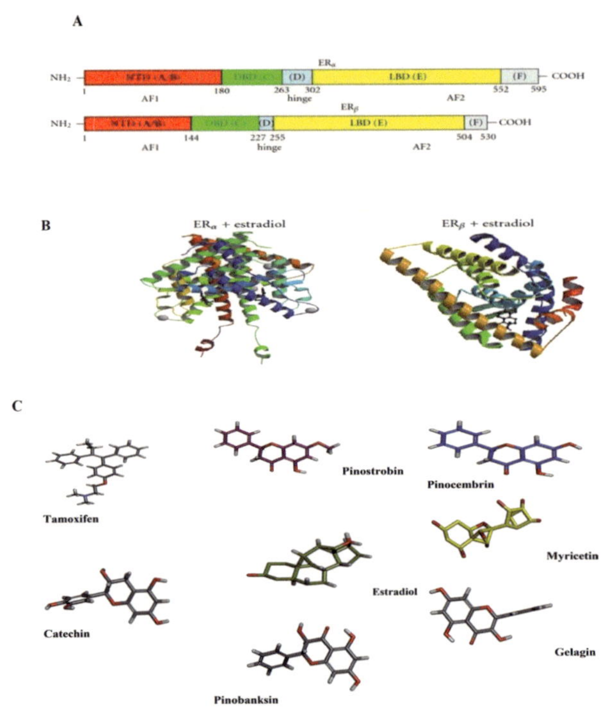

Figure 1.
Sequence organization of estrogen receptors, ER_{α} and ER_{β} (A and B) and the 3D structures of studied ligands (C). (A) Shows different domains highlighted in different colors: NTD = amino terminal domain (in red); DBD = DNA binding domain (in green); hinge region in blue; LBD = ligand-binding domain (in yellow); F region located towards the C-terminal end (in gray). Amino acid sequence position is given for each domain. (B) Shows 3-dimensional structures of ER_{α} (left) and ER_{β} (right) bound to estradiol (PDB structures 1A52 [5] and 3OLS [6]. (C) Shows 3D structures of all studied ligands.

to be less toxic [9] which can destabilize and/or downregulate the commonly implicated estrogen receptor (hERα) in a bid to intercept the complicated crosstalks [10].

There are critical steps in the development of effective pharmacotherapy, with many phases and stages within each of them. The first step which is discovery and development involve target discovery and validation, lead refinement as well as preclinical development. This is often followed by preclinical research, which tests the new drug on non-human subjects for efficacy, toxicity, and pharmacokinetic (PK) information with unrestricted dosages. Preclinical research involves *in vivo*, *in vitro*, *ex vivo* and *in silico* assays. The next step is the clinical development and involves clinical trials and volunteer studies to fine-tune the drug for human use before submitting for a holistic FDA review. The final critical step is the FDA post-market safety monitoring. It cost so much before a suitable drug candidate finally gets to the market and failure which frequently taunts the process can better be imagined than experienced.

Several promising drug candidates have failed to reach the market due to their poor pharmacokinetic properties. Many compounds with promising pre-clinical medicinal properties may not even stand a chance of being tried because of their non-drug-likeness except after rigorous improvement which may end up increasing toxicity. Today, with the advancement in medical and pharmaceutical sciences, computational techniques has proven useful for early prediction of the absorption, distribution, metabolism, excretion and toxicity (ADMET) profile of potential drug molecules before subjecting them to rigorous pre-clinical and clinical testings [11]. *In silico* approaches like molecular docking has been successfully applied in the screening and selection of potent drugs in the treatment of diseases [12]. These techniques are now extensively employed by pharmaceutical companies for screening for lead compounds to facilitate entrance of potential drug molecules with good drug-like-properties into the market while eliminating molecules with poor profile [13]. The purpose of this study was to investigate the pharmacokinetic properties and drug-likeness of the selected small molecules and investigate its inhibitory potential to the ERα, with the view of mitigating this sex hormone's receptor extranuclear signaling.

2. Materials and methods

2.1 Computer hardware and software

The molecular docking simulation was performed on the Lenovo Precision workstation 6.1.7600 running Intel® Core™ i5 Duo Processor, 4.0GB RAM, 436 GB hard disk and AMD Radeon graphics card (Lenovo PC HK Limited, China). The 3D structures of the small molecules were obtained from the National Centre for Biotechnology Information, Pubchem database www.ncbi.nlm. nih.gov/ pccompound) in SDF format and prepared with Maestro, using ligprep version 3.6 (LigPrep 2015). The solution x-ray crystal structure of the human ERα (3UUD, 1.60 Å resolution) was retrieved from the protein databank (**www.rcsb.org**) using Discovery Studio visualizer 4.5 (Accelryls, USA). Protein-ligand docking simulation was performed using the Schrodinger molecular docking suite version 2018-4.

2.2 Preparation of ligands and protein

The ligands were prepared using LigPrep, a utility of Schrodinger software suit that combines tools for generating 3D structures from 1D (Smiles) and 2D (SDF) representation. Molecular mechanics force fields, optimized potentials for liquid simulations-2005 (OPLS_2005) with default settings were employed for the ligand minimization and the ligands were thereafter filtered for computational studies.

The crystal structure of hERα (3UUD) was prepared using Schrodinger protein preparation wizard tool (Glide), which performed the following steps: assigning of bond orders, addition of hydrogens, optimization of hydrogen bonds by flipping amino side chains, correction of charges and minimization of the protein complex. All the bound water molecules, ligands and cofactors were removed (preprocess) from the protein and the output file was saved in maestro format. The idle side chains were neutralized before restrained minimization of co-crystallized complex, which reoriented side chain hydroxyl groups and alleviated potential steric clashes. The complex obtained was minimized using OPLS_2005 force field with Polack-Ribiere Conjugate Gradient (PRCG) algorithm. The minimization was terminated when the energy gradient converged below 0.05 kcal/mol [14].

2.3 Prediction of pharmacokinetic properties and drug-likeness

The molecular weight, number of hydrogen bond donor, number of hydrogen bond acceptor and octanol–water partition coefficients were used to verify the compounds adherence to Lipinski's rule of five which qualifies their drug-likeness. To nominate drug candidates, certain pharmacokinetics descriptors that portray their drug-likeness [15] were investigated using the QikProp module of the Schrodinger Suite, a program designed by Professor William L. Jorgensen [16]. In addition to predicting physically significant and pharmaceutically relevant molecular descriptors, QikProp also provides ranges for comparing predicted descriptors of each compound with those of 95% of drugs known for oral use. The pharmacokinetic descriptors evaluated were: molecular weight(Mwt), total solvent accessible surface area (SASA), Donor hydrogen bond (DonorHB), number of acceptable hydrogen bond (Accept HB), predicted octanol/water partition coefficient (QPlogPo/w), predicted aqueous solubility (QPlogS), predicted apparent Caco-2 cell permeability (QPPCaco), predicted brain/blood partition coefficient (QPlogBB), number of likely metabolic reactions(#metab), human oral absorption, van der Waals surface area of polar nitrogen and oxygen atoms (PSA) and prediction of plasma protein binding(Khsa). Cytochrome P450 inhibitory promiscuity and inhibition of the human either-a-go-go-ralted gene was also accessed via admerSAR web server. The analysis in the present study was run on QikProp at the normal processing mode with default settings (QikProp 2018). The prepared ligands were used as input structures and their pharmacokinetics profiles with respect to properties shared by 95% of drugs known for oral use were evaluated. Compliance or deviant of the tested potential drug candidates to the Lipinski's rule of five was also examined before they were considered drug-like [17].

2.4 Docking studies

Docking studies were carried out using Glide XP of the Schrodinger Suite (Maestro Version 11.8 and Glide version 8.0, 2018-4) docking program following the reported standard procedures [18]. Each ligand was individually docked onto the LBD of the hERα using Glide extra precision (XP) mode. In the course of the docking, several binding poses were generated for each ligand and the best binding pose was selected at the end of the docking process.

2.5 Calculation of ligand free energy of binding with the hERα using the MM-GBSA approach prime energy analysis

The Prime MM-GBSA or 'molecular mechanics energies combined with the generalized Born and surface area continuum solvation' approach was used in the post-assessment of free energy of binding of ligands-hERα complex [19]. This approach uses the OPLS_2005 all-atom force field for protein residues, ligands and cofactors [20, 21]. The input structures for these calculations were taken from a pose viewer file Glide output after the docking study.

The following descriptors were generated by the prime MM-GBSA approach:

1. MM-GBSA_ΔG_bind (ligand binding energy (ΔG_{bind}))
2. MM-GBSA_E_complex (energy of the complex ($G_{complex}$))
3. MM-GBSA_E_protein (energy of the receptor without the ligand ($G_{protein}$)) and
4. MM-GBSA_E_ligand (energy of the unbound ligand (G_{ligand})).

The total free energy (ΔGbind) of binding is expressed as:

$$\Delta G_{bind} = G_{complex} - \left(G_{protein} + G_{ligand}\right) \tag{1}$$

The other parameters for the complex were:

1. Prime Coulomb energy (ΔG_{bind} coulomb)
2. Prime Van der Waals energy (ΔG_{bind} vdW)
3. Prime Hydrogen Bond (ΔG_{bind} H-bond)

The MM-GBSA scoring and experimental binding affinity data of the binding site for the molecules on hERα were recorded.

3. Results

3.1 The structures of the protein and studied ligands

The 3D structures of the studied ligands are as shown in **Figure 1c**. Complete X-ray structure of of the hERα (**Figure 2A**) and its binding amino acids depicted with green sticks are as shown in **Figure 2B** above.

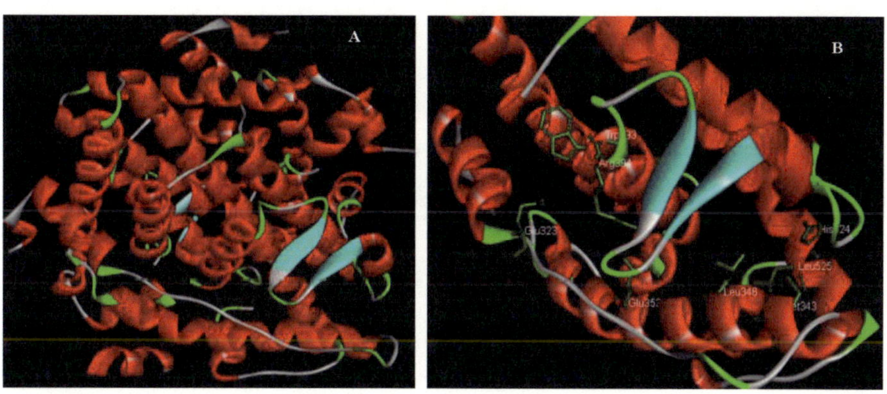

Figure 2.
(A) Complete X-ray structure of hERα shown as ribbon (B) active amino acids shown in green sticks at the catalytic site of hERα.

Compounds	MW[A]	SASA[B]	Donor HB[C]	AcceptHb[D]	QPlogPo/w[E]	QPlogS[F]	QPPCaco[G]	QPlog BB[H]	#metab[I]	Human Oral Absorption (%)[J]	PSA[K]	KHSA[L]	Rule of Five[M]
Myricetin	318.239	522.36	5	6	−0.279	−2.557	7.666	−2.817	6	28.186	161.312	−0.493	1
Estradiol	272.386	510.237	2	2.45	4.00	−4.672	1221.948	−0.366	4	100	43.693	0.438	0
Catechin	290.272	513.734	5	5.45	0.466	−2.648	53.247	−1.904	7	60.572	115.499	−0.42	0
Pinobanksin	272.257	492.522	2	4.95	1.472	−3.088	211.884	−1.171	5	77.194	97.055	−1.68	0
Pinocembrin	256.257	486.989	1	3.25	2.383	−3.684	431.998	−0.83	5	88.067	77.67	0.136	0
Gelangin	270.241	488.021	2	3.75	1.791	−3.296	193.621	−1.221	3	78.363	95.964	−0.041	0
Pinostrobin	270.284	509.441	0	3.25	3.084	−3.844	1427.908	−0.351	5	100	63.409	0.181	0
Tamoxifen	371.521	725.086	0	2.75	6.525	−5.833	2203.131	0.366	3	100	11.493	−7.4	1

Range for 95% known drugs: A (Molecular weight = 130.0–725.0); B (Total solvent accessible surface area = 300.0–1000.0); C (Donor HB = 0.0–6.0); D (Accept HB = 2.0–20.0); E (Predicted octanol/water partition coefficient = −2.0-6.5); F (Predicted aqueous solubility = −6.5-0.5); G (Predicted apparent Caco-2 cell permeability = < 25 poor, >500 great); H (Predicted brain/blood partition coefficient = −3.0-1.2); I (Number of likely metabolic reactions = 1–8); J (% Human oral absorption = > 80% → High, < 25% → Poor); K (van der Waals surface area of polar nitrogen and oxygen atoms = 7.0–200.0); L (Human serum albumin = −1.5-1.5); M (Number of violations of Lipinskis Rule of Five; mol MW < 500, QPlogPo/w < 5, donor HB ≤ 5, accpt HB ≤10. Compounds that satisfy these rules are considered drug-like.

Table 1.
Pharmacokinetic properties of studied ligands.

3.2 Pharmacokinetic profile of tested ligands

All the tested compounds obeyed the Lipinski's rule of five (see **Table 1**). From the result of cell permeability using the caco-2 model, estradiol, pinostrobin and tamoxifen showed a great permeability prediction while moderate permeation was observed with catechin, pinobankskin, pinocembrin and gelagin (**Table 1**). Myrecetin, on the other hand showed very poor predicted cell permeability. All studied ligands had good predicted aqueous solubility (log S), and their blood brain barrier prediction, surface area of solvent absorption, predicted number of possible metabolic transformations, as well as polar surface area was within the range set for orally available drugs (see **Table 1**). For the prediction of plasma protein binding, tamoxifen had a score of −7.4, which was not within the stipulated range of −1.5-1.5, howbeit, other ligands had a good plasma protein prediction. Pinostrobin, tamoxifen, estradiol and pinocembrin had high predicted oral bioavailabilities

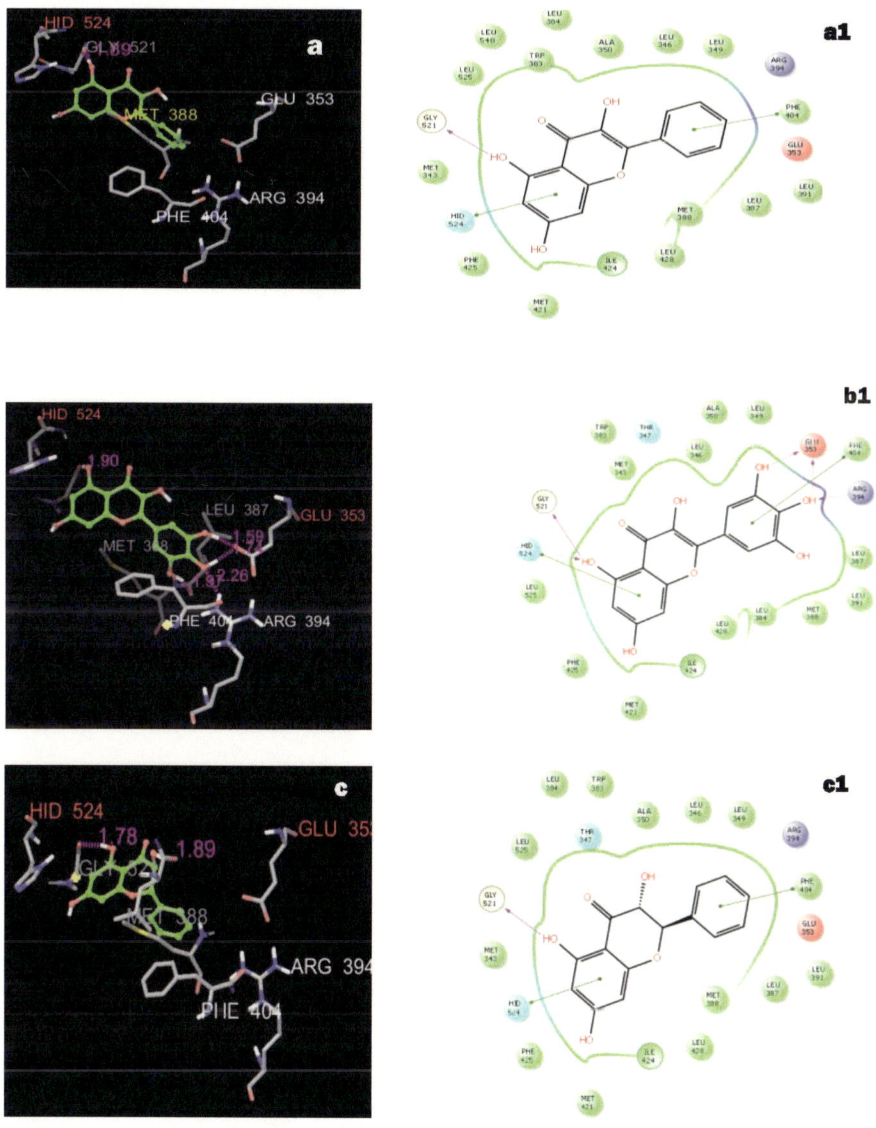

Figure 3.
3D and 2D molecular interaction of gelagin (a, a1), myrecetin (b, b1) and pinobanksin (c, c1) with crucial amino acids at the ligand binding domain of hERα.

while moderate oral bioavailabilities were observed with Gelagin, pinobanksin, and catechin. Myricetin had the least predicted human oral availability.

3.3 Protein-ligand interactions

Structurally, each of the studied ligand contained the basic flavone skeleton linked by a three-carbon chain forming a closed pyran ring. Considering hydrogen bond interactions of the studied molecules with active amino acids of the estrogen receptor, from the results, the 7-OH of gelagin (**Figure 3 (a & a1)**) formed one hydrogen bond with Glycin 521 at a distance of 1.89 Å and a π-cation interactions with phenylalnine 404 and histidine 524. The 3^1- OH and 4^1- OH groups of myricetin each established 1H bond with glutamic acid 353 residue at distances of 1.59 Å and 1.74 Å respectively. A firm interaction was also observed with Arginine 394 by the 4^1- OH of myricetin at distances of 1.97 Å and 2.26 Å. The 8- OH of myricetin also established 1H bond with histidine 524 and glycin 521 at 1.90 Å. There was also a π-interaction of this ligand with phenylalanine 404 and histidine 524 (**Figure 3 (b & b1)**). In **Figure 3 (c & c1)** 1H bond each was established between the 8- OH of

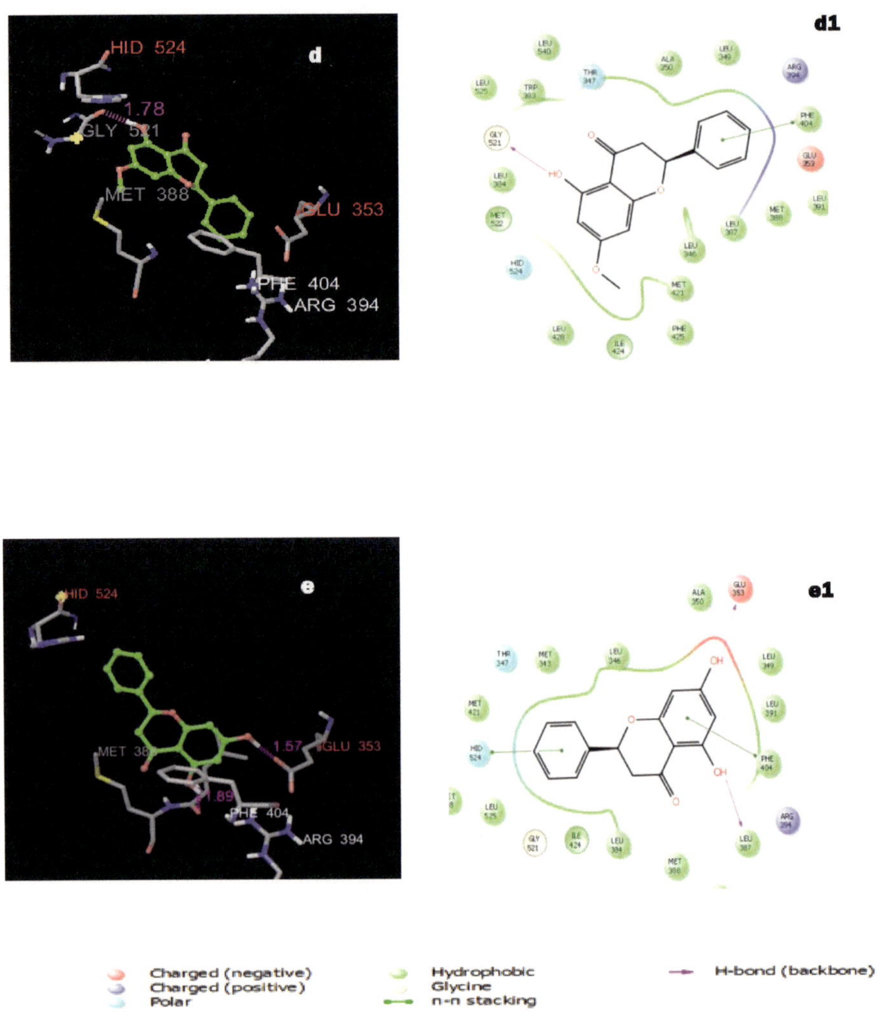

Figure 4.
3D and 2D molecular interaction of pinostrobin (d, d1), pinocembrin (e, e1) and with crucial amino acids at the ligand binding domain of hERα.

pinobankskin and Glycine 521 and Methionine 388 at distances of 1.78 Å and 1.89 Å respectively. A pi-pi interaction was also observed between the ligand and phenyalanine 404 as well as histidine 524. A pi-pi interaction was formed between pinostrobin and phenyalanine 404 of the hERα while its 8- OH group formed one hydrogen bond with glycine 521 at 1.78Å (**Figure 4** (**d** & **d1**)). Pinocembrin (**Figure 4** (**e** & **e1**)) established a pi-cation interaction with phenylalanine 404 and histidine 524 while its 5-OH group formed 1H bond with leucine 387 at 1.89 Å. A strong interaction was observed between its 8- OH group and glutamate 353 at 1.57 Å. Tamoxifen, on the other hand, established 1H bond with Arginine 394 at 2.34 Å and a pi-cation interaction with phenylalanine 404 and histidine while estradiol, the native ligand had 1H bond each with glutamate 353 and histidine 524 at distances of 1.80Å and 2.04Å respectively (**Figure 5** (**f** and **g**)). A pi-pi interaction was also observed with histidine 524 and phenylalanine 404.

3.4 Post docking prime analysis of studied ligands

From the prime energy calculations, the quantity of free energy of binding, ΔG_{bind} calculated from Eq. (1) was in the following order: estradiol>myricetin>catechin>gelagin>pinobankskin>pinocembrin>pinostrobin (**Figure 6**). Other components which contributed to the electrostatic interaction like the quantity of prime coulomb energy of the complex (ΔG_{bind} coulomb), prime van der Waals energy of the complex interaction (ΔG_{bind} vdW), the quantity of prime hydrogen bonding interaction are as presented in **Table 2**.

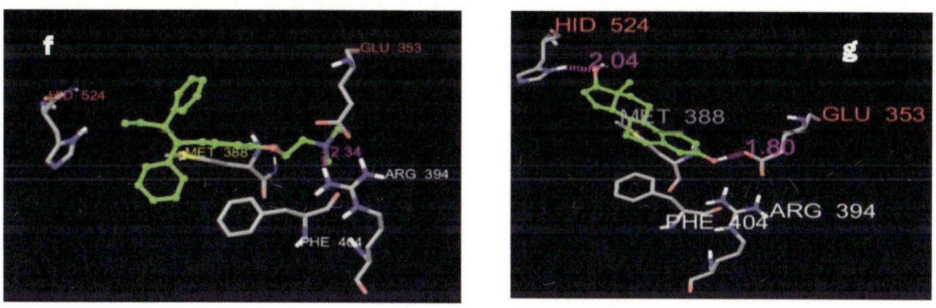

Figure 5.
Molecular interaction of tamoxifen (f) and estradiol (g) with crucial amino acids at the ligand binding domain of hERα.

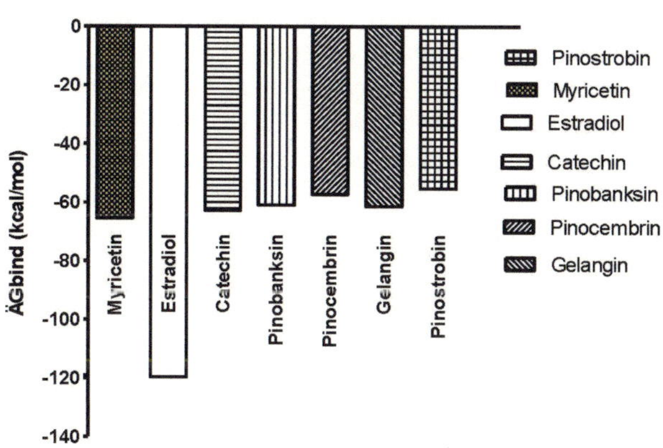

Figure 6.
The free energy of binding ΔGbind (kcal/Mol) for the studied ligands with the hERα binding site.

Molecules	ΔGbind Coloumb	ΔGbind Hbond	ΔGbind lipophilic	ΔGbind vdW
Myricetin	−34.6588	−2.2352	−34.5106	−33.2389
Estradiol	−20.0967	−2.04811	−66.6318	−47.0585
Catechin	−28.643	−2.94963	−39.0821	−23.3243
Pinobanksin	−13.6085	−0.092	−36.3471	−35.5581
Pinocembrin	−14.97	−0.99013	−36.5651	−26.7548
Gelangin	−9.44593	−0.16506	−34.4349	−37.5343
Pinostrobin	−5.32169	−0.2392	−41.3577	−25.8845

Table 2.
Output properties from a prime MM-GBSA calculation for the studied ligands.

4. Discussion

Estrogen, a major sex hormone plays an important role in mammary gland development and in the initiation and progression of breast cancer. The activities of estrogen are being mediated via its unique receptors, ERα and ERβ. The former (ERα), is the major ER subtype in the mammary epithelium. Upon activation of the hERα following its occupation, the receptor translocates to the nucleus, where it interacts with the target gene promoters of estrogen response element to mediate nuclear as well as extranuclear signaling [8, 22]. This results in the regulation of numerous critical cellular processes and is implicated in the dilemma of breast cancer. Research reveals that ERα extranuclear pathways, which are incited by undue activation of hERα have the potential to activate gene transcription, modulate cytoskeleton, and promote tumor cell proliferation, survival, as well as metastasis. The expression of extranuclear components ERα is deregulated in tumors, thus, serving as an important target for tumorigenic and metastatic control. Resistance to available endocrine therapies provokes metastasis and frustrates the management of this disease, thus, reducing the survival rate of patients bearing such tumors [23, 24]. This study evaluated the inhibitory potential of the reported small molecules from nature against hERα in a bid to suppress its downstream signaling.

The high attrition rate of new chemical entities has been attributed majorly to poor pharmacokinetic profile [25]. The reported ligands have been shown to be drug-like, having satisfied the Lipinski's rule of five [17] and also possess pharmaceutically relevant properties when compared to 95% of orally available drugs [16]. Hence, these compounds are fit in their current state to be developed into drugs without any modification/optimization except myricetin. Myricetin showed poor human absorption when examining its caco-2 permeability and human oral bioavailability. This observed poor absorption of myricetin will retard how quickly and how much of it will reach its intended target (site) of action. Hence, this phytoconstituent will require optimization to prevent its failure in the market [26].

Aqueous solubilities and human oral absorption are critical for oral dosage formulation and their *in silico* prediction had been reported to correlate well with *in vivo* bioavailabilities [27]. According to Bergström 2005 [28], aqueous solubility and intestinal permeability are the two rate-limiting barriers for oral drug absorption while the therapeutic potential of a drug is dependent on its bioavailabilty [29]. All the tested compounds showed positive human intestinal absorption.

Following absorption, the drug or intended drug molecule will circulate through the body, permeating different tissues at varying speed, depending on its ability to cross membranes. Some drugs migrate very slowly from the bloodstream because they get tightly bound to proteins circulating in the blood. Others quickly leave the bloodstream and enter other tissues because they are less tightly bound to blood proteins. There are also possibilities for virtually all molecules of a drug to bind tightly to blood proteins. It is worthy of note that irrespective of how promising a drug molecule is, its efficacy will be lost if its maximum concentration gets bound to plasma proteins. This will eventually result in the decrease of effective concentration at the site of action in the tissues, as only unbound drugs can be available for pharmacological activity [14]. To predict the distribution of the studied ligands, their plasma protein binding and blood brain barrier penetration was investigated. Unlike all compounds which showed good distribution, tamoxifen, however, did not comply within the range, indicating its high potential binding to albumin. This observation was in line with previous report on the high binding affinity of tamoxifen to serum albumin [30, 31]. Considering blood brain barrier permeation, studied compounds showed no tendency of crossing it. This can be explained by the lipophobicity of the studied ligands. It therefore means that they will not provoke any significant central effect that will result in subsequent toxicity.

Another key parameter is metabolism, which is responsible for the elimination of drugs from the body. Through metabolism, drug molecules can also be converted into pharmacologically more active substrates. In this study, the molecules were investigated to predict their possible number of biotransformation which could point to potential toxicities [32, 33]. From the results, all the compounds complied with the range of metabolic reactions displayed by 95% of orally available drugs. Some of the phytoligands were predicted to possess cytochrome P450 (CYP 450) inhibitory promiscuity, revealing their capacity to bind to and decrease or diminish the activity of multiple different CYP 450 isoform enzymes [34]. It should be noted that all the molecular descriptors predicted by qikprop are exclusively for drugs intended for oral delivery. This route of drug administration is still the most preferred route for new chemical entities (NCEs) in spite of advances in drug delivery methods. Oral mode of drug delivery is convenient, cheap and has high patient compliance. Using the *in silico* prediction of pharmacokinetics-related profile of intended drug molecules helps to reduce the rate of attrition of new chemical entities in clinical trial and reduces the cost of bringing a candidate drug to the market.

In modern drug discovery, molecular docking has been gainfully employed in the screening and selection of potent inhibitors [35] especially when the anticancer target has been identified. In this study, structurally similar phytochemicals from plant origin were used to probe for binding interaction with the human estrogen receptor α. As a prerequisite, the molecular docking protocol was validated. From the results, the redocked binding pose of the native ligand was correctly reproduced within the root mean square tolerance of 2 Å. This distance is an indication of an appropriate reproducibility for a docking experiment [36, 37]. This reproducibility of the redocked native ligand was similar to the poses of the docking control reported by Hocker *et al.* (2013) [38].

Inhibiting hERα is a valid approach in ameliorating the progression of breast cancer. This study revealed strong binding affinities of the investigated compounds to the hERα. This interaction which was depicted in their free energy of binding was greatly influenced by the vicinal diol groups. The residues of estrogen receptor which partook in this binding interaction was earlier reported to play critical roles in the inhibition of the ligand binding domain of the hERα [39, 40]. The interaction of these compounds with the binding domain of hERα, created a conformational change in the receptor, inducing its dimerization, thus, interrupting its downstream signaling as well as crosstalks [41]. The conformational change observed in the estrogen receptor upon interaction with the studied ligands will also impair phosphorylation on hERα specific residues, impairing ligand-independent estrogen receptor activation. It is promising that these interactions with the sex hormone's receptor, hERα with provoke breast cancer cell death, thus halting its progression to immortality [42].

5. Conclusion

The potential of the studied drug-like small molecules to inhibit estrogenic signaling is a vital approach that should be exploited in the management of metastatic breast cancers.

Conflict of interest

The authors declare no conflict of interest.

Author details

Imaobong Etti[1]*, Chukwuemeka Nwafor[2] and Grace Essien[1]

1 Department of Pharmacology and Toxicology, University of Uyo, Uyo, Nigeria

2 Department of Pathology, University of Uyo, Uyo, Nigeria

*Address all correspondence to: ettiimaobong@gmail.com; imaobongetti@uniuyo.edu.ng

References

[1] Song, P., Li Y, Dong Y. Estrogen receptor β inhibits breast cancer cells migration and invasion through CLDN6-mediated autophagy. Journal of experimental and clinical cancer research 2019; **38**: 354.

[2] Heldring, N., Pike, A., Andersson S Matthews, J., Cheng, G., Hartman, J., Tujague, M., Ström, A., Treuter, E., Warner, M., Gustafsson, JÅ. Estrogen receptors: how do they signal and what are their targets. Physiological reviews 2007; **87**: 905-31.

[3] Kuiper, G., Enmark, E., Pelto-Huikko, M., Nilsson, S., Gustafsson, J. Cloning of a novel estrogen receptor expressed in rat prostate and ovary. Proceedings of the National Academy of Sciences 1996; **91**: 5925-30.

[4] Cowley, S., Hoare, S., Mosselman, S., Parker, M. Estrogen receptors alpha and beta form heterodimers on DNA. Journal of biological chemistry 1997; **272**: 19858-62.

[5] Tanenbaum, D., Wang, Y., Williams, S., Sigler, P. Crystallographic comparison of the estrogen and progesterone receptor's ligand binding domains. Proceedings of the National Academy of Sciences 1998; **95**: 5998-6003.

[6] Mocklinghoff, S., Rose, R., Carraz, M., Visser, A., Ottmann, C., Brunsveld, L. Synthesis and crystal structure of a phosphorylated estrogen receptor ligand binding domain. *Chembiochem* 2010; **11**: 2251-4.

[7] Berger CE, Qian Y, Liu G, Chen H, Chen X. p53 , a Target of Estrogen Receptor (ER) α , Modulates DNA Damage-induced Growth Suppression in ER-positive Breast Cancer Cells. The Journal of Biological Chemistry 2012; **287**: 30117-27.

[8] Cortez V, Mann M, Brann D, Vadlamudi R. Extranuclear Signaling by Estrogen: Role in Breast Cancer Progression and Metastasis. *Minerva ginecol*, 2010.

[9] Etti IC, Abdullah R, Kadir Hashim M, Yeap SK, Imam MU, Ramli F, Malami I, Lam KL, Etti U, Waziri P, Rahman M. The molecular mechanism of the anticancer effect of Artonin E in MDA-MB 231 triple negative breast cancer cells. PLoS ONE 2017; **12**: 1-20.

[10] Fan, W., Chang, J., Fu, P. Endocrine therapy resistance in breast cancer: current status, possible mechanisms and overcoming strategies. Future medicinal chemistry 2015; **7**: 1511-9.

[11] Grime K, Barton P, MCGinnity D. Application of In Silico, In Vitro and Preclinical Pharmacokinetic Data for the Effective and Efficient Prediction of Human Pharmacokinetics. Molecular pharmaceutics 2013; **10**: 1191-206.

[12] Pinzi L, Rastelli G. Molecular Docking: Shifting Paradigms in Drug Discovery. International journal of molecular sciences 2019; **20**: 4331.

[13] Josh M., Pradeep S, Adarsh VK Vijayalekshmi K, Sudha R, Balachandran S, Sreejith M, Jaleel U. In silico evidences for the binding of phthalates onto human estrogen receptor α , β subtypes and human estrogen-related receptor γ. Molecular Simulation 2014; **40**: 408-17.

[14] Kaminski G, Friesner R, Tirado-Rives J, Jorgensen W. Evaluation and reparametrization of the OPLS-AA force field for proteins via comparison with accurate quantum chemical calculations on peptides. Journal of physical chemistry 2001; **28**: 6474-87.

[15] Dong, J., Wang, N., Yao Z. ADMETlab: a platform for systematic

ADMET evaluation based on a comprehensively collected ADMET database. Journal of chemical informatics 2018; **10**: 29.

[16] Jorgensen WL, Duffy EM. Prediction of drug solubility from structure. Advanced Drug Delivery Reviews 2002; **54**: 355-66.

[17] Lipinski C., Lombardo F, Dominy B, Feeney P. Experimental and computational approaches to estimate solubility and permeability in drug discovery and development settings. Advanced drug delivery reviews 2001; **46**: 3-26.

[18] Etti I, Abdullah R, Hashim NM Kadir A, Abdul AB, Etti C, Malami I, Waziri P, How CW. Artonin E and structural analogs from Artocarpus species abrogates estrogen receptor signaling in breast cancer. Molecules 2016; **21:**839.

[19] Salgado-Moran G, Ramirez-Tagle R, Glossman-Mitnik D Ruiz-Nieto S, Kishore-Deb P, Bunster M, Lobos-Gonzalez F. Docking studies of binding of Ethambutol to the C terminal domain of the Arabinosyltransferase *Mycobacterium tuberculosis*. Virology and Mycology 2015; **4**: 141.

[20] Genheden S, Ryde U. The MM/PBSA and MM/GBSA methods to estimate ligand-binding affinities. Expert opinion on drug discovery 2015; **5**: 449-61.

[21] Vijayakumar B, Umamaheswari A, Puratchikody A, Velmurugan D. Selection of an improved HDAC8 inhibitor through structure-based drug design. Bioinformation 2011; **7**: 134-41.

[22] McDonnell D, Norris J. Connections and regulation of the human estrogen receptor. Science 2002; **296**: 1642-4.

[23] Andruska ND, Zheng X, Yang X, Mao C, Cherian MM, Mahapatra L. Estrogen receptor α inhibitor activates the unfolded protein response , blocks protein synthesis , and induces tumor regression. Proceedings of the National Academy of Sciences 2015; **112**: 4737-42.

[24] Jiang Q, Zheng S, Wang G. Development of new estrogen receptor-targeting therapeutic agents for tamoxifen-resistant breast cancer. Future medicinal chemistry 2013; **9**.

[25] Kiriiri GK, Njogu PM, Mwangi A. Exploring different approaches to improve the success of drug discovery and development projects: a review. Future journal of pharmaceutical science 2020; **6**: 27.

[26] Kim MT, Sedykh A, Chakravarti S. Critical Evaluation of Human Oral Bioavailability for Pharmaceutical Drugs by Using Various Cheminformatics Approaches. Pharmaceutical Research 2014; **31**: 1002-14.

[27] Veber DF, Stephen R, Johnson H, Cheng B, Smith KW, Kenneth DK. Molecular Properties That Influence the Oral Bioavailability of Drug Candidates. Journal of medicinal chemistry 2002; **12**: 2615-23.

[28] Bergström CAS. In silico Predictions of Drug Solubility and Permeability: Two Rate-limiting Barriers to Oral Drug Absorption. Basic and clinical pharmacology and therapeutics 2005; **96**: 156-61.

[29] Alavijeh MS, Chishty M, Qaiser MZ, Palmer AM. Drug Metabolism and Pharmacokinetics, the Blood-Brain Barrier, and Central Nervous System Drug Discovery. The Journal of the American Society for Experimental NeuroTherapeutics 2005; **2**: 554-71.

[30] Maciążek-Jurczyk,M., Maliszewska, J., Równicka-Zubik, PJ., Sułkowska G, Gora A. Tamoxifen and curcumin binding to serum albumin. Spectroscopic study. Journal

of Molecular Structure 2013; **1044**: 194-200.

[31] Paterson SC, Lim CK, Smith KD. Analysis of the interaction between alpha-1-acid glycoprotein and tamoxifen and its metabolites. Biomedical chromatoghraphy 2003; **17**: 143-8.

[32] Ntie-Kang F. An in silico evaluation of the ADMET profile of the StreptomeDB database. SpringerPlus 2013; **2**: 353.

[33] Onguéné PA, Ntie-Kang F, Mbah JA Lifongo LL, Ndom JC, Sippl W, Mbaze, L M. The potential of anti-malarial compounds derived from African medicinal plants, part I: a pharmacological evaluation of alkaloids and terpenoids. Malaria journal 2013; **12**: 449.

[34] Liao C, Sitzmann M, Pugliese A, Nicklaus MC. Software and resources for computational medicinal chemistry. Future medicinal chemistry 2011; **3**: 1057-85.

[35] López-Vallejo F, Caulfield T, Martínez-Mayorga K, Giulianotti MA, Nefzi A, Houghten RA M-FJ. Integrating virtual screening and combinatorial chemistry for accelerated drug discovery. Combinatorial Chemistry and High Throughput Screening 2011; **6**: 475-87.

[36] Abd-Elzaher MM, Labib AA, Mousa HA, Moustafa SA, Ali MM, El-Rashedy AA. Synthesis, anticancer activity and molecular docking study of Schiff base complexes containing thiazole moiety. Beni-Suef University Journal of Basic and Applied Sciences 2016; **5**: 85-96.

[37] Kishore,P., Maillabaram, Rao,R., Rao, M. Antiinflammatory Evaluation and Docking Studies of Some New Thienopyrimidines. Asian Journal of Chemistry 2013; 25: 10583-7.

[38] Hocker HJ, Cho K-J, Chen C-Y Rambahal N, Sagineedu S R, Shaari K, Stanslas J, Hancock JF, Gorfe, A. Andrographolide derivatives inhibit guanine nucleotide exchange and abrogate oncogenic Ras function. Proceedings of the National Academy of Sciences of the United States of America 2013; **110**: 10201-6.

[39] Desai N, Mahto MK, Alekhya B, Naveen CR, Bhaskar PM. Comparative docking studies of estrogen receptor inhibitors and their binding interaction analysis. International Journal of Pharmaceutical Sciences Review and Research 2012; **16**: 91-5.

[40] Celik L, Lund J, Schiøtt B. Exploring Interactions of Endocrine-Disrupting Compounds with Different Conformations of the Human Estrogen Receptor α Ligand Binding Domain: A Molecular Docking Study. Chemical Research in Toxicology 2008; **21**: 2195-206.

[41] Le Dily F, Beato M. Signaling by Steroid Hormones in the 3D Nuclear Space. International journal of molecular sciences 2018; **19**: 2.

[42] Etti I, Abdullah R, Kadir A, Apoptosis inducing effect of Artonin E. In: Yusuf Tutar,,editors. Current understanding of Apoptosis-programmed cell death, 1st ed. London:IntechOpen: 2018. p.21-32. DOI: 10.5772/intechopen.71637..

Chapter 9

Non-Reproductive Effects of Estradiol: Hydromineral Homeostasis Control

Gislaine Almeida-Pereira, Lucila L.K. Elias and José Antunes-Rodrigues

Abstract

The hydromineral homeostasis is fundamental to survival due to maintenance constant the osmotic properties of the plasma and proper tissue perfusion pressure, being maintained primarily through the regulation of the ingestion and urinary excretion of water and electrolytes, mainly sodium. The Renin-Angiotensin System (RAS) plays an essential role in the maintenance of hydromineral homeostasis by eliciting sodium and water intake and by inducing sodium urinary retention through aldosterone release and hemodynamic effect via angiotensin II a key component of the RAS. The hypothalamus-pituitary system also plays a fundamental role in the maintenance of body fluid homeostasis by secreting vasopressin (AVP) and oxytocin (OT) in response to osmotic and non-osmotic, and volemic stimuli. Furthermore, some studies report that besides reproductive function and sexual behavior, ovarian gonadal hormones, mainly 17β-estradiol (E2), modulate other non-reproductive functions such as cardiovascular system, body fluid balance, mood, mental state, memory, and cognition. Estradiol is known to mediate hydromineral homeostasis and blood pressure mainly by attenuating RAS actions. On the other hand, estradiol modulates neurohypophysial hormones secretion in many different ways. In this chapter, we will discuss the main non-reproductive effects of E2 on the control of hydromineral homeostasis, focusing on ingestive behavior and neurohypophyseal hormonal release.

Keywords: angiotensin II, cell signaling, thirst, sodium appetite, vasopressin, oxytocin

1. Introduction

Because sodium is the most abundant cation in the extracellular fluid (ECF) and is an osmotically effective ion, sodium body content is the pivotal determinant of ECF volume. Then, when sodium moves between extracellular and intracellular compartments, water moves together in favor of the osmotic gradient. The osmolality and volume of body fluids are maintained, respectively, through the regulation of the ingestion (gain) and urinary excretion (loss) of water and electrolytes, mainly sodium (for review see [1]). The constancy of the sodium concentration and the osmolality of extracellular body fluid are essential to hydromineral homeostasis and are therefore fundamental to survival since is very important for proper tissue perfusion pressure and osmotic gradient across the cellular membrane [1].

1.1 Renin-Angiotensin System role on the hydromineral homeostasis

The Renin-Angiotensin System (RAS) plays an essential role in the maintenance of the hydromineral homeostasis by eliciting sodium and water intake and by inducing sodium urinary retention through aldosterone release and hemodynamic effect via angiotensin II a key component of the RAS [2, 3]. The octapeptide hormone angiotensin II (ANGII) induces its effects on body fluids control mainly by acting on its angiotensinergic receptor type 1 (AT1) [4, 5]. The AT1 receptor is a member of the G-protein (heterotrimeric guanine nucleotide-binding protein)-coupled receptor (GPCR) superfamily of integral membrane proteins and is coupled to the Gq. Then, its stimulation leads to the activation of phospholipase C, protein kinase C (PKC), and members of the mitogen-activated protein kinase family (MAPK) as extracellular signal-regulated kinases 1 and 2 (ERK1/2), p38 MAPK and c-Jun N-terminal Kinase (JNK) (for review see [6]). Hines et al. [7] showed that the activation of MAPKs, mediated by AT1, can be PKC dependent or independent according to the activated conformations that the receptor may adopt. Recently, some studies have postulated that these intracellular signaling pathways from the AT1 receptor are involved in different ingestive behavioral responses. In this context, ANGII-induced sodium intake requires the PKC-independent ERK1/2 signaling pathway while water intake requires PKC, JNK, and the mechanistic target of the rapamycin complex 1 (mTORC1) signaling pathways [8–10].

ANGII induces rapid and prominent water and sodium intake when injected centrally even in normohydration animals, as well in response to hypovolemic and hyponatremic stimuli [3]. In the brain, peripheral and central ANGII induces sodium and water intake by binding to AT1 in important forebrain structures involved in the generation of fluid intakes, such as the organum vasculosum of the lamina terminalis (OVLT), the median preoptic nucleus (MnPO), and the subfornical organ (SFO) [11, 12]. The SFO is a key sensory circumventricular organ (CVO) involved in the control of body fluids homeostasis, that receives, integrates, and responds to both blood-borne and central nervous system (CNS) signals [5]. The CVOs are specialized structures of CNS, comprising the SFO, area postrema, OVLT, median eminence, and neurohypophysis, which lack the normal blood–brain barrier and thus provide essential communication between the circulation and the CNS [13]. The increase in the circulating and central ANGII levels enhances the neural activity of the SFO, which sends axonal projections to the anteroventral third ventricle region (AV3V), particularly the OVLT and MnPO ventral, and to the hypothalamus as the supraoptic nucleus (SON), and the paraventricular nucleus (PVN) (for review see [5]).

1.2 Hypothamalo-neurohypophysial system role on the hydromineral homeostasis

Magnocellular neurosecretory neurons of the PVN and the SON synthesize vasopressin (AVP) and oxytocin (OT) which are released into the circulation from the neurohypophysis [14]. OT, beyond its classic effects on uterine contraction and myoepithelial cells of the breast alveoli, participates in body fluid control by eliciting natriuresis and sodium appetite inhibition [15–17]. The antidiuretic action of AVP is the main physiological effect of this hormone on body fluid control, exerting an important role in osmolality urinary regulation. The hypothalamo-neurohypophysial system plays a fundamental role in the maintenance of hydromineral homeostasis by secreting AVP and OT in response to osmotic and non-osmotic, and volemic stimuli (for review see [11]). Furthermore, in response to AT1 receptor activation, SFO efferent angiotensinergic projections increase the excitability of vasopressinergic and oxytocinergic neurons in the PVN and SON, leading to AVP and OT secretion [18]. ANGII also can directly increase AVP and OT secretion by acting on its AT1 receptor expressed in the PVN [19]. Concerning the ANGII signaling pathway in neurohypophysial secretion, Felgendreger et al. [20] showed that the ERK1/2 activation induced by endogenous ANGII is not involved in AVP and OT secretion in male rats. However, PKC involvement was not analyzed in this study.

1.3 Interaction of body fluid balance with blood pressure control

The balance of body fluid involves a close correlation with blood pressure control, and thus, disturbances in one of these imply adjustments in the other. The proper maintenance of cardiovascular functions, such as peripheral vascular tone, cardiac activity, and, consequently, blood pressure involves orchestrated activities of the sympathetic and parasympathetic nervous system. The sympathetic activity also exerts an important control renal function in the regulation of plasma volume and osmolality, which influence cardiovascular function [11]. Moreover, some of the key brain regions that are involved in the control of hydromineral homeostasis also promote adjustments in the neuroendocrine and autonomic mechanisms of blood pressure control. For example, the peripheral portion of the SFO sends projections to areas important for fluid balance (magnocellular neurosecretory neurons in the PVN and SON) while the core projects to areas involved in blood pressure control (parvocellular presympathetic neurons in the PVN) [5]. Thus, during disturbances of hydromineral homeostasis that lead to increased peripheral and central ANGII results in activation of neurosecretory and presympathetic neurons in the PVN, via afferent projections from the SFO, inducing an increased systemic AVP release and renal sympathetic outflow which act together to restore hydromineral balance [11]. AVP from neurosecretory neuronal populations also modulates sympathetic outflow and consequently blood pressure by increasing the activity of the presympathetic neurons within the PVN that project to the rostral ventrolateral medulla, a region responsible for the sympathetic system control on the cardiovascular function [21]. In addition, both circulating ANGII and AVP modulate blood pressure through its effects on peripheral vascular tone, inducing potent vasoconstriction and consequently increased total peripheral resistance [6, 11].

Taken together, SFO and hypothalamus, particularly PVN, play an important role in the generation of integrative homeostatic responses through orchestrated activities of neuroendocrine and autonomic networks [5, 11, 22]. An imbalanced interaction among these circuits results in maladaptive responses that can lead to an increased risk of developing cardiovascular disease, such as hypertension [23].

1.4 Estradiol regulation of the hydromineral homeostasis

It is well known that besides reproductive function and sexual behavior, ovarian gonadal hormones, mainly 17β-estradiol (E2), modulate other non-reproductive functions such as cardiovascular function, body fluid balance, feeding, sleep cycles, temperature regulation, mood, mental state, memory, and cognition [3, 24–30]. Nevertheless, in this chapter, we will discuss the main non-reproductive effects of estradiol on the control of hydromineral homeostasis, focusing on ingestive behavior and neurohypophyseal hormonal release.

Mounting evidence reports changes in the hydromineral balance associated with the different phases of the reproductive cycle, gestation period, and reproductive senescence [3, 31, 32]. Receptor for estrogens (ER) is expressed in several tissues that play pivotal roles in hydromineral homeostasis, comprising the kidney, adrenal gland, blood vessels, and brain structures such as lamina terminalis (i.e., OVLT, MnPO, and SFO), and hypothalamus (PVN and SON) (for review see [33]). ER expression in the tissues that are involved in body fluid control supports the hypothesis that estrogens modulate hydromineral homeostasis control. Thus, the study of the influence of E2 on hydromineral homeostasis has been widely appreciated in recent decades, although the precise mechanism of its control is not always in agreement.

1.5 Estrogen receptor signaling

Upon entering the cell, due to their lipophilic character, estrogens bind to their classical intranuclear receptors, which are classified as ER type alpha (ERα) and beta (ERβ), and mediate the regulation of genes and transcription factors, comprising their classic genomic signaling pathway. However, several studies have shown that estrogens can also trigger non-genomic events by binding plasmatic membrane-associated ER (mER), inducing rapid effects [34, 35]. In addition to other proteins, ER stimulation activates members of the MAPK family, such as ERK1/2, JNK, and p38 MAPK [30, 36, 37] as well increases PKC and PKA activities [38].

Importantly, most evidence supports that ERα and ERβ are trafficked to the membrane and also activated membrane estradiol cell signaling. Moreover, there are estrogen membrane-binding proteins that mediate estradiol non-genomic signaling, such as G protein-coupled estrogen receptor (GPER/GPR30), a putative receptor (ER-X), and splice variants of ERα and/or ERβ receptors (for review see [35]). However, the role of these mERs in estradiol signaling and effects remain to be better characterized.

2. Estradiol effects on the fluid intake

Thirst and sodium appetite and the water and sodium intake resulting comprise motivated behaviors involved in the regulation of the hydromineral and cardiovascular homeostasis [3]. A number of epidemiological, clinical, and genetic studies in humans and animals have been showing a link between chronically high salt consumption and the development of hypertension (for review see [24]). Although the involved mechanisms are not fully understood, it is known that occurs increased in the sympathetic and RAS activities, besides be associated with a reduced ability of the kidney to excrete large amounts of salt [23, 24]. Nevertheless, women during their reproductive period have a lower incidence of hypertension than age-matched men [39, 40]. On the other hand, women and females tend to have salt sensitivity and increased blood pressure at postmenopausal or reproductive senescence, suggesting sex differences in body fluid balance and blood pressure regulation [3, 24]. In fact, E2 is known to mediate hydromineral homeostasis and blood pressure mainly by attenuating RAS activity (**Figure 1**). E2 replacement therapy decreases ANGII-induced water and sodium intake [3, 9, 41]; blood pressure increased induced by ANGII and development of hypertension in spontaneously hypertensive rats (for review see [40, 42]); angiotensin-converting enzyme (ACE) and renin activities [43–45]; AT1 mRNA expression, ANGII-AT1 binding, and ANGII-induced Fos immunoreactivity in the OVLT and SFO [28, 46–48]. Moreover, women during reproductive period have lower (pro)renin and renin plasma levels than men [49]. In rats, females at proestrus and estrus respond less to RAS activation and ANGII administration than at other stages of the cycle [3, 50].

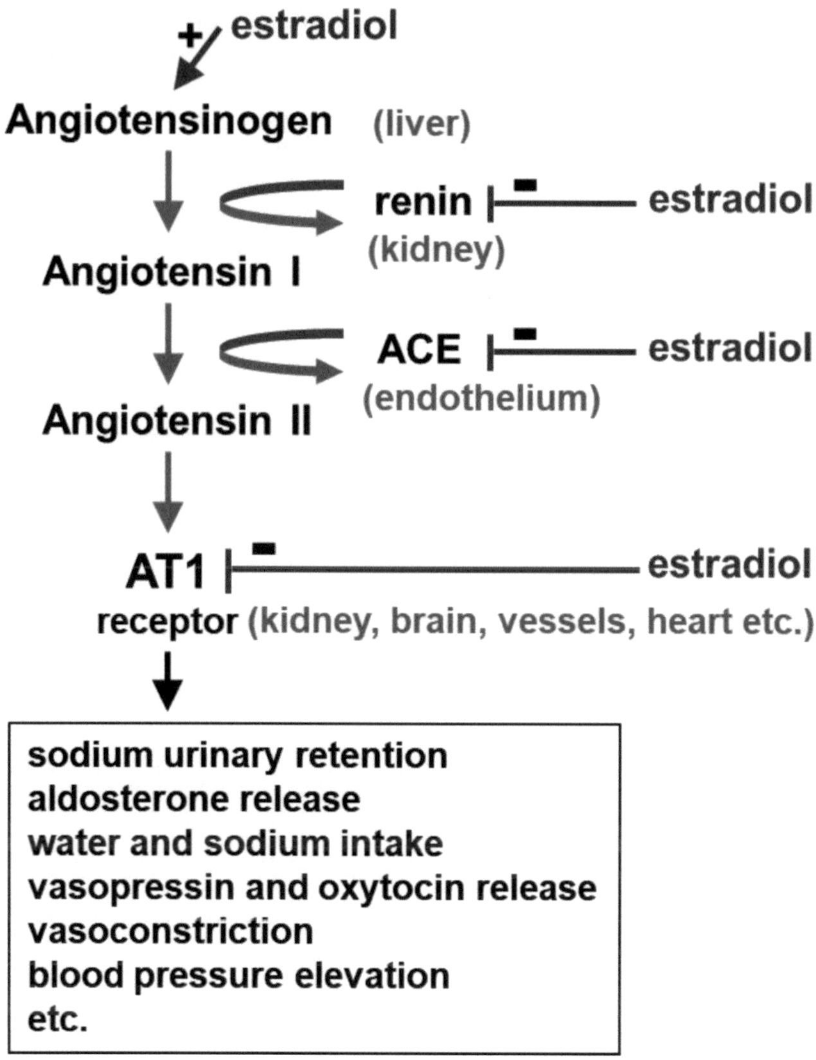

Figure 1.
Schematic summary displays the cascade leading to peripheral ANGII formation and subsequent AT1 receptor activation and the E2 influence on RAS components. Importantly, all these RAS components are also expressed within the brain, leading to central ANGII formation [19].

Although E2 and progesterone have complementary actions in reproductive function, regarding RAS, studies have shown that progesterone has an opposite effect of E2 [43, 51] and is not involved in water regulation in response to ANGII [52].

2.1 Interaction between E2 and ANGII signaling on the fluid intake

Interestingly, in ovariectomized (OVX) rats and during their period of most active, i.e., at night, both water and sodium intakes induced by ANGII require p38 MAPK, JNK, and PKC signaling pathways. ANGII-induced sodium intake also requires ERK1/2 signaling pathway PKC-independent in female [9, 41]. These observations corroborate with Coble et al. [53], which also showed that PKC is involved in both ANGII-induced water and sodium intake in the SFO in male mice. However, Daniels et al. [8] showed that PKC signaling is exclusively involved in ANGII-induced water intake in male rats. Thus, these divergent results suggest a sexually dimorphic aspect to the AT1 signaling pathway involved in fluid intake induced by ANGII. Indeed, several studies report that the RAS is differentially regulated in males and females [3, 39, 40, 42].

In the brain, ERα is extensively distributed in the neurons of the nuclei of the basal forebrain, such as lamina terminalis. SFO neurons have been shown to express both AT1 and ERα [5, 33]. Evidence from our group showed that E2 impairs ANGII signaling [9, 41, 54] besides decreased AT1 mRNA expression in the SFO [28]. For example, E2 attenuates JNK phosphorylation as well as prevents p38 MAPK phosphorylation induced by ANGII in the lamina terminalis. Moreover, E2 attenuates ANGII-induced ERK1/2 phosphorylation within the SFO. These mechanisms can explain, at least in part, the E2 inhibitory effect on the fluid intake induced by ANGII.

An important feature of GPCRs is that they are rapidly phosphorylated by specific GPCR kinases (GRKs) in their serine and threonine residues within the intracellular loop and carboxyl-terminal tail domains. GRK family members selectively phosphorylate agonist activated GPCRs, promoting the binding with cytosolic cofactor proteins termed arrestins, which uncouple GPCRs from G proteins, interrupting the signaling pathway. This process is referred to as desensitization, which occurs within seconds to minutes (for review see [55, 56]). Nevertheless, it is currently known that arrestins can also act as scaffolds to recruit signaling molecules, such as ERK1/2 and JNK, to increase the repertoire of receptor responses. When β-arrestin binds to the AT1 receptor that is phosphorylated by GRK5 or GRK6, it functions as an intracellular signaling adapter leading to robust ERK1/2 activation [57, 58]. In this context, evidence from our group showed that E2 reduced the expression of GRK5 in the lamina terminalis [54]. This observation suggests that E2 may also impair the ANGII signaling pathway by decreasing the activation of ERK1/2 via negative regulation of the GRK5, which can be relevant to the inhibitory effect of E2 on sodium intake induced by ANGII.

Furthermore, Almeida-Pereira et al. [9] showed that the inhibitory effect of E2 on ANGII-induced water and sodium intake requires the ERK1/2 and JNK signaling pathways. Because these inhibitory effects of E2 were quickly reversed by the central inhibition of ERK1/2 and JNK activities, suggesting that there is the involvement of a non-genomic effect of ER agonism. E2 replacement therapy also induces ERK1/2 and JNK phosphorylation in the lamina terminalis [9], and these proteins are involved in the AT1 receptor desensitization process [59, 60]. These observations point to the idea that ERK1/2 and JNK activation from E2 signaling may contribute to the AT1 receptor desensitization process in the lamina terminalis.

Regarding PKC signaling, central PKC inhibition maintains the inhibitory effect of E2 on ANGII-induced fluid intake, and when analyzing PKC activation, E2 induced an increase in PKC (specifically alpha isoform) translocation to the plasmatic membrane in the lamina terminalis structures. Thus, perhaps PKC is not involved in the inhibitory effect of E2 on fluid intake induced by ANGII or E2 may change other protein activation from the sequence of PKC signaling cascade. Indeed, E2 prevents p38 MAPK phosphorylation induced by ANGII and does not activate p38 MAPK in the lamina terminalis [41]. In addition, as already described, E2 attenuates ERK1/2 and JNK phosphorylation in response to ANGII. Lastly, besides GRK, it is known that PKC also phosphorylates the AT1 receptor, exposed or not to agonists, inducing its desensitization [56]. Taken together, these findings lead to the hypothesis that E2 can modulate AT1 desensitization by PKC activation in the lamina terminals. A summary of all these signaling interactions is provided in **Figure 2**.

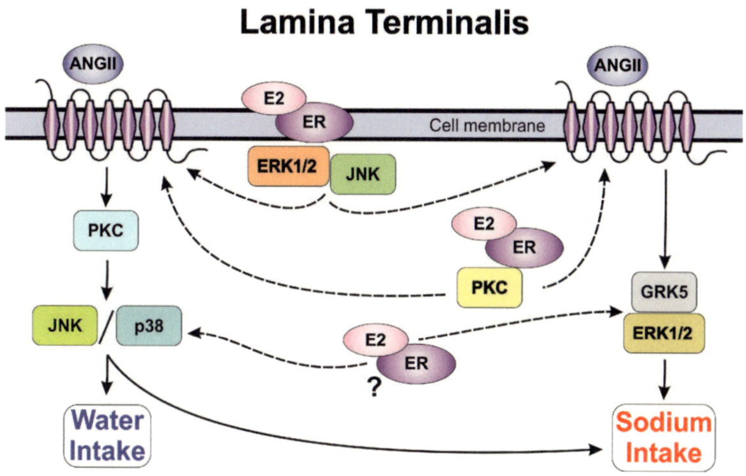

Figure 2.
Schematic summary of the proposed interaction between E2 and ANGII signaling within lamina terminalis structures involved in water and sodium intake. E2 impairs MAPKs phosphorylation in response to ANGII by inducing AT1 desensitization, reduced GRK5 expression, and (or) phosphatase activation (not identified), which leads to ANGII-induced fluid intake reduction. A possible explanation for the E2-induced AT1 desensitization is through ER-mediated ERK1/2 and (or) JNK signaling. Another is through PKC activation mediated by ER inducing AT1 phosphorylation and, consequently, its desensitization. Legend: continuous arrow indicates stimulation and dashed arrow indicates inhibition.

3. Estradiol effects on the neurohypophysial hormone release

It is widely known that OT plays a pivotal role in parturition and lactation by inducing contractions of the uterus and myoepithelial cells of the breast alveoli. In addition, OT participates in the hydromineral balance as a regulator of blood volume by eliciting natriuresis and sodium appetite inhibition [15–17]; and participates in the blood pressure control through its vascular and cardiac relaxation effects [61, 62]. In the central nervous system, OT acts as a neurotransmitter involved in sex and maternal behavior (for review see [63]).

The plasma hyperosmolality is the major stimulus for AVP secretion following by hypotension or decreased blood volume [64]. Thus, through its main antidiuretic effect, AVP plays a fundamental role in hydromineral homeostasis as a regulator of plasma osmolality [11]. Regarding blood pressure control, as described previously, AVP increases sympathetic outflow and peripheral vascular tone by eliciting vasoconstriction and increase consequently the blood pressure [11, 21].

In situ hybridization studies reported a wide distribution of mRNA expression for ERβ in the brain of rats, including in the neurons of SON and the parvo and magnocellular divisions of PVN [65, 66]. Hrabovszky et al. [67] showed that OT and AVP neurons from PVN and SON co-express mRNA for ERβ. These findings provide a neuroendocrine basis for E2 influence on the hypothalamo-neurohypophysial system by acting directly on the PVN and SON neurons. Importantly, E2 can also regulate neurohypophysial hormone release through ERα activation present in the lamina terminal structures and via connections with PVN and SON [33]. In this context, E2 is known to modulate OT release positively, besides increases mRNA expression for OT in the PVN and SON [68–70]. Conversely, the influence of E2 on AVP secretion is complex with controversial data in the literature. Nevertheless, in general, studies point out that there is a positive correlation between AVP secretion and E2 plasma levels associated with body water retention. Moreover, E2 decreases the osmotic threshold for AVP stimulation during dehydration without affect renal free water clearance, suggesting that E2 may alter renal sensitivity to AVP or even interfere with AVP action in the kidney [71–73].

3.1 Interaction between E2 and ANGII signaling on the OT and AVP secretion

A decrease in blood volume and increased renal sympathetic outflow stimulate renin release from the kidney, which results in increased circulating levels of ANGII [3, 11]. Furthermore, during hypovolemia and hypotension, AVP secretion is stimulated mainly by neural (from cardiac baroreceptors and afferent inputs from the brainstem that project to the SON and PVN) and humoral (i.e., ANGII) signals. In dehydration and hyperosmolality conditions, both AVP and OT secretion are stimulated by an osmoregulatory circuit comprising osmoreceptors activation and axonal projections from the basal forebrain to the PVN and SON besides the intrinsic osmosensitivity of magnocellular neurons of the PVN and SON [11, 64]. Thus, hypovolemia (from hemorrhage or dehydration) and hyperosmolality (from dehydration) stimulate RAS activation as well as AVP and OT secretion.

Evidence from our group provides interesting insights that neurohypophysial secretion in response to ANGII involves distinct signal transduction pathways in OVX rats. We reported for the first time that PKC/p38 MAPK signaling is involved in ANGII-induced OT release while AVP release requires ERK1/2 and p38 MAPK signaling PKC-independent [9, 41]. However, Felgendreger et al. [20] showed that the ERK1/2 activation induced by endogenous ANGII is not involved in AVP secretion in male rats. These divergent results suggest a sexually dimorphic aspect to the AT1 signaling pathway involved in ANGII-induced AVP secretion. As already described, several studies reported that the RAS is differentially regulated in males and females, which can be attributed to differences in gonadal and steroid profiles [3, 39, 40, 42].

Concerning E2 modulation on ANGII-induced AVP and OT release, it was observed that E2 inhibits AVP and OT secretion in response to ANGII by impairing ERK1/2 and p38 MAPK phosphorylation, respectively, in the PVN and SON [9, 41]. MAPK proteins are inactivated by phosphatases, such as mitogen-activated protein kinase phosphatases (MKPs). MPKs are dual-specificity protein phosphatases (also known as DUSPs) that dephosphorylate both tyrosine and threonine residues on MAPK members [74]. MAPK phosphatase 1 (MKP-1) was the first of the MKPs to be characterized and is known for dephosphorylating all three major classes of MAPK (ERK, p38 MAPK, and JNK) being expressed in the brain besides many others tissues [75]. MKP-1 is under the positive regulation of E2 in the PVN and SON and thereby can participate in the inhibitory effect of E2 by eliciting ERK1/2 and p38 MAPK dephosphorylation [9]. In addition, it was hypothesized that E2 inhibits ANGII-induced AVP release via PKC-mediated MKP-1 induction and consequent ERK1/2 dephosphorylation, involving E2 non-genomic signaling [54]. A summary is provided in **Figure 3**.

Importantly, ANGII can also stimulate AVP and OT release by acting in the lamina terminalis structures which send angiotensinergic projections to magnocellular neurons of the PVN and SON [5, 13]. Thus, E2 can indirectly modulate AVP and OT release induced by ANGII via afferent inputs from the basal forebrain that project to the SON and PVN. Nevertheless, as E2 increases MKP-1 specifically in the PVN and SON and not in lamina terminalis structures, it is suggested that E2 plays an important direct modulation on AVP and OT release induced by ANGII in hypothalamic nuclei [9, 41]. In the same sense, Vilhena-Franco et al. [76] showed that E2 modulates AVP secretion in response to water deprivation via a direct mechanism mediated by ERβ expressed in the SON and PVN. Additionally, others studies have

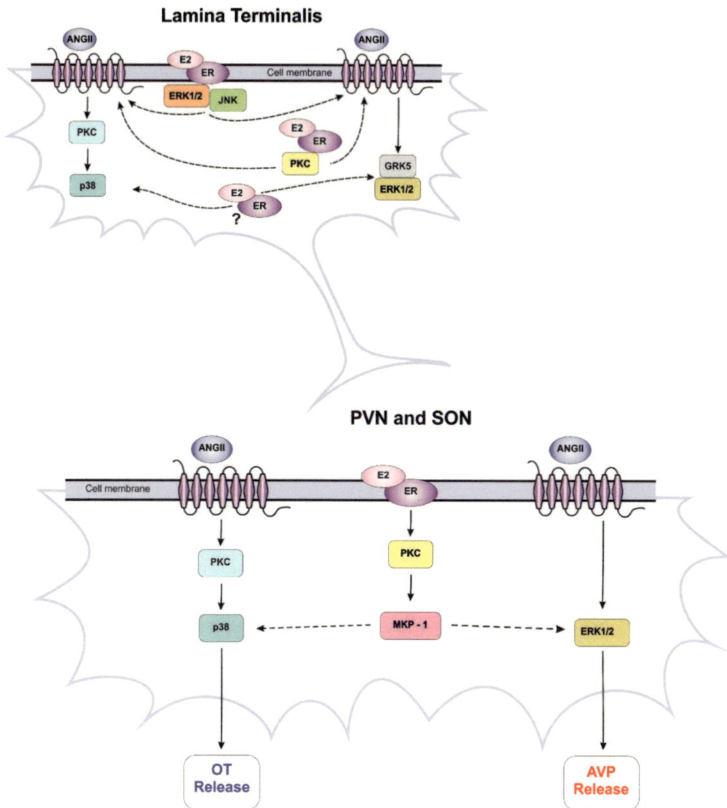

Figure 3.
Schematic summary of the regulatory mechanisms of E2 proposed on ANGII-induced OT and AVP release. Top: E2 can indirectly modulate AVP and OT release induced by ANGII via angiotensinergic afferent inputs from the lamina terminalis structures that project to the SON and PVN. E2 impairs ANGII signaling in neurons of the lamina terminalis leading thereby to the OT and AVP neurons decreased activity in the SON and PVN. Bottom: E2 directly acts in OT and AVP neurons in the PVN and SON, preventing MAPKs phosphorylation through PKC/MKP-1 signaling pathway. Legend: continuous arrow indicates stimulation and dashed arrow indicates inhibition.

demonstrated that E2 modulates OT and AVP release directly via its ERβ or mER (mainly AVP release) in magnocellular neurons of the PVN and SON [77–79].

3.2 Interaction between ovarian hormones, phoenixin and AVP release

A novel peptide, conserved across species, was recently described and named phoenixin (PNX). PNX is produced in the brain and heart binding selectively in the pituitary gland, ovary, and brain. The hypothalamus was identified to produce the most PNX of all tissues examined as well as presented the highest binding of labeled PNX [80]. PNX has been implicated to play an important role in the hypothalamic–pituitary-gonadal axis control by increasing the gonadal release hormone (GnRH) expression and its receptor in the hypothalamus besides increasing luteinizing hormone (LH) release [80, 81]. Using a deductive ligand-receptor matching strategy (U.S. Patent #9, 146, 240, B2), the orphaned G protein-coupled receptor (GPR)173 was identified to be a candidate PNX receptor [82].

The novel reproductive neuropeptide PNX and its receptor, GPR173, were also identified in magnocellular neurons of the PVN and SON, suggesting the participation of PNX on the hypothalamo-neurohypophysial system control and hence of the hydromineral homeostasis. [80, 82]. In fact, Gasparini et al. [83] demonstrated that PNX induces AVP release through its candidate receptor, GPR173, besides depolarizes magnocellular neurons of the PVN. Interestingly, PNX does not modulate OT release. Despite there are no differences between males and females on PNX-induced AVP release, a potential estrogen response element (ERE) upstream of PNX was identified, suggesting that ovarian hormones, especially E2, can modulate PNX [80, 83]. Consistent with this idea, ovarian failure induced by OVX induces downregulation of PNX compared with intact females in the hypothalamus [84].

Circulating levels of ovarian steroids progesterone, and, mainly 17β-estradiol, increase throughout the pregnancy, reaching maximum values at the end of pregnancy in women [85, 86]. On the other hand, in rats, peripheral plasma levels of estradiol increase across pregnancy with a concomitant decrease in progesterone [87]. However, in both humans and animals, it is observed changes in hydromineral homeostasis over the pregnancy, such as blood volume expansion and low osmolality associated with a reduced threshold for hyperosmotic stimulation of AVP secretion. Thus, AVP secretion is paradoxically elevated during this hypervolemic and hyponatremic state of the pregnancy [32, 88] although is important to maintain water homeostasis offsetting AVP that is metabolized by vasopressinase in humans [89]. A dysfunction in the metabolism of vasopressinase and AVP can predispose women to develop cardiovascular diseases associated with hydromineral imbalance, as pregnancy-induced hypertension, that occurs after the second trimester of pregnancy [89, 90].

In this context, our group demonstrated upregulation of GPR173 during late post-puberty in the PVN, and importantly, upregulation during the last third of pregnancy in the hypothalamus. Moreover, it was observed an increase in the hypothalamic levels of PNX and AVP across pregnancy compared with levels present during diestrus with a positive correlation between both peptides [84]. Thus, these results suggest an important role of PNX on AVP release during late pregnancy, which can help to provide potential pharmacological targets for preventing the development of cardiovascular diseases across pregnancy.

4. Conclusions

Estradiol replacement therapy initiated at the time of or prior to menopause is usually employed for decreasing the risk of cardiovascular and neurodegenerative diseases [91–93]. Nowadays, the high composition of salt in the contemporary diet constitutes an important public health concern, since uncontrolled sodium consumption increases the risk of hypertension [24], particularly in women in later menopause, who have a greater risk of developing cardiovascular disease [3, 24]. The increased central and peripheral RAS activity is involved in the pathophysiology of hypertension. Given the wide complexity of the crosstalk signaling pathways, cellular and molecular studies are important to better elucidate the mechanisms of the interaction between E2 and ANGII signaling as well as mapping out the potential benefits of E2 replacement and its action on the central nervous system. In this context, advanced evidence has been contributed to the further understanding of E2 and ANGII interaction in the hydromineral homeostasis, which can reveal potential pharmacological targets to prevent cardiovascular diseases, with uncontrolled salt consumption as a predisposing factor, during female reproductive senescence. Taken together, E2 impairs ANGII signaling besides induces the downregulation of AT1 receptor. E2 attenuates MAPKs phosphorylation involved in ANGII physiological actions in the lamina terminalis structures and hypothalamic nuclei, namely, PVN and SON.

Acknowledgements

This study was supported by the Sao Paulo Research Foundation, Brazil (FAPESP, grant #2012/04620-0, #2014/25005-8, #2017/22140-0 from Gislaine Almeida-Pereira, and #2013/09799-1 from José Antunes-Rodrigues), Brazilian Council for Scientific and Technological Development (CNPq) and the Brazilian Federal Agency for Support and Evaluation of Graduate Education (CAPES). The authors thank Santo Oliani Junior for his help in drawing the figures.

Author details

Gislaine Almeida-Pereira*, Lucila L.K. Elias and José Antunes-Rodrigues
Department of Physiology, Medical School of Ribeirao Preto of Sao Paulo University, Ribeirao Preto, Brazil

*Address all correspondence to: g.almeidapereira@gmail.com

References

[1] Cannon WB. 1929. Organization for physiological homeostasis. Physiology Review, 4(3):399-431.

[2] Hollenberg NK. 1984. The renin-angiotensin system and sodium homeostasis. Journal of Cardiovascular Pharmacology, 6: S176–S183.

[3] Fitzsimons JT. 1998. Angiotensin, thirst, and sodium appetite. Physiological Reviews, 78: 583-686.

[4] Beresford MJ and Fitzsimons JT. 1992. Intracerebroventricular angiotensin II-induced thirst and sodium appetite in rat are blocked by the AT1 receptor antagonist, losartan (DuP 753), but not by the AT2 antagonist, CGP 42112B. Experimental Physiology, 77: 761-764.

[5] Coble JP, Grobe JL, Johnson AK, Sigmund CD. 2015. Mechanisms of brain renin angiotensin system-induced drinking and blood pressure: importance of the subfornical organ. American Journal of Physiology: Regulatory, Integrative and Comparative Physiology, 308: R238–R249.

[6] Mehta PK and Griendling KK. 2007. Angiotensin II cell signaling: physiological and pathological effects in the cardiovascular system. American Journal of Physiology: Cell Physiology, 292: C82–C97.

[7] Hines J, Fluharty SJ, Yee DK. 2003. Structural determinants for the activation mechanism of the angiotensin II type 1 receptor differ for phosphoinositide hydrolysis and mitogen-activated protein kinase pathways. Biochemical Pharmacology, 66: 251-262.

[8] Daniels D, Yee DK, Fluharty SJ. 2007. Angiotensin II receptor signalling. Experimental Physiology, 92: 523-527.

[9] Almeida-Pereira G, Coletti R, Mecawi AS, Reis LC, Elias LLK, Antunes-Rodrigues J. 2016. Estradiol and angiotensin II crosstalk in hydromineral balance: role of the ERK1/2 and JNK signaling pathways. Neuroscience, 322: 525-538.

[10] Muta K, Morgan DA, Grobe JL, Sigmund CD, Rahmouni K. 2016. mTORC1 signaling contributes to drinking but not blood pressure responses to brain angiotensin II. Endocrinology, 157: 3140-3148.

[11] Antunes-Rodrigues J, de Castro M, Elias LLK, Valença MM, McCann SM. 2004. Neuroendocrine control of body fluid metabolism. Physiological Reviews, 84: 169-208.

[12] Morris MJ, Wilson WL, Starbuck EM, Fitts DA. 2002. Forebrain circumventricular organs mediate salt appetite induced by intravenous angiotensin II in rats. Brain Research, 949(1-2):42-50.

[13] Ferguson AV and Bains JS. 1996. Electrophysiology of the circumventricular organs. Frontiers in Neuroendocrinology, 17: 440-475.

[14] Leng G, Brown CH, Russell JA. 1999. Physiological pathways regulating the activity of magnocellular neurosecretory cells. Progress in Neurobiology, 57:625-655.

[15] Stoeckel ME, Freund-Mercier MS, Falacios JM, Richard P, Porte A. 1987. Autoradiographic localization of binding sites for oxytocin and vasopressin in the rat kidney. Journal of Endocrinology, 113: 179-182.

[16] Tribollet E, Barberis C, Jard S, Dubois-Dauphin M, Dreifuss JJ. 1988. Localization and pharmacological characterization of high affinity binding sites for vasopressin and oxytocin

in the rat brain by light microscopic autoradiography. Brain Research, 442: 105-118.

[17] Amico JA, Morris M, Vollmer RR. 2001. Mice deficient in oxytocin manifest increased saline consumption following overnight fluid deprivation. American Journal Physiology, 281:1368-73.

[18] Ferguson AV and Renaud LP. 1986. Systemic angiotensin acts at subfornical organ to facilitate activity of neurohypophysial neurons. American Journal of Physiology: Regulatory, Integrative and Comparative Physiology, 251: R712–R717.

[19] Lenkei Z, Palkovits M, Corvol P, Llorens-Cortes C. 1997. Expression of angiotensin type-1 (AT1) and type-2 (AT2) receptor mRNAs in the adult rat brain: a functional neuroanatomical review. Frontiers in Neuroendocrinology, 18: 383-439.

[20] Felgendreger LA, Fluharty SJ, Yee DK, Flanagan-Cato LM. 2013. Endogenous angiotensin II-induced p44/42 mitogen-activated protein kinase activation mediates sodium appetite but not thirst or neurohypophysial secretion in male rats. Journal of Neuroendocrinology, 25 (2):97-106.

[21] Son SJ, Filosa JA, Potapenko ES, Biancardi VC, Zheng H, Patel KP, Tobin VA, Ludwig M, Stern JE. 2013. Dendritic peptide release mediates interpopulation crosstalk between neurosecretory and preautonomic networks. Neuron, 78(6):1036-1049.

[22] Swanson LW and Sawchenko PE. 1980. Paraventricular Nucleus: A site for the Integration of Neuroendocrine and Autonomic Mechanisms. Progress in Neuroendocrinology, 31: 410-417.

[23] Toney GM and Stocker SD. 2010. Hyperosmotic activation of CNS sympathetic drive: implications for cardiovascular disease. Journal Physiology, 588.18: 3375-3384.

[24] Meneton P, Jeunemaitre X, de Wardener HE, MacGregor GA. 2005. Links between dietary salt intake, renal salt handling, blood pressure, and cardiovascular diseases. Physiological Reviews, 85: 679-715.

[25] Fink G, Sumner B, Rosie R, Wilson H, McQueen J. 1999. Androgen actions on central serotonin neurotransmission: relevance for mood, mental state and memory. Behavioural Brain Research, 105(1): 53-68.

[26] Panay N and Studd JW. 1998. The psychotherapeutic effects of estrogens. Gynecology Endocrinology, 12.5: 353-365.

[27] Hay M. 2016. Sex, the brain and hypertension: brain oestrogen receptors and high blood pressure risk factors. Clinical Science (Lond), 130(1): 9-18.

[28] Almeida-Pereira G, Rorato R, Reis LC, Elias LLK, Antunes-Rodrigues J. 2013. The role of estradiol in adrenal insufficiency and its interaction with corticosterone on hydromineral balance. Hormones and Behavior, 64: 847-855.

[29] Almeida-Pereira, G. 2018. Non-Reproductive Effects of Estradiol: Brain Behavior. EC Psychology and Psychiatry, 7.5: 261-262.

[30] Micevych PE and Kelly MJ. 2012. Membrane estrogen receptor regulation of hypothalamic function. Neuroendocrinology, 96: 103-110.

[31] Antunes-Rodrigues J and Covian MR. 1963. Hypothalamic control of sodium chloride and water intake. Acta Physiology Latin American, 13: 94-100.

[32] Brunton PJ, Arunachalam S, Russell JA. 2008. Control of

neurohypophysial hormone secretion, blood osmolality and volume in pregnancy. Journal Physiology Pharmacology, 59(8):27-45.

[33] Somponpun, SJ. 2007. Neuroendocrine Regulation of Fluid and Electrolyte Balance by Ovarian Steroids: Contributions from Central Oestrogen Receptors. Journal of Neuroendocrinology, 19:809-818.

[34] Toran-Allerand CD. 2004. Estrogen and the brain: beyond ER-a and ER-b. Experimental Gerontology, 39:1579-1586.

[35] Micevych P and Dominguez R. 2009. Membrane estradiol signaling in the brain. Front Neuroendocrinol, 30(3):315-327.

[36] Feng W, Webb P, Nguyen P, Liu X, Li J, Karin M, Kushner PJ. 2001. Potentiation of estrogen receptor activation function 1 (AF-1) by Src/JNK through a serine 118-independent pathway. Molecular Endocrinology, 15(1):32-45.

[37] Sétáló Jr. G, Singh, M, Guan, X, Toran-Allerand, CD. 2002. Cellular localization of estradiol-induced phospho-ERK1/2 in mouse cerebral cortical explants: the roles of heat shock protein 90 (Hsp90) and MEK2. Journal of Neurobiology, 50:1-12.

[38] Qiu, J, Bosch, MA, Tobias, SC, Grandy, DK, Scanlan, TS, Rønnekleiv, OK, Kelly, MJ. 2003. Rapid signaling of estrogen in hypothalamic neurons involves a novel G protein-coupled estrogen receptor that activates protein kinase C. Journal of Neuroscience, 23:9529-9540.

[39] Cutler JA, Sorlie PD, Wolz M, Thom T, Fields LE, Roccella EJ. 2008. Trends in hypertension prevalence, awareness, treatment, and control rates in United States adults between 1988-1994 and 1999-2004. Hypertension, 52:818-827.

[40] Sandberg K and Ji H. 2012. Sex differences in primary hypertension. Biology of Sex Differences, 3: 7.

[41] Almeida-Pereira G, Vilhena-Franco T, Coletti R, Cognuck SQ, Silva HVP, Elias LLK, Antunes-Rodrigues J. 2019. 17β-Estradiol attenuates p38MAPK activity but not PKCα induced by angiotensin II in the brain. Journal of Endocrinology, 240(2):345-360.

[42] Fischer M, Baessler A, Schunkert H. 2002. Renin angiotensin system and gender differences in the cardiovascular system. Cardiovascular Research, 53: 672-677.

[43] Oelkers WKH. 1996. Effects of estrogens and progestogens on the renin-aldosterone system and blood pressure. Steroids, 61:166-171.

[44] Schunkert H, Danser AH, Hense HW, Derkx FH, Kürzinger S, Riegger GA. 1997. Effects of estrogen replacement therapy on the renin-angiotensin system in postmenopausal women. Circulation, 95(1):39-45.

[45] Gallagher PE, Li P, Lenhart JR, Chappell MC, Brosnihan KB. 1999. Estrogen regulation of angiotensin-converting enzyme mRNA. Hypertension, 33:323-328.

[46] Kisley LR, Sakai RR, Fluharty SJ. 1999. Estrogen decreases hypothalamic angiotensin II AT1 receptor binding and mRNA in the female rat. Brain Research, 844: 34-42.

[47] Tanaka J, Miyakubo H, Okumura T, Sakamaki K, Hayashi Y. 2001. Estrogen decreases the responsiveness of subfornical organ neurons projecting to the hypothalamic paraventricular nucleus to angiotensin II in female rats. Neuroscience Letters, 307(3):155-158.

[48] Krause EG, Curtis KS, Stincic TL, Markle JP, Contreras RJ. 2006. Oestrogen and weight loss decrease isoproterenol-induced Fos immunoreactivity and angiotensin type 1 mRNA in the subfornical organ of female rats. Journal of Physiology, 573: 251-262.

[49] Danser AH, Derkx FH, Schalekamp MA, Hense HW, Riegger GA, Schunkert H. 1998. Determinants of interindividual variation of renin and prorenin concentrations: evidence for a sexual dimorphism of (pro)renin levels in humans. Journal of Hypertension, 16(6):853-862.

[50] Findlay AL, Fitzsimons JT, Kucharczyk J. 1979. Dependence of spontaneous and angiotensin-induced drinking in the rat upon the oestrous cycle and ovarian hormones. Journal of Endocrinology, 82(2):215-225.

[51] Nickenig G, Strehlow K, Wassmann S, Bäumer AT, Albory K, Saucr H, Böhm M. 2000. Diffcrcntial effects of estrogen and progesterone on AT(1) receptor gene expression in vascular smooth muscle cells. Circulation, 102(15):1828-1833.

[52] Kisley LR, Sakai RR, Ma LY, Fluharty SJ. 1999. Ovarian steroid regulation of angiotensin II-induced water intake in the rat. American Journal Physiology, 276(1):R90-R96.

[53] Coble JP, Johnson RF, Cassell MD, Johnson AK, Grobe JL, Sigmund CD. 2014. Activity of protein kinase C-α within the subfornical organ is necessary for fluid intake in response to brain angiotensin. Hypertension, 64: 141-148.

[54] Almeida-Pereira G, Elias LLK, Antunes-Rodrigues J. 2020. SUN-248 Estradiol Changes Angiotensin II-Induced ERK1/2 Phosphorylation by Different Pathways in the Hypothalamus and Lamina Terminalis. Journal of the Endocrine Society, 4. Issue Supplement 1.

[55] Lefkowitz RJ. 1998. G protein-coupled receptors. III. New roles for receptor kinases and beta-arrestins in receptor signaling and desensitization. Journal of Biological Chemistry, 273(30):18677-18680.

[56] Ferguson SS. 2001. Evolving concepts in G protein-coupled receptor endocytosis: the role in receptor desensitization and signaling. Pharmacology Review, 53: 1-24.

[57] Kim J, Ahn S, Ren XR, Whalen EJ, Reiter E, Wei H, Lefkowitz RJ. 2005. Functional antagonism of different G protein-coupled receptor kinases for beta-arrestin-mediated angiotensin II receptor signaling. Proceedings of the National Academy of Sciences U S A, 102(5):1442-1447.

[58] Shenoy SK, Lefkowitz RJ. 2011. β-Arrestin-mediated receptor trafficking and signal transduction. Trends in Pharmacological Sciences, 32(9):521-533.

[59] Wei H, Ahn S, Barnes WG, Lefkowitz RJ. 2004. Stable interaction between beta-arrestin 2 and angiotensin type 1A receptor is required for beta-arrestin 2-mediated activation of extracellular signal-regulated kinases 1 and 2. Journal of Biological Chemistry, 279(46):48255-48261.

[60] Vento PJ and Daniels D. 2012. Mitogen-activated protein kinase is required for the behavioural desensitization that occurs after repeated injections of angiotensin II. Experimental Physiology, 97(12):1305-14.

[61] Jankowski M, Hajjar F, AL Kawas S, Mukaddam-DaherS,HoffmanG,McCann S M, Gutkowska J. 1998. Proceedings of

the National Academy of Sciences USA, 95:14558-14563.

[62] Jankowski M, Wang D, Hajjar F, Mukaddam-Daher S, McCann SM, Gutkowska J. 2000. Oxytocin and its receptors are synthesized in the rat vasculature. Proceedings of the National Academy of Sciences USA, 97(11):6207-6211.

[63] Argiolas A and Gessa GL. 1991. Neuroscience & Biobehavioral Reviews, 15:217-231.

[64] Stricker EM and Sved AF. 2002. Controls of vasopressin secretion and thirst: similarities and dissimilarities in signals. Physiology Behavior, 77(4-5):731-6.

[65] Simerly RB, Chang C, Muramatsu M, Swanson LW. 1990. Distribution of androgen and estrogen receptor mRNA-containing cells in the rat brain: an in situ hybridization study. Journal of Comparative Neurology, 294:76-95.

[66] Shughrue PJ, Lane MV, Merchenthaler I. 1997. Comparative distribution of estrogen receptor-alpha and -beta mRNA in the rat central nervous system. Journal of Comparative Neurology, 388:507-525.

[67] Hrabovszky E, Kallo I, Hajszan T, Shughrue PJ, Merchenthaler I, Liposits Z. 1998. Expression of estrogen receptor-beta messenger ribonucleic acid in oxytocin and vasopressin neurons of the rat supraoptic and paraventricular nuclei. Endocrinology, 139: 2600-2604.

[68] Yamaguchi K, Akaishi T, Negoro H. 1979. Effect of estrogen treatment on plasma oxytocin and vasopressin in ovariectomized rats. Endocrinol Jpn, 26:197-205.

[69] Van Tol HH, Bolwerk EL, Liu B, Burbach JP. 1988. Oxytocin and vasopressin gene expression in the hypothalamo-neurohypophyseal system of the rat during the estrous cycle, pregnancy, and lactation. Endocrinology, 122:945-951.

[70] Nomura M, McKenna E, Korach KS, Pfa. DW, Ogawa S. 2002. Estrogen receptor-beta regulates transcript levels for oxytocin and arginine vasopressin in the hypothalamic paraventricular nucleus of male mice. Molecular Brain Research, 109:84-94.

[71] Forsling ML, Strömberg P, Akerlund M. 1982. Effect of ovarian steroids on vasopressin secretion. Journal of Endocrinology, 95(1):147-151.

[72] Peysner K and Forsling ML. 1990. Effect of ovariectomy and treatment with ovarian steroids on vasopressin release and fluid balance in the rat. Journal of Endocrinology, 124(2):277-284.

[73] Stachenfeld NS. 2008. Sex hormone effects on body fluid regulation. Exercise and Sport Sciences Reviews, 36(3):152-9.

[74] Salojin K and Oravecz T. 2007. Regulation of innate immunity by MAPK dual-specificity phosphatases: knockout models reveal new tricks of old genes. Journal of Leukocyte Biology, 81: 860-869.

[75] Caunt CJ and Keyse SM. 2012. Dual-specificity MAP kinase phosphatases (MKPs): shaping the outcome of MAP kinase signaling. FEBS Journal, 280: 489-504.

[76] Vilhena-Franco T, Mecawi AS, Almeida-Pereira G, Lucio-Oliveira F, Elias LLK, Antunes-Rodrigues J. 2019. Oestradiol acts through its beta receptor to increase vasopressin neuronal activation and secretion induced by dehydration. Journal of Neuroendocrinology, 2019: e12712.

[77] Swenson KL and Sladek CD. 1997. Gonadal steroid modulation of vasopressin secretion in response to osmotic stimulation. Endocrinology, 138: 2089-2097.

[78] Somponpun S and Sladek CD. 2002. Role of estrogen receptor-beta in regulation of vasopressin and oxytocin release in vitro. Endocrinology, 143: 2899-2904.

[79] Somponpun SJ, Holmes MC, Seck JR, Russell JA. 2004. Modulation of oestrogen receptor-b mRNA expression in rat paraventricular and supraoptic nucleus neurones following adrenal steroid manipulation and hyperosmotic stimulation. Journal of Neuroendocrinology, 16: 472-482.

[80] Yosten GL, Lyu RM, Hsueh AJ, Avsian-Kretchmer O, Chang JK, Tullock CW, Dun SL, Dun N, Samson WK. 2013. A novel reproductive peptide, phoenixin. Journal of Neuroendocrinolody, 25(2):206-215.

[81] Treen AK, Luo V, Belsham DD. 2016. Phoenixin Activates Immortalized GnRH and Kisspeptin Neurons Through the Novel Receptor GPR173. Molecular Endocrinology, 30(8):872-888.

[82] Stein LM, Tullock CW, Mathews SK, Garcia-Galiano D, Elias CF, Samson WK, Yosten GL. 2016. Hypothalamic action of phoenixin to control reproductive hormone secretion in females: importance of the orphan G protein-coupled receptor Gpr173. American Journal Physiology Regulatory Integrative Comparative Physiology, 311(3):R489-496.

[83] Gasparini S, Stein LM, Loewen SP, Haddock CJ, Soo J, Ferguson AV, Kolar GR, Yosten GLC and Samson WK. 2018. Novel regulator of vasopressin secretion: phoenixin. American Journal Physiology Regulatory Integrative Comparative Physiology, 314:R623-R628.

[84] Haddock CJ, Almeida-Pereira G, Stein LM, Yosten GLC, Samson WK. 2020. A novel regulator of thirst behavior: phoenixin. American Journal Physiology Regulatory Integrative Comparative Physiology, 318: R1027–R1035.

[85] Dörr HG, Heller A, Versmold HT, Sippell WG, Herrmann M, Bidlingmaier F, Knorr D. 1989. Longitudinal study of progestins, mineralocorticoids, and glucocorticoids throughout human pregnancy. The Journal of Clinical Endocrinology and Metabolism, 68(5):863-868.

[86] Kuijper EA, Ket JC, Caanen MR, Lambalk CB. 2013. Reproductive hormone concentrations in pregnancy and neonates: a systematic review. Reproductive BioMedicine Online, 27(1):33-63. Erratum in: Reprod Biomed Online. 2013 Oct;27(4):448-449.

[87] Wilson L Jr, Stanisc D, Khan-Dawood F, Dawood MY. 1982. Alterations in reproductive tissue prostaglandins E and F, 6-keto prostaglandin F1 alpha and thromboxane B2 with gestational age in the rat. Biology of Reproduction, 27(5):1207-1215.

[88] Tkachenko O, Shchekochikhin D, Schrier RW. 2014. Hormones and hemodynamics in pregnancy. International Journal of Endocrinology and Metabolism, 12(2):e14098.

[89] Krege JH and Katz VL. 1990. A proposed relationship between vasopressinase altered vasopressin and preeclampsia. Medical Hypotheses, 31(4):283-287.

[90] Cornelius DC. 2014. Copeptin: a new biomarker that is specific for preeclampsia? Hypertension, 64(6):1189-1191.

[91] Bold MLK. 1999. Estrogen, natriuretic peptides and

renin-angiontesin system. Cardiovascular Research, 41(3):524-531.

[92] Bowling M, Oparil S, Hage F, Hilgers R, Xing D. 2012. Sex Hormones and Vascular Function. Chapter 1, Sex Hormones, Raghvendra K. Dubey, IntechOpen. Available from: https://www.intechopen.com/books/sex-hormones/sex-hormones-and-vascular-function.

[93] Arevalo MA, Azcoitia I, Garcia-Segura LM. 2015. The neuroprotective actions of oestradiol and oestrogen receptors. Nature Reviews Neuroscience, 16(1):17-29.

Section 4

Kisspeptin

Chapter 10

Kisspeptin: Role in Female Infertility

Abdulsamed Kükürt, Mushap Kuru, Ömer Faruk Başer and Mahmut Karapehlivan

Abstract

Kisspeptin is a neuropeptide encoded by the kisspeptin gene (Kiss1) and located in different brain regions, primarily in the hypothalamus. Kisspeptin and its receptor G-protein-coupled receptor-54 (GPR54), are also found in behavioural brain regions such as the hippocampus and cortex. Kisspeptin, a very powerful neuropeptide that stimulates the secretion of follicle-stimulating hormone (FSH) and luteinizing hormone (LH) from the pituitary, does this by increasing gonadotropin-releasing hormone (GnRH) levels. In recent studies, it has been noted that kisspeptin is effective on reproductive functions. Globally 8 to 12% of couples have infertility problems, and the majority are residents of developing countries. Approximately 70% of infertility cases are caused by fertility problems in women. The frequency of infertility in women continues to increase every year and the underlying factors require further research. Bearing this problem in mind, this review examines the possible role of kisspeptin in female infertility. In doing so, it aims to find out how future application of kisspeptin may potentially unravel the neural reproductive disorder.

Keywords: kisspeptin, metastin, GPR54, Kiss1, Kiss1r, infertility, nitric oxide, sex streoid, progesterone, GnRH, LH, FSH

1. Introduction

Infertility is the inability to get pregnant despite regular sexual intercourse for one year or more (without contraception or the impairment of a person's or a couple's fertility) [1]. Fertility and pregnancy rates decrease due to ageing in women. For this reason, it is recommended that women aged 35 and above start receiving infertility treatment after 6 months of conception attempt. After the age of 40, this period should not be waited for treatment. Many factors cause female infertility. These can be listed as medical history (family history, previous treatments, menstrual history, sexual history, etc.), physical factors (weight, body mass index, etc.), diminished ovarian reserves, ovulatory dysfunction (hypothalamic–pituitary axis (HPG axis) disorders, ovarian disorders, thyroid disorders and hyperprolactinemia, etc.), tubal factors, uterine factors and unexplained causes [2, 3]. More than 186 million people worldwide suffer from infertility, and the majority of them are residents of developing countries [4].

Kisspeptin was discovered in 1996 as the product of the kisspeptin gene (Kiss1), which is a metastatic tumour suppressor gene; therefore, it was initially called metastin [5]. Kisspeptins are a family of neuropeptides in RF-Amide structure [(neuropeptides containing arginine-phenylalanine (Arg-Phe) at the C-terminal are defined as RF-Amides)] [6]. Two years later, the connection between kisspeptin-54 and G-protein-coupled receptor-54 (GPR54) was shown for the first time [7]. In 2003, inactivating mutations of GPR54 were found in people with hypogonadotropic hypogonadism [8]. The respective receptor was previously called the GPR54, it is also identified as the kisspeptin receptor (Kiss1r) nowadays [9].

The detection of the role of the kisspeptin receptor mutation in leading to idiopathic hypogonadotropic hypogonadism paved the way for further investigations about the roles played by the kisspeptin, Kiss1, and Kiss1r systems in the field of reproductive endocrinology [10]. Many studies have shown that kisspeptin plays key roles in the regulation of different aspects of reproduction [11–17]. This review examines the possible role of kisspeptin in female infertility. In doing so, it aims to find out how future application of kisspeptin may potentially unravel the neural fertility disorder.

2. Kisspeptin

The Kiss1 gene encodes the neuropeptide kisspeptins. They, originally identified as metastasis suppressors, were later found to play a central regulatory role in reproduction [18]. The gene is located on human chromosome 1q32. This gene contains 2 non-expressed and 2 partially expressed regions and four exons, assembling the leader peptide consisting of 145 amino acids [19]. This precursor protein transforms into various active forms of kisspeptin with lengths of 54, 14, 13, and 10 amino acids through various post-translational modifications (**Figure 1**) [20]. These forms belong to the RF-amide peptide hormone family, which is closely associated with energy metabolism and reproduction. The members of the RF-amide peptide hormone family contain the common Arg-Phe-NH_2 moiety at the C-terminal [21].

Kisspeptin receptors were first discovered in 2001 in studies about cancer, and they were named as the GPR54. Today, they are identified as the Kiss1r [9]. Kiss1r is a 396-amino acid receptor and a member of G protein-coupled receptors. The minimum length required to activate GPR54 is a 10-amino acid carboxyl terminal sequence (Kisspeptin-10) [22].

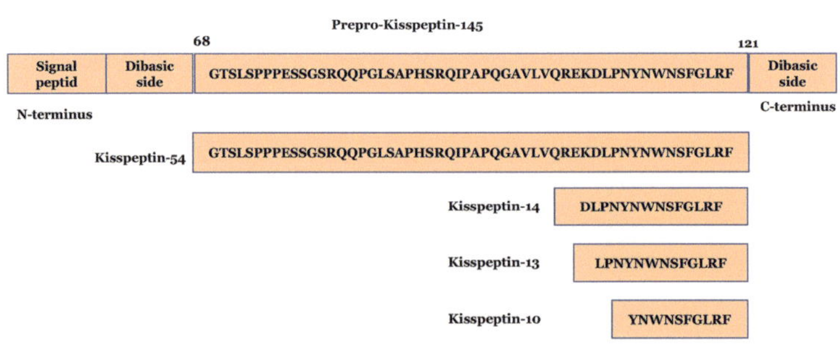

Figure 1.
Amino acids sequence of human kisspeptin isoforms [23, 24].

3. Kisspeptin's mechanism of action

As a result of the kisspeptin binding to the GPR54/Kiss1r receptor, activates the G-protein (G_q/11) and phospholipase-C (PLC). Subsequently, diacylglycerol and

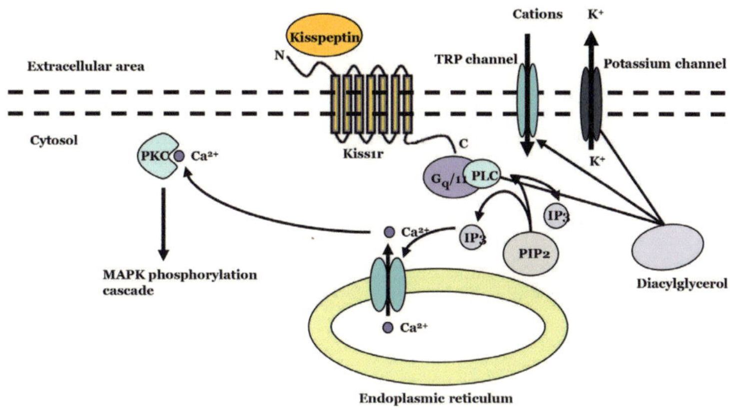

Figure 2.
Cellular action mechanism of kisspeptins [27].

inositol trisphosphate (IP3) are formed from phosphatidylinositol bisphosphate (PİP2), resulting in elevated Ca^{+2} concentrations. Activation of this mechanism results in the closure of the potassium channels and opening of the cation channels (TRP channels), leading to the depolarization of GnRH neurons. Consequently, GnRH neurons start secreting hormones [25]. Kisspeptin increase apoptosis and decrease cell proliferation and metastasis by stimulating the mitogen-activated protein kinase pathway (MAPK) via protein kinase C (PKC) and the extracellular signal-regulated kinase (ERK) pathway (**Figure 2**) [26].

4. Distribution of kisspeptin neurons and effects on the HPG axis

Kisspeptin gene neurons are involved in several actions including steroid hormone feedback, metabolic signalling, and photoperiodic information regulation. It is suggested that, compatibly with their mediator role in steroid hormone feedback mechanisms, Kiss1 neurons are involved in the expression of estrogen receptors (ERα and ERβ) and progesterone receptors [21].

Kiss1 neurons are located in the periventricular nucleus (PeN), arcuate nucleus (ARC) and anteroventral periventricular nucleus (AVPV) which are located in the preoptic area of the hypothalamus (POA) in the brain and which are the regions that regulate the secretion of the GnRH hormone in mouse [28]. Kisspeptins are secreted by these nuclei. However, AVPV displays sexual dimorphism. Kiss1 mRNA expression is higher in AVPV in females compared to males. This indicates that the role of kisspeptin neurons in AVPV varies by gender [29].

The different patterns of Kiss1 mRNA regulation in the forebrain nuclei are important in the emergence of the different physiological effects of Kiss1 on the HPG axis. ARC acts as the negative feedback regulation centre for the GnRH and gonadotropin secretion, while AVPV acts as the positive feedback regulation centre responsible for the LH surge in females. ERα, ERβ, and progesterone receptors are abundant in AVPV. When these receptors bind to their ligands; they increase LH secretion, resulting in the LH surge. Furthermore, Kiss1 neurons in AVPV synapse with GnRH neurons; Kiss1 mRNA expression in AVPV peaks simultaneously with the GnRH/LH release, and the estrogen-dependent Kiss1 mRNA induction in females is involved in the GnRH/LH surge during preovulation [30]. While gonadal steroids inhibit Kiss1 neurons in ARC (negative feedback), they stimulate Kiss1 neurons in AVPV (positive feedback) [23]. Signals arising from kisspeptin

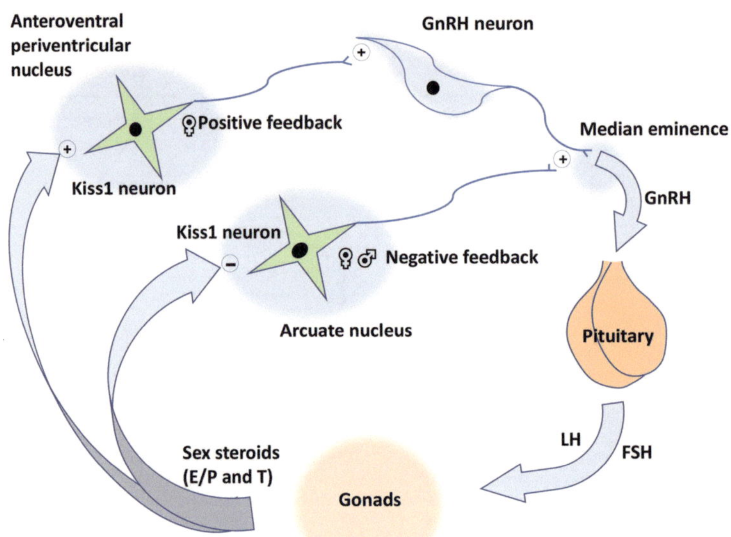

Figure 3.
Kiss1 signalling in mouse brain [32].

binding to GPR54 receptors of the hypothalamic GnRH neurons induce the release of GnRH to the pituitary circulation. GnRH induces the release of gonadotropins (FSH, LH) from the pituitary by binding to the GnRH receptors in the pituitary gland (**Figure 3**) [31, 32].

The molecular mechanisms underlying the different effects of estrogen on the Kiss1 expression in ARC and AVPV is yet to be known. However, progesterone receptors are also thought to be involved in this phenomenon. Kiss1 neurons are colocalized with or stand very close to progesterone neurons in mouse. Tyrosine hydroxylase and Kiss1 mRNAs are colocalized in AVPV but not in ARC. Consequently, it is thought that dopamine is also involved in the induction of estrogen-dependent Kiss1 expression in AVPV [33].

In mouse, ARC Kiss1 neurons synthesize Tachykinin (TAC), neurokinin-B (NKB), and dynorphin (Dyn) in variable quantities depending on species; therefore, they are also known as KNDy (Kisspeptin/Neurokinin/Dynorphin) neurons. NKB and Dyn have been shown to mutually act on kisspeptin neurosecretion [34].

5. The effect of kisspeptin on puberty

The detection of the role of the kisspeptin receptor mutation in leading to idiopathic hypogonadotropic hypogonadism paved the way for studies to further investigate the other roles played by the Kisspeptin, Kiss1, and Kiss1r systems in the field of reproductive endocrinology [10]. The direct/indirect effects of kisspeptin on GnRH neurons leave no doubt that kisspeptin plays a critical role in pubertal activation. Indeed, studies on various species have shown that the Kiss1 and/or Kiss1r expression increases significantly with the onset of puberty [21]. In a study on mice, it was shown that the Kiss1 mRNA expression significantly increased in AVPV during puberty [35]. Also, centrally or peripherally administered kisspeptin in juvenile female rats shortened the timing of vaginal opening by stimulating LH release and ovulation [36, 37]. Similarly, the increase in kisspeptin-54 signal frequency in primates occur at the beginning of puberty, supporting the findings associated with the pubertal increase in kisspeptin secretion [38]. Kiss1 mRNA expression increases in ARC during puberty along with an associated increase in LH secretion in Rhesus monkeys [39].

Kisspeptin receptor damage impair normal sexual development and to result in the failure of starting puberty. Despite the synthesis of GnRH at normal levels in the hypothalamic GnRH neurons, LH/FSH secretions do not occur and pituitary gonadotropic cells remain unresponsive to externally administered GnRH in such cases [40]. The emergence of problems in the process of starting puberty in the presence of kisspeptin deficiencies has led to the idea that kisspeptin may be an important factor for the start of sexual maturation. This idea has been confirmed by significantly increased levels of released GnRH via kisspeptin injections in mammals and by the acceleration of pubertal start via repeated Kisspeptin injections in juvenile rats. Thus, it has been proven that Kisspeptin certainly participates in pubertal development [41].

A cerebral antibody binds and inactivates kisspeptin in the female rats, impairing or even stopping reproductive functions. Also, the administration of kisspeptin in fasted rats sustains the release of GnRH and that mammals suspend their reproductive functions during states of long-term hunger in order to spend energy only enough to maintain physiological requirements. Nonetheless, the administration of kisspeptin reverses this natural process and restarts reproductive functions [42].

Nitric oxide (NO) is another potential mediator that can affect the onset of puberty since it is a mediator involved in several vital functions such as gonadotropin release, steroidogenesis, folliculogenesis, ovulation, luteal development, luteolysis, and pregnancy [43, 44]. Neuronal nitric oxide synthase (nNOS) is one of the three forms of an enzyme that oxidizes L-arginine to L-citrulline and NO. nNOS neurons in mice and rats contain high densities of ERα [45]. In rats, NO stimulates LH and GnRH release. In mice, deletion of nNOS causes infertility and hypogonadism [46]. Furthermore, recent evidence suggests that kisspeptin may directly act on the release of NO. In adult female mice, kisspeptin close-contacts to nNOS neurons have been observed in the ARC and preoptic region; however, Kiss1r is expressed only from nNOS neurons in the preoptic region [47].

6. Kisspeptin in female infertility

Kisspeptin and neurokinin-B agonists can be used to stimulate the HPG axis in conditions associated with infertility due to central nervous system causes if the system of GnRH neurons is intact. Kisspeptin and neurokinin-B may offer a novel therapeutic approach to treat failures associated with increased/reduced gonadotropin pulsatile secretion. Kisspeptins may be associated with a lower risk of ovarian hyperstimulation syndrome (OHSS) compared to human chorionic gonadotropin (hCG) injections [48]. In polycystic ovary syndrome (PCOS), kisspeptin antagonists can help normalize LH hypersecretion along with ovulation and follicular development [49].

In a study on patients with unexplained infertility (UI), PCOS, and male factor infertility (MFI); In PCOS group kisspeptin levels were measured and found to be significantly higher compared to the MFI and UI groups. The investigators suggested that IU can be treated with kisspeptin injections and that high kisspeptin levels can be a reliable indicator to estimate the antral follicle count (AFC) and to diagnose PCOS [50].

In women with functional hypothalamic amenorrhea (HA) due to low body weight, the administration of kisspeptin-54 acutely stimulates secretion of gonadotropin and that the effect on gonadotropin secretion is significant after the first injection but diminishes considerably (tachyphylaxis) after injections for two weeks [51]. Nevertheless, the frequency of injections was changed from twice a day to twice a week in another study, and gonadotropin response was sustained [52]. Eight-hour intravenous infusion of kisspeptin-54 has been shown to temporarily increase LH pulse frequency and amplitude in women with hypothalamic amenorrhea [53].

Hyperprolactinemia is one of the leading causes of female infertility as it causes hypogonadotropic anovulation [54]. Since kisspeptin neurons have recently been shown to express prolactin receptors, kisspeptin has been identified as the key mediator involved in this system [55]. In mice, hyperprolactinemia causes anovulation through decreased gonadotropin and GnRH secretion and low levels of kisspeptin expression. Kisspeptin administration in these mice repairs ovarian cycle and gonadotropin secretion. It suggests that kisspeptin neurons have a role in hyperprolactinemic anovulation [56].

Endometriosis is a disease that causes infertility in women [57]. A study conducted in 2012 about endometriosis reported that Kiss1 expression could not be detected in any sample taken from endometriosis patients [58]. In one study, researchers found that the level of Kiss1 expression was statistically significantly higher in endometriosis lesions compared to the level determined in eutopic glandular endometrium and concluded that Kiss1 might have a possible role in the pathogenesis of endometriosis [59]. Another study reported that Kiss1r mRNA levels were statistically significantly higher in the cumulus cells of endometriosis patients compared to healthy oocyte donors. In consequence, researchers argue that the increased Kiss1r expression may be one of the many factors involved in the root cause of endometriosis and related infertility [60].

A study in women suffering from infertility, investigating the genetic association between the neurokinin (TAC3/TAC3R) systems and kisspeptin (Kiss1/Kiss1r) and investigating the expression of these systems, found that the expression of Kiss1, TAC3, and TAC3R was downregulated in the cumulus cells. Similarly, these three genes have been reported to be downregulated in older women with age-related infertility [60]. In that study, these findings could only be attributed to age because infertile patients were significantly older than healthy donors and because the endometriosis patients were younger and showed just an opposite expression profile compared to all other patients, including patients with age-related infertility and low responders [61].

7. Conclusion

This review has examined the association of kisspeptin with female infertility and concluded that kisspeptin has a key role in the HPG axis and can be potentially used for the treatment of reproductive disorders including hypogonadism, ovarian hyperstimulation syndrome (OHSS), polycystic ovary syndrome (PCOS), unexplained infertility (UI), male factor infertility (MFI), hypothalamic amenorrhea (HA), and endometriosis. The literature review revealed that no adverse effects were reported after kisspeptin administration in healthy individuals and patients. Therefore, kisspeptin can be used safely in both healthy and infertile individuals. Especially its positive effects on GnRH and its key role in the initiation of physiological events in the hypothalamic–pituitary-gonadal axis (HPG axis) show that kisspeptin has a say in fertility. For this reason, kisspeptin is an option that should be focused on in the solution of infertility cases that develop in mammals (humans and especially livestock) and are one of the diseases of the age.

Author details

Abdulsamed Kükürt[1*], Mushap Kuru[2], Ömer Faruk Başer[3]
and Mahmut Karapehlivan[3]

1 Department of Biochemistry, Faculty of Veterinary Medicine, Kafkas University, Kars, Turkey

2 Department of Obstetrics and Gynecology, Faculty of Veterinary Medicine, Kafkas University, Kars, Turkey

3 Department of Biochemistry, Faculty of Medicine, Kafkas University, Kars, Turkey

*Address all correspondence to: samedkukurt@gmail.com

References

[1] Definitions of infertility and recurrent pregnancy loss: a committee opinion. Fertil Steril. 2020;113(3):533-5.

[2] Aflatoonian A, Baghianimoghadam B, Partovi P, Abdoli A, Hemmati P, Tabibnejad N, et al. A new classification for female infertility. Clinical and Experimental Obstetrics & Gynecology. 2011;**38**(4):379-381

[3] Breitkopf DM, Hill M. Infertility Workup for the Women's Health Specialist. Obstet Gynecol. 2019;**133**(6):e377-e384

[4] Inhorn MC, Patrizio P. Infertility around the globe: new thinking on gender, reproductive technologies and global movements in the 21st century. Human Reproduction Update. 2015;**21**(4):411-426

[5] Lee J-H, Miele ME, Hicks DJ, Phillips KK, Trent JM, Weissman BE, et al. KiSS-1, a Novel Human Malignant Melanoma Metastasis-Suppressor Gene. JNCI J Natl Cancer Inst. 1996;**88**(23):1731-1737

[6] Kuohung W, Kaiser UB. GPR54 and KiSS-1: Role in the regulation of puberty and reproduction. Reviews in Endocrine & Metabolic Disorders. 2007;7(4):257-263

[7] Muir AI, Chamberlain L, Elshourbagy NA, Michalovich D, Moore DJ, Calamari A, et al. AXOR12, a Novel Human G Protein-coupled Receptor, Activated by the Peptide KiSS-1. The Journal of Biological Chemistry. 2001;**276**(31):28969-28975

[8] de Roux N, Genin E, Carel J-C, Matsuda F, Chaussain J-L, Milgrom E. Hypogonadotropic hypogonadism due to loss of function of the KiSS1-derived peptide receptor GPR54. Proceedings of the National Academy of Sciences. 2003;**100**(19):10972-10976

[9] Kirby HR, Maguire JJ, Colledge WH, Davenport AP. International Union of Basic and Clinical Pharmacology. LXXVII. Kisspeptin receptor nomenclature, distribution, and function. Pharmacological Reviews. 2010;**62**(4):565-578

[10] Tena-Sempere M. Kisspeptin signaling in the brain: Recent developments and future challenges. Molecular and Cellular Endocrinology. 2010;**314**(2):164-169

[11] Funes S, Hedrick JA, Vassileva G, Markowitz L, Abbondanzo S, Golovko A, et al. The KiSS-1 receptor GPR54 is essential for the development of the murine reproductive system. Biochemical and Biophysical Research Communications. 2003;**312**(4):1357-1363

[12] Seminara SB, Messager S, Chatzidaki EE, Thresher RR, Acierno JS, Shagoury JK, et al. The GPR54 Gene as a Regulator of Puberty. The New England Journal of Medicine. 2003;**349**(17):1614-1627

[13] Castellano JM, Gaytan M, Roa J, Vigo E, Navarro VM, Bellido C, et al. Expression of KiSS-1 in Rat Ovary: Putative Local Regulator of Ovulation? Endocrinology. 2006;**147**(10):4852-4862

[14] Kauffman AS, Clifton DK, Steiner RA. Emerging ideas about kisspeptin– GPR54 signaling in the neuroendocrine regulation of reproduction. Trends in Neurosciences. 2007;**30**(10):504-511

[15] Votsi E, Roussos D, Katsikis I, Karkanaki A, Kita M, Panidis D. Kisspeptins: a multifunctional peptide system with a role in reproduction, cancer and the cardiovascular system. Hippokratia. 2008;**12**(4):205-210

[16] Xu Z, Kaga S, Mochiduki A, Tsubomizu J, Adachi S, Sakai T, et al.

Immunocytochemical localization of kisspeptin neurons in the rat forebrain with special reference to sexual dimorphism and interaction with GnRH neurons. Endocrine Journal. 2012;**59**(2):161-171

[17] Zhang P, Tang M, Zhong T, Lin Y, Zong T, Zhong C, Zhang B, Ren M, Kuang H. Expression and Function of Kisspeptin during Mouse Decidualization. Wang H, editor. PLoS One. 2014;9(5):e97647.

[18] Pinilla L, Aguilar E, Dieguez C, Millar RP, Tena-Sempere M. Kisspeptins and Reproduction: Physiological Roles and Regulatory Mechanisms. Physiological Reviews. 2012;**92**(3):1235-1316

[19] West A, Vojta PJ, Welch DR, Weissman BE. Chromosome Localization and Genomic Structure of the KiSS-1 Metastasis Suppressor Gene (KISS1). Genomics. 1998;**54**(1):145-148

[20] Hameed S, Jayasena CN, Dhillo WS. Kisspeptin and fertility. The Journal of Endocrinology. 2011;**208**(2):97-105

[21] Clarkson J, Han S-K, Liu X, Lee K, Herbison AE. Neurobiological mechanisms underlying kisspeptin activation of gonadotropin-releasing hormone (GnRH) neurons at puberty. Molecular and Cellular Endocrinology. 2010;**324**(1-2):45-50

[22] Kotani M, Detheux M, Vandenbogaerde A, Communi D, Vanderwinden J-M, Le Poul E, et al. The Metastasis Suppressor Gene KiSS-1 Encodes Kisspeptins, the Natural Ligands of the Orphan G Protein-coupled Receptor GPR54. The Journal of Biological Chemistry. 2001;**276**(37):34631-34636

[23] Roseweir AK, Millar RP. The role of kisspeptin in the control of gonadotrophin secretion. Human Reproduction Update. 2008;**15**(2):203-212

[24] Ke R, Ma X, Lee LTO. Understanding the functions of kisspeptin and kisspeptin receptor (Kiss1R) from clinical case studies. Peptides. 2019;**120**:170019

[25] Colledge WH. Kisspeptins and GnRH neuronal signalling. Trends in Endocrinology and Metabolism. 2009;**20**(3):115-121

[26] Castaño JP, Martínez-Fuentes AJ, Gutiérrez-Pascual E, Vaudry H, Tena-Sempere M, Malagón MM. Intracellular signaling pathways activated by kisspeptins through GPR54: Do multiple signals underlie function diversity? Peptides. 2009;**30**(1):10-15

[27] d'Anglemont de Tassigny X, Colledge WH. The Role of Kisspeptin Signaling in Reproduction. Physiology. 2010;**25**(4):207-217

[28] Gottsch ML, Cunningham MJ, Smith JT, Popa SM, Acohido BV, Crowley WF, et al. A Role for Kisspeptins in the Regulation of Gonadotropin Secretion in the Mouse. Endocrinology. 2004;**145**(9):4073-4077

[29] Gottsch ML, Clifton DK, Steiner RA. Kisspepeptin-GPR54 signaling in the neuroendocrine reproductive axis. Molecular and Cellular Endocrinology. 2006;**254-255**:91-96

[30] Adachi S, Yamada S, Takatsu Y, Matsui H, Kinoshita M, Takase K, et al. Involvement of Anteroventral Periventricular Metastin/Kisspeptin Neurons in Estrogen Positive Feedback Action on Luteinizing Hormone Release in Female Rats. The Journal of Reproduction and Development. 2007;**53**(2):367-378

[31] Seminara SB. Metastin and its G protein-coupled receptor,

GPR54: Critical pathway modulating GnRH secretion. Frontiers in Neuroendocrinology. 2005;**26**(3-4):131-138

[32] Oakley AE, Clifton DK, Steiner RA. Kisspeptin Signaling in the Brain. Endocrine Reviews. 2009;**30**(6):713-743

[33] Robertson JL, Clifton DK, de la Iglesia HO, Steiner RA, Kauffman AS. Circadian Regulation of Kiss1 Neurons: Implications for Timing the Preovulatory Gonadotropin-Releasing Hormone/Luteinizing Hormone Surge. Endocrinology. 2009;**150**(8):3664-3671

[34] Maguire CA, Song YB, Wu M, León S, Carroll RS, Alreja M, et al. Tac1 Signaling Is Required for Sexual Maturation and Responsiveness of GnRH Neurons to Kisspeptin in the Male Mouse. Endocrinology. 2017;**158**(7):2319-2329

[35] Han S-K. Activation of Gonadotropin-Releasing Hormone Neurons by Kisspeptin as a Neuroendocrine Switch for the Onset of Puberty. The Journal of Neuroscience. 2005;**25**(49):11349-11356

[36] Matsui H, Takatsu Y, Kumano S, Matsumoto H, Ohtaki T. Peripheral administration of metastin induces marked gonadotropin release and ovulation in the rat. Biochemical and Biophysical Research Communications. 2004;**320**(2):383-388

[37] Navarro VM, Castellano JM, Fernández-Fernández R, Barreiro ML, Roa J, Sanchez-Criado JE, et al. Developmental and Hormonally Regulated Messenger Ribonucleic Acid Expression of KiSS-1 and Its Putative Receptor, GPR54, in Rat Hypothalamus and Potent Luteinizing Hormone-Releasing Activity of KiSS-1 Peptide. Endocrinology. 2004;**145**(10):4565-4574

[38] Keen KL, Wegner FH, Bloom SR, Ghatei MA, Terasawa E. An Increase in Kisspeptin-54 Release Occurs with the Pubertal Increase in Luteinizing Hormone-Releasing Hormone-1 Release in the Stalk-Median Eminence of Female Rhesus Monkeys in Vivo. Endocrinology. 2008;**149**(8):4151-4157

[39] Shahab M, Mastronardi C, Seminara SB, Crowley WF, Ojeda SR, Plant TM. Increased hypothalamic GPR54 signaling: A potential mechanism for initiation of puberty in primates. Proceedings of the National Academy of Sciences. 2005;**102**(6):2129-2134

[40] Meczekalski B, Podfigurna-Stopa A, Genazzani AR. Why kisspeptin is such important for reproduction? Gynecological Endocrinology. 2011;**27**(1):8-13

[41] Dhillo WS. Kisspeptin: A Novel Regulator of Reproductive Function. Journal of Neuroendocrinology. 2008;**20**(8):963-970

[42] Zhou Q, Chen H, Yang S, Li Y, Wang B, Chen Y, et al. High-fat diet decreases the expression of Kiss1 mRNA and kisspeptin in the ovary, and increases ovulatory dysfunction in postpubertal female rats. Reproductive Biology and Endocrinology. 2014;**12**(1):127

[43] Kükürt A, Kuru M, Karapehlivan M. Nitrik Oksit, Nitrik Oksit Sentaz ve Dişi Üreme Sistemindeki Rolleri. In: Evereklioğlu C, editor. Sağlık Bilimleri Alanında Akademik Çalışmalar - II. Gece Kitaplığı. 2020;**2**:113-123

[44] Kuru M, Kükürt A, Oral H, Öğün M. Clinical Use of Progesterone and Its Relation to Oxidative Stress in Ruminants. In: Drevenšek G, editor. Sex Hormones in Neurodegenerative Processes and Diseases. InTech; 2018. pp. 303-327

[45] Bedenbaugh MN, O'Connell RC, Lopez JA, McCosh RB, Goodman RL, Hileman SM. Kisspeptin,

gonadotrophin-releasing hormone and oestrogen receptor α colocalise with neuronal nitric oxide synthase neurones in prepubertal female sheep. Journal of Neuroendocrinology. 2018;**30**(1):e12560

[46] Gyurko R, Leupen S, Huang PL. Deletion of exon 6 of the neuronal nitric oxide synthase gene in mice results in hypogonadism and infertility. Endocrinology. 2002;**143**(7):2767-2774

[47] Hanchate NK, Parkash J, Bellefontaine N, Mazur D, Colledge WH, d'Anglemont de Tassigny X, et al. Kisspeptin-GPR54 Signaling in Mouse NO-Synthesizing Neurons Participates in the Hypothalamic Control of Ovulation. The Journal of Neuroscience. 2012;**32**(3):932-945

[48] Abbara A, Jayasena C, Comninos A, Nijher M, Christopoulos G, Izzi-Engbeaya C, et al. Kisspeptin: a novel physiological trigger for oocyte maturation in in-vitro fertilisation treatment. Lancet. 2014;**383**:S17

[49] Skorupskaite K, George JT, Anderson RA. The kisspeptin-GnRH pathway in human reproductive health and disease. Human Reproduction Update. 2014;**20**(4):485-500

[50] Kaya C, Alay İ, Babayeva G, Gedikbaşı A, Ertaş Kaya S, Ekin M, et al. Serum Kisspeptin levels in unexplained infertility, polycystic ovary syndrome, and male factor infertility. Gynecological Endocrinology. 2019;**35**(3):228-232

[51] Jayasena CN, Nijher GMK, Chaudhri OB, Murphy KG, Ranger A, Lim A, et al. Subcutaneous Injection of Kisspeptin-54 Acutely Stimulates Gonadotropin Secretion in Women with Hypothalamic Amenorrhea, But Chronic Administration Causes Tachyphylaxis. The Journal of Clinical Endocrinology and Metabolism. 2009;**94**(11):4315-4323

[52] Jayasena CN, Nijher GMK, Abbara A, Murphy KG, Lim A, Patel D, et al. Twice-Weekly Administration of Kisspeptin-54 for 8 Weeks Stimulates Release of Reproductive Hormones in Women With Hypothalamic Amenorrhea. Clinical Pharmacology and Therapeutics. 2010 Dec 27;**88**(6):840-847

[53] Jayasena CN, Comninos AN, Narayanaswamy S, Bhalla S, Abbara A, Ganiyu-Dada Z, et al. Acute and chronic effects of kisspeptin-54 administration on GH, prolactin and TSH secretion in healthy women. Clinical Endocrinology. 2014;**81**(6):891-898

[54] Molitch ME. Can prolactinomas be cured medically? Nature Reviews. Endocrinology. 2010;**6**(4):186-188

[55] Kokay IC, Petersen SL, Grattan DR. Identification of Prolactin-Sensitive GABA and Kisspeptin Neurons in Regions of the Rat Hypothalamus Involved in the Control of Fertility. Endocrinology. 2011;**152**(2):526-535

[56] Sonigo C, Bouilly J, Carré N, Tolle V, Caraty A, Tello J, et al. Hyperprolactinemia-induced ovarian acyclicity is reversed by kisspeptin administration. The Journal of Clinical Investigation. 2012;**122**(10):3791-3795

[57] Fuldeore MJ, Soliman AM. Prevalence and Symptomatic Burden of Diagnosed Endometriosis in the United States: National Estimates from a Cross-Sectional Survey of 59,411 Women. Gynecologic and Obstetric Investigation. 2017;**82**(5):453-461

[58] Alian S, Ahangarkani F, Arabsheybani S. A Case of Orf Disease Complicated with Erythema Multiforme and Bullous Pemphigoid-Like Eruptions. Case Rep Infect Dis. 2015;**2015**:1-4

[59] Timologou A, Zafrakas M, Grimbizis G, Miliaras D, Kotronis K, Stamatopoulos P, et al.

Immunohistochemical expression pattern of metastasis suppressors KAI1 and KISS1 in endometriosis and normal endometrium. European Journal of Obstetrics, Gynecology, and Reproductive Biology. 2016;**199**:110-115

[60] Blasco V, Pinto FM, Fernández-Atucha A, González-Ravina C, Fernández-Sánchez M, Candenas L. Female infertility is associated with an altered expression of the neurokinin B/ neurokinin B receptor and kisspeptin/ kisspeptin receptor systems in ovarian granulosa and cumulus cells. Fertility and Sterility. 2020;**114**(4):869-878

[61] Chatzicharalampous C. A genetic association study of kisspeptin 1/ neurokinin B systems in patients with infertility: Is it that simple? Fertility and Sterility. 2020;**114**(4):762-763

Section 5

Pregnancy

Chapter 11

Neuroendocrinology of Pregnancy: Participation of Sex Hormones

Luz Irene Pascual Mathey

Abstract

Pregnancy is characterized by hormonal changes, critical for the mother's physiological adaptation, exercising a role in the fetus's development, maintenance, protection, and nutrition. Since born, the neuroendocrine system's involvement is necessary to prevent the embryo from being rejected by the mother's immune system. These changes are regulated by fluctuations in hormones such as Progesterone, Testosterone, Androstenedione, Dehydroepiandrosterone, Estradiol, Prolactin, human Placental Lactogen, human Chorionic Gonadotropin, and Thyroid hormones, which promote the mother's development and the fetus (maternal-fetal development). Therefore, given the great importance of these hormones during pregnancy, this chapter will explain the preclinical and clinical participation of sex hormones in maternal-fetal development.

Keywords: pregnancy, hormonal changes, maternal-fetal development

1. Introduction

During pregnancy, the neuroendocrine system undergoes significant hormonal fluctuations determined by stimulatory and inhibitory inputs from the mother and fetus to maintain the internal environment (milieu). This process is regulated mainly by both the maternal brain and the placenta, acting through the maternal-placental-fetal unit (MPFU). It also serves as a protection system against stress and immune responses [1, 2].

Interestingly, the neuroendocrine responses generate a feedback circuit regulated by the placenta. This organ begins its development in days six-seven after conception. It has been considered a passive organ for many years, acting as a barrier between the mother and the fetus, provide nourishing and eliminate metabolism products such as urea, uric acid, and creatinine. However, the placenta is a neuroendocrine organ that can synthesize and release hormones, neuroactive factors, and other mediators, allowing the proper development of the fetus's maternal tissues to ensure an optimal pregnancy, allowing the fetus to adapt and survive under conditions of stress, infections, hypoxia, and malnutrition [3, 4]. This neuroendocrine mechanism involves at least three different endocrine axes; the hypothalamus-pituitary-gonads axis (HPG), the hypothalamus-pituitary–adrenal gland axis (HPA), and the hypothalamus-pituitary-thyroid axis (HPT), to ensure optimal maternal-fetal development [1].

Specifically, the HPG axis, which is the central axis involved in regulating the reproductive function in vertebrates by a releasing pulsing of GnRH at the hypothalamus and placenta, has a decisive role in the different stages of pregnancy. In this sense, it plays a central role in regulating MPFU development through positive and negative regulation of sex hormones [1].

2. Gonadotropin-releasing hormone (GnRH), FSH, and LH, primary mediators of sex hormones releasing

The GnRH is a hormone synthesized by the hypothalamic neurons. It travels through the portal-pituitary-system to bind to its receptors (GnRHR-I) in pituitary cells (gonadotrophs), activating the synthesis of FSH (Follicle-stimulating hormone) and LH (Luteinizing hormone). These hormones are released into the systemic circulation to act on sex organs regulating both oogenesis and spermatogenesis. Interestingly, GnRH isoforms (GnRH-I and GnRH-II) have also been identified in other tissues, including the testicles, prostate, mammary gland, endometrium, and placenta. In these organs, it has been shown that GnRH-II acts by binding to GnRHR-II receptors [5].

The functions associated with these isoforms are the production of the β-human chorionic gonadotropin (β-hCG) by the syncytiotrophoblast in the early stages of pregnancy. Here, β-hCG intervenes in at least two vital functions, avoiding luteolysis and ensuring Progesterone's production (P4) until the placenta is implanted. Thus, specific conditions that interfere with this endocrine axis before weeks seven to nine of gestation would culminate in pregnancy loss [5].

Moreover, recent evidence indicates that GnRH is involved in the maternal-fetal environment's remodeling (milieu) that allows the fetus's correct implantation. This process is accompanied by increased proliferation of trophoblasts, which invade the decidua and form the outer and inner layers of syncytiotrophoblast, directly contacting maternal tissue. In this condition, the expression of specific metalloproteinases (MMP) is affected. Preclinical studies have shown that both isoforms (GnRH-I and GnRH-II) modify cellular matrix metalloproteinases' expression. Two of them, MMP-2 and MMP-9, are the most directly involved in the migration and invasion of trophoblasts [5].

In addition to the above, it has been shown that both isoforms can produce proangiogenic cytokines, playing a central role in the rerouting of immune system cells involved in the restructuring of the arteries in the maternal-fetal interface [5]. Therefore, GnRH's direct participation is vital for all physiological, hormonal, and structural changes that will culminate in the fetus's correct implantation.

On the other hand, GnRH causes the stimulation of the pituitary hormone's LH and FSH to regulate the sexual function. However, preclinical studies showed that both hormones are inhibited because of Progesterone and Estrogen increased production during pregnancy. Moreover, FSH and LH level rises on day ten after birth, which correlates to the decrease in sex hormones. In this sense, it has been established that the reduction of sex hormones after delivery performs negative feedback, which can achieve the complete reestablishment of reproductive function two months later after birth [6].

Interestingly, these data provide information valuable in understanding the positive and negative feedback mechanisms that play the sexual hormones during the pregnancy to maintain the MPFU.

3. Progesterone, the "pregnancy hormone"

Progesterone (P4) is considered the "pregnancy hormone" because it is critical for gestational maintenance [3]. During this stage, P4 is produced mainly by the ovary's luteal body until the twelfth week of pregnancy. After that, its release is principally maintained by the placenta, reaching levels of up to 3 μg/g, while blood concentrations range from 100 to 500 nM, being four to six times its basal levels [7, 8]. These values rise significantly as gestational age progresses. It is involved in both the maintenance and development of the endometrium and inhibiting the uterus' smooth muscle from preventing premature contractions (spontaneous abortion) [8].

Interestingly, the increase in this hormone's levels seems to be regulated by an independent mechanism that generally restricts the synthesis of this hormone, being produced by the placental trophoblast cells in response to the stimuli produced in the uterine-fetal microenvironment [9]. At this level, its synthesis is carried out by converting the maternal cholesterol to the pro-hormone pregnenolone into the mitochondrial cytochrome P450. After that, by the action of 3-β-hydroxysteroid dehydrogenases (HSD), it is metabolized to Progesterone. Of the total synthesized Progesterone, 90% go into the maternal circulation, and the remaining 10% goes into fetal circulation [10].

Placental P4 plays an essential role in establishing a pregnancy, as it is responsible for inhibiting uterine contractions that occur at the myometrium's smooth muscle. In this context, the deficiency of this hormone during the luteal phase has been widely related to infertility and loss of the pregnancy, presenting abortion, a situation that can occur at any stage of pregnancy [8, 9]. Besides, it is involved in the formation of decidua (a layer that coats the endometrium). In this sense, P4 is involved in the structural changes that the uterus undergoes during this period by increasing blood vessels' permeability and endometrial density. Moreover, it has been suggested that the increase in decidual density is related to a lower likelihood of miscarriage. Also, P4 ensures the integrity of the fetus-maternal interface during the process of trophoblastic invasion and placenta formation [8, 11, 12]. What is more, P4 blocks the early production of T-cell lymphopoiesis protective role intrauterine environment's immune system (milieu). For that reason, it has been suggested that Progesterone acts as an immunosteroid since a satisfactory pregnancy depends on maternal tolerance to the fetal 'semi-allograft' [8].

Similarly, it has been suggested that the increase in P4 levels induces changes in gene expression in the uterine endometrium, indirectly favoring embryo growth [12]. Furthermore, it is a crucial factor between the endocrine and immune system since it has been shown that this hormone is involved in the implantation of tissue, preventing it from being rejected by the mother, a mechanism that appears to be mediated by Th cells (helper T cells), as well as by the interleukins (IL) IL-3, IL-4, IL-5, and IL-10, in such a way, it has been suggested that through inhibition of Th 1 cells and increased production of interleukins, Progesterone is involved in the implantation of the fetus and its maintenance [7, 8].

On the other hand, P4 is involved in regulating the expression of uterine dendritic cells. These are known as antigen-presenting cells (APCs) involved in innate immune response and tolerance maintenance. However, in immature stages, these cells have a tolerogenic phenotype characterized by the low expression of co-stimulating molecules and pro-inflammatory cytokines. Thereby, it has been shown that in the early stages of pregnancy, Progesterone prevents dendritic cells' maturation. All these previous actions contributed to the maintenance of pregnancy [8].

More interesting, it has been shown that P4 is also involved in reducing gestational stress. In this sense, it has been shown that it can over-express the mPRα gene, which encodes for a membrane receptor present in Cytolytic T lymphocytes CD8 + T cells, and whose increase has been linked to a protective effect against stress-induced abortion [7].

Finally, it is known that P4 levels decrease at the end of pregnancy, a phenomenon that is related to the onset of labor. Hence, an excellent regulatory mechanism of P4 (both at the endocrine and immunological level) from the beginning to the culmination of pregnancy, it is necessary to the implantation, maintenance, and completion of this [12, 13].

4. The modulatory hormones in pregnancy; testosterone (T), androstenedione (A4), and dehydroepiandrosterone (DHEA)

The androgenic hormones T, A4, and DHEA, plays a central role in regulating reproductive processes in many mammalian species. Besides, the presence of androgen receptors has also been demonstrated in different tissues such as the ovary, the myometrium, and placenta, where they are known to participate in implanting the fetus and placentation. In this sense, it has been shown that, once pregnancy occurs, androgen synthesis takes place in the small luteal cells (SLC) of the corpus luteum by stimulation of the human chorionic gonadotrophin (hCG) [3, 14]. In addition to the above, once the placenta has been established, it becomes an independent androgen production source [14]. In this aspect, placental syncytiotrophoblast uses the circulating DHEA, provided by the maternal and fetal adrenal glands, turning it into A4 and T. Which, in turn, as will be discussed later, can be converted to estrogens by different routes to regulate embryonic development [3, 15]. Interestingly, it has been suggested that myometrium could be another important source of androgens during pregnancy; a recent *in vitro* study showed that this tissue could also produce T and A4 [15].

Suppressively, these hormones are coordinated synthesized during pregnancy. Specifically, it has been shown that T levels increase in the first trimester of pregnancy, reaching a plateau in the second trimester, to later decrease slightly, rising considerably in the last month of pregnancy [14, 15]. Concerning A4, the study carried out by Satué et al. (2018) in mares shows that this hormone rises during gestation, from the second month of pregnancy, reaching a peak maximum in the first stage of pregnancy, and, in the second state, it reduces significantly, reaching its lowest levels in the last month of gestation. However, a clinical study conducted by Makieva et al. (2014) showed that A4 remains stable throughout pregnancy without significant fluctuations. About DHEA, it increases progressively from the first to the fifth month of pregnancy, reaches its highest levels, then begins to decrease between months 6 and 7, reaching its lowest levels in the last month of pregnancy in mares, which is agree with the observed in pregnant women, with levels up to 50% lower than those observed in non-pregnant women, an effect associated with negative E2 feedback to the maternal adrenal glands [14, 15].

The fluctuations in these hormones have specific functions during pregnancy. The significant increase observed in the first months of gestation is associated with the function of the corpus luteum, which uses T for estrogens' production (analyzed in the next topic), regulating the implantation and decidualization. Later, the decrease observed in the middle of the gestation is related significantly to the development of the fetal gonads, providing the necessary substrates for the synthesis of placental estrogens. So, the primary site of estrogen synthesis at this stage could be the fetus. Finally, T's elevation in the last stage of pregnancy, but not of A4 and DHEA, could be associated with the restructuring that the cervix must undergo to be prepared for the moment of delivery. At this stage, it has been shown that the cervix can convert T into another metabolite, Dihydrotestosterone (DHT), through the action of 5-alpha-reductase. This androgen is involved in restructuring the cervix's extracellular matrix tissue, including the structural changes that allow the myometrium's contractility [14, 15].

Therefore, these interesting data confirm the surprising interrelation and interdependence between estrogens and androgens produced by MPFU to protect and ensure pregnancy's proper development.

5. Estrogens in pregnancy, an orchestral regulatory mechanism

Estrogens are a group of four different steroid hormones: Oestrone (E1), 17β-Oestradiol (E2), Oestriol (E3), and Oesterol (E4), cyclically synthesized in response to changes during the ovarian cycle, specifically during the pre-ovulation phase, favoring folliculogenesis. However, estrogens also play a central role in the growth of the uterus and mammary gland. It increases the blood flow indispensable for transporting nutrients between the uterus and the fetus [16]. During pregnancy and up to the time of delivery, significant amounts of estrogens are released by the maternal-fetus-placental unit, formed by the luteal body, placenta, and the fetal adrenal cortex [3], suffering significant adjustments between the weeks seven to nine of pregnancy, reaching its highest levels at the time of delivery [17, 18].

17β-Oestradiol (E2) is the most abundant hormone synthesized during pregnancy. In connection with this, until the third month of pregnancy, significant levels of E2 are released by the luteal body, a period from which the primary site of estrogen production is the placenta [3]. It should be noted that the placenta has no autonomic innervation, so these increases occur in response to close communication between the mother and the fetus, where the hormone acts in an autocrine-paracrine form in the development of the mammary gland and uterus, as well as in the development of sexual characteristics in the fetus. This connection allows the placenta and fetus to exchange and share steroid precursors, thus achieving their hormonal self-regulation [18].

Several studies have shown that the increase in estrogen levels is the result of a mutual exchange between the mother and placenta, in which the placenta uses the circulating androgen DHEA produced by the adrenal glands of the MPFU, where it is converted to Testosterone and Androstenedione and then metabolized to E1 and E2 with the help of the cytochrome cyp450 aromatase enzyme [3, 7]. In such a way, both the mother and the fetus contribute to the increase in estrogen synthesis, regulating their production. In addition to this, and due to the high maintenance of this hormone throughout pregnancy, there is sufficient evidence to suggest that regulation in levels of this hormone could also be at the neural level, where E2 could act as a trigger factor of the HPA gland axis. So, the adaptive changes that occur in the mother-fetus are regulated by a positive feedback mechanism, in which the binding of E2 to their receptors at the brain could be sending signals to the adrenal glands for producing a more significant amount of DHEA, thus maintaining their constant levels [19]. Therefore, it seems clear that estrogen levels regulation during pregnancy occurs both locally, by an interaction of the placental-fetal unit and in an autonomic way, with the direct participation of the Central Nervous System.

Concerning its functions, estrogen has been shown to act through binding to nuclear receptors, participating in multiple processes to ensure the maintenance of pregnancy having different roles: in human endometrial explant cultures, they are involved in uterine vascular restructuring by binding to their nuclear receptors present in epithelial and stromal cells of the cervix and endometrium, acting regulating the expression of different genes that control intrauterine growth, maturation of vital organs such as mammary glands for breastfeeding and childbirth [16–18, 20]. Besides, it promotes the processes of angiogenesis and vasodilation that allow the transfer and exchange of nutrients and oxygen between the placenta and the fetus through uterine and fetal circulation, a process associated with an increase in endothelial production of nitric oxide [3, 21].

On the other hand, in the primary culture of endometrial-epithelial cells (ESC), it has been found that E2 plays an essential role at the beginning of pregnancy by acting in processes such as differentiation and cell proliferation through the secretion of insulin growth factor type 1 (IGF-1) [22]. Also, it increases the rate at which the fertilized egg travels through the fallopian tube, so low estrogen levels promote ectopic pregnancies because the egg stays longer in the fallopian tube [23].

In addition to the above, estrogens E1, E3, and E4, also, play a central role in pregnancy. E1 is the most abundant conjugated estrogen (estrone sulfate) during pregnancy; it increases from the first trimester of pregnancy, reaching its maximum peak in the 35th week of gestation; among its functions, the decrease of estrogenicity has been indicated in the time of delivery [24]. E3 (Oestriol) is also considered a derivative of estradiol, whose primary role during pregnancy is increased utero-placental blood flow during pregnancy. However, a specific function has also been suggested in the induction of myometrial cells' contractions through the increase of connexin-4, allowing the restructuring of the myometrium that will trigger the initiation of labor [3]. On the other hand, Oesterol (E4) has an uncertain function during pregnancy since it is produced exclusively by the fetal liver starting up from the ninth week of pregnancy, reaching its significantly elevated levels after week 30, with a peak at week 40. Although its function is unclear, preclinical studies have shown that it can bind to estrogen and progesterone receptors at the uterus, producing histological structural changes and biochemical fluctuations, essential during the differentiation of endometrial cells in pregnancy and delivery [25].

Therefore, during pregnancy, the hyperestrogenic state plays a significant role in maternal-fetal development, being a key piece in fetal growth. Hence, all these actions make the estrogen pleiotropic essential hormones in pregnancy.

6. Prolactin in pregnancy, more than a lactation hormone

Prolactin (PRL) is a protein hormone synthesized by the lactotroph cells of the anterior pituitary gland. Unlike other pituitary hormones, its release is inhibited by Dopamine (DA), a hypothalamic factor produced by dopaminergic neurons located in the arcuate nucleus, which has not only been shown to be able to regulate the release of PRL but can act at the lactotrophic cells, regulating their proliferation [1]. In addition, PRL can control its release, directly stimulating dopaminergic neurons and through direct and indirect mechanisms regulated by E2 [23].

In this sense, a preclinical rat model study showed that in the different reproductive stages, PRL intervenes in a coordinated manner with E2 and Dopamine in regulating the proliferative activity of lactotrophic cells. In this collaborative process, these cells' activity is elevated in the estrus and delivery stages. But it is decreased during the early stages of pregnancy and lactation, even though PRL levels are increased in all these reproductive stages. In this context, it has been suggested that E2 participates in stimulating the release of PRL during the early stages of pregnancy and lactation by acting at the hypothalamic level regulating both the increase in prolactin levels and the activity of the lactotroph cells when DA is not present, play a dual role in the release of this hormone [23, 26].

Evermore, during pregnancy, essential adaptations occur to allow the release of significant amounts of this hormone by the stimulation caused by the mammary gland and the luteal body [27], with substantial elevations from the twentieth week of pregnancy, until after childbirth [26]. Specifically, PRL has been shown to play a vital role in regulating IL-10 and IL-12 interleukins (essential regulators of immune responses during inflammatory processes). On the one hand, IL-12 interleukin has a pro-inflammatory function, activating itself in response to situations such as stress. On the other hand, IL-10 is an anti-inflammatory cytokine, which intervenes in the regulation of the expression of IL-12. In this sense, it has been shown that, during pregnancy, PRL increases the concentration of IL-10, an effect suggested is associated with the proper maintenance of this [28].

At the clinical level, this hormone has been shown to provide luteotropic support to the luteal body by intervening in the biosynthesis of P4 for its maintenance in the first three months of pregnancy, having an indirect function in the implantation of fetus in the uterus, as well as in the induction of vascular factors necessary for the increase in the volume of the luteal body [1, 29]. On the other hand, it acts directly on the mammary gland, determining the growth and development of alveoli, promoting the expression of genes related to milk synthesis and lactopoiesis. It also helps maintain the luteal body's integrity and decidual cell survival [30]. Moreover, it is involved in the synthesis of relaxin, a hormone responsible for dilating the cervix during labor, thus facilitating the fetus's expulsion [27].

PRL, it has been shown to play an essential role in regulating leptins expression in the gestational stage [31]. Leptins are hormones produced mostly by adipocytes, whose central role is related to the regulation of body weight, appetite, and energy homeostasis. The increase in their plasma levels is associated with the rise in the amount of body fat. However, during the gestational stage, vast quantities of leptins are released by the ovary and placenta, remaining constant throughout pregnancy, intervening in the regulation of fetal weight and growth, and with the development of gestational diabetes [32]. In this sense, the increase in PRL levels has been suggested to inhibit the receptor to leptins (LepR), thus blocking the signaling pathways that regulate the development of gestational diabetes [31].

Finally, it has a central role in mother–child recognition by increasing the generation of neurons at the olfactory bulb level, which is essential for such recognition [29]. For that reason, PRL recognizes like a multifaceted hormone, with dual actions during and after delivery.

7. Human placental lactogen, an exclusive metabolic hormone in pregnancy

The human placental lactogen hormone (hPL), known as human Chorionic somatomammotropin, is a polypeptide hormone elevated during pregnancy and is produced exclusively by the placenta [3]. hPL levels are detected between the first and second weeks of placenta gestation. However, it is released into the maternal circulation between the third to sixth week of pregnancy, being possible its detection, which increases until reaching its constant levels with a significant increase at the end of pregnancy with substantial effects after delivery [3].

Although there is controversy regarding its participation during pregnancy, it has been suggested that its primary function is the regulation of maternal metabolism of lipids and carbohydrates, being crucial to maintaining energy homeostasis between mother and fetus. In this sense, at the preclinical level, it has been shown that it stimulates the production of the IGF-1 factor in maternal hepatocytes. It modulates intermediate metabolism by increasing food intake (orexigenic drive), which favors the increase in glucose available for transfer to the fetus and prevents the development of gestational diabetes caused by peripheral resistance, typical at this stage [1, 3].

Moreover, it has been suggested that it has a central role in intrauterine growth because more than 50% of neonates with stunted growth have shown a deficiency in hPL levels. It is also believed that, by stimulating the uptake of glucose, glycerol, and free fatty acids, it could significantly participate in fat deposits, serving as an energy-saving mechanism for the fetus [1, 3].

Furthermore, it is well documented that in a normal state of pregnancy, insulin sensitivity decreases with the advance of the gestational state, which allows the fetus to maintain energy, an effect caused by a joint inhibitory action of peptide hormones (C-reactive protein, leptins, and hPL) on insulin levels causing dysfunction of pancreatic β-cells, named "diabetogenic condition." However, a clinical study conducted by Ngala et al. (2017) showed that, throughout pregnancy, important maternal factors could predict the development of gestational diabetes mellitus (GDM) in addition to the already known factors of obesity and family history. In this sense, the levels of glucose, insulin, glycosylated hemoglobin (GHb), and hPL, among others, are increased in pregestational pregnant women, an effect not observed in non-diabetic pregnant women. Interestingly, under this condition, E2 and P4 levels decreased in pre-diabetic women, while in healthy women, the levels of both hormones are increased. On the other hand, between weeks 24–28 of gestation, an increase in Progesterone, Estradiol, Leptins, GHb, and Fasting blood glucose (FBG) was observed in developing GMD, an effect associated with the increased insulin resistance. Controversially, although there is little information linking hPL with the development of GDM, it is believed that the decrease in the levels of this hormone after delivery is associated with the reduction in glucose resistance and with the increased risk of diabetes-prediabetes in nursing mothers [33, 34].

Interestingly, hPL participates in lactation by stimulating the breast epithelium, facilitating breast development during the gestational stage. In this process, both hormones (hPL and PRL) act in maternal behavior, suppressing stress responses in the last stage of pregnancy and lactation [1]. In this sense, it has been shown that dopaminergic neurons' activity can be maintained by hPL [23].

All these results confirm the metabolic action of hPL in pregnancy and lactation, alone or together to other placental and maternal hormones.

8. Human chorionic gonadotropic (hCG), the placental essential hormone

HCG is considered one of the essential hormones during gestational development, having similarities with other members of the same family of glycoproteic proteins such as LH and pituitary FSH. Its synthesis is regulated by the luteal body and placenta, exercising a pleiotropic role during gestation by autocrine and paracrine mechanisms [3]. It is possible to detect significant levels from day eight after fertilization, reaching its maximum levels around the tenth week of development. After which, it maintains at constant levels when the placenta is fully developed. At this point, the luteal body's secretions are no longer necessary [3].

It participates in the process of steroidogenesis and in the restoration-maintenance of the luteal body, where it acts as a relay system, whose purpose is to prevent menstruation by increasing the synthesis of P4, allowing that the embryo can be implanted in the uterine endometrium, ensuring pregnancy until placental production of Progesterone is well established [3].

The hCG has also been shown to have a structure like Thyroid stimulating hormone (TSH) to bind to the same receptors, having implications for regulating thyrotropic activity. Preclinical studies have shown that maternal TSH decreases at the end of the third trimester of pregnancy. This decrease correlates with increased placental hCG and fetal thyroxine-binding globulin (TGB) [1]. *In vitro* studies have shown that it can have angiogenic effects; it increases vascular-endothelial growth factor (VEGF) and placental microvascular endothelial cells [3].

Moreover, clinical studies have shown that it is also involved in the differentiation of cytotrophoblast in syncytiotrophoblast, constituting an essential factor in the secretion of relaxing decidual production of PRL. On the other hand, it has androgenic properties. It can promote the synthesis of DHEA by the fetal adrenal cortex, regulating both testicular function and fetal male differentiation during the first weeks of gestation [35]. In addition, it has been suggested that it has participated in other functions; in the immune system, stimulates the production of the anti-inflammatory interleukins IL-8 and IL-10, and inhibits lymphocyte response, preventing rejection of the fetus, suggesting an immunosuppressive role of hCG during pregnancy; it stimulates testicular Leydig cells for testosterone production and provides nutrients and hormones for optimal maintenance of intrauterine microenvironment [3, 35]. So, the metabolic implications of this hormone suggested it like a metabolic hormone in pregnancy.

9. Cortisol and glucocorticoids; is it just stress in pregnancy?

The secretion of cortisol levels during pregnancy is regulated by the placenta, which, by secreting the corticotropin-releasing hormone (CRH), produces an exponential increase in cortisol from the eighth week of gestation up to three times above systemic values [5, 36]. It is present in both the maternal and fetal phases but at different levels; under normal conditions, cortisol levels reach 200 ng/ml at the end of pregnancy, while fetal levels range from around 20 ng/ml [37]. These differences are due to the presence of a natural barrier that prevents maternal cortisol, whose molecular composition can cross the placenta, quickly reaches fetal space [38, 39].

This barrier corresponds to the uterus/fetus interface and is mainly com posed of maternal decidua and fetal placenta chorion. Here the regulation of cortisol is carried out through placental glycoprotein P, as well as the enzyme 11-β-hydroxysteroid-dehydrogenase (11-β-HSD) type 2 of trophoblastic and fetal cells, which inactivates cortisol by converting it into cortisone to avoid exposure of the fetus to high levels of cortisol [37, 40]. However, because of its role in organ maturation and labor, fetal cortisol increases towards the end of pregnancy by several mechanisms: a) decrease of 11-β-HSD type 2 in fetal tissues, b) increased synthesis of cortisol by the fetal adrenal gland, and c) increased 11-β-HSD type 1 in fetal tissues, which converts cortisone, into active cortisol [41].

As for the functions of cortisol during pregnancy, glucocorticoids (GC) have been described as participating in the processes of implantation and formation of decidua, as well as in fetal development and maturation, and initiation of childbirth [17, 36, 42]. Elevated levels of GC present during pregnancy are involved in the suppression of inflammation of the uterus, placenta, and fetal membranes, which contributes to maintaining the homeostasis necessary for the maintenance of pregnancy [42]. Moreover, recent evidence suggests that significant increases in cortisol levels play a critical role in the baby's growth in the postnatal stage [43]. In this sense, studies have shown that high concentrations of cortisol during the fetal phase positively correlated with weight gain within the first five years of postnatal growth, indicating that the higher increase in placental cortisol levels, the more significant weight gain can be observed in children during this stage, suggesting that hormonal changes within the maternal-fetal environment have repercussions in post-birth stages, a highly relevant endocrinological aspect [43].

Conversely, cortisol is also involved in developing pregnancy complications, being responsible for the so-called "Hypothalamic Stress Amenorrhea," whose consequence is the generation of miscarriages [8, 44]. On the one hand, it has been shown that low maternal cortisol levels compromise the placenta's structure. In contrast, elevated levels can lead to miscarriages, uterine contractions from placental CRH deregulation, the elevation of fetal cortisol levels, and obstetric alterations by activation of the HPA gland axis [14, 36, 38, 45]. In this sense, two main axes, the HPA, and the sympathetic nervous system-adrenal medulla exerts a negative effect on the reproductive system when activated in stressful situations. In this feedback mechanism, the CRH that is produced at the pituitary can act, in a short negative feedback mechanism, directly inhibiting GnRH at the hypothalamus.

Even more, cortisol act at the pituitary to inhibit the release of LH and FSH, and, consequently, inhibits steroidal ovarian hormones, Estrogen, and P4, resulting in abortion. It has been confirmed in preclinical and clinical studies, where exposure to stressors, such as noise, has been verified to induce miscarriages, with a significant decrease in P4 levels [8, 44]. More interesting, stress increases the excitability of the sympathetic nervous system, resulting in a decrease in blood flow supply to the placenta caused placental hypoxia and increased generation of reactive oxygen species, causing damage to trophoblasts; the outer layer of the blastocyst, responsible for providing nourishing to the embryo [44].

Finally, it has also been suggested that high cortisol levels could mediate a disbalance in T helper cells Th 1 and Th 2, with a specific impact in the decrease of adaptative immune system responses that allow the fetus's maintenance. However, more studies are needed to confirm this [44]. So, it is evident that cortisol is not just a "stress hormone"; it has several functions supporting the MPFU.

10. Thyroid hormones in pregnancy; regulation by sex hormones?

During pregnancy, high estrogens and corticosteroids induce an increase in TGB levels in the liver, which is significant from week twenty of gestation, reaching its maximum level from week twenty to twenty-four. The rise in TGB during the first half of pregnancy is related to further deiodination of the inner ring of the hormones T4 (Thyroxine) and T3 (Triiodothyronine) at the placenta, which is responsible for the physiological effect attributed to them [46, 47].

As far as the fetus is concerned, it has been shown that there are at least two mechanisms for it to contribute to thyroid hormones: the development of the fetal thyroid gland and the maternal thyroid gland. More interesting, the increase in concentrations of T4 in the first half of pregnancy and the expression of receptors to thyroid hormones in the brain, suggesting its participation in the development of brain structures of the fetus. Moreover, from weeks twelve-fourteen, in which the fetal thyroid begins to synthesize T4, its levels increase progressively, until reaching its maximum levels between week thirty-four to thirty-six, remaining elevated until the delivery time [46].

About iodine levels begin to be detected from ten to eleven weeks of gestation, a stage in which the fetal thyroid can concentrate. Around the twelfth week, the pituitary starts to produce and synthesize TSH and TRH (Thyrotropin-releasing hormone) by the hypothalamic neurons [46].

Before the fetal thyroid develops, the placenta has a particular involvement in maternal-fetal thyroid regulation. It is responsible for exchanging thyroid hormones to the fetus, suggesting an essential role in early fetal growth. Among the functions attributed to thyroid hormones are the brain's development and the acceleration of fetal pulmonary maturation. The effect has been demonstrated in preclinical and clinical models in which fetal pulmonary growth has been shown to increase after intraamniotic injection of T3 or T4. On the other hand, the effect at the brain level has been demonstrated in intrauterine hypothyroidism conditions. It is related to irreversible damage to the brain and mental disability in children born under these conditions [46, 47].

Interestingly, clinical studies conducted in children whose mothers suffered from hypothyroidism, a condition that occurs in 0.05–0.02% during pregnancy, have shown that these irreversible changes specifically affect neurodevelopment. In this sense, it has been demonstrated that any situation that leads to the development of clinical hypothyroidism (generally associated with Graves' disease) and hypothyroxinemia (associated with overtreatment of antithyroid drugs) that can occur during the first trimester of pregnancy can lead to a cognitive delay in children, learning disorders, maturational delay, encephalopathy, and seizures among other conditions [48].

Significantly, the increase in TSH, T3, and T4 during pregnancy could have protective effects against fetal anemia because it has been suggested that they may have cardiotonic effects by direct activation of the sympathetic-adrenal nervous system, in addition to being shown to stimulate the production of erythropoietin, which is involved in the production of red blood cells and therefore in the release of oxygen to tissues [47].

In this sense, it is fascinating to understand that sex hormones regulate the release of thyroid hormones and the vital functions involved, like brain development, being crucial during pregnancy and childhood.

11. Conclusions

Pregnancy is a physiological state characterized by critical hormonal changes. Collective participation of the endocrine system is necessary to carry out adequate development and maintenance of both the mother and the fetus. This system is responsible for generating an optimal environment that provides an adequate microenvironment of communication between the maternal-placental-fetal unit, facilitating the exchange of nutrients, hormones, and oxygen, essential throughout the gestational period. These neuroendocrine processes are produced thanks to the synchronous and fluctuating production of sex hormones regulated by endocrine, paracrine, and autocrine mechanisms. Their function is essential before, during, and after the gestational period to ensure the fetus's correct development and growth.

Acknowledgements

The author thanks the National Council of Science and Technology (CONACyT) for the supporting founding.

Conflict of interest

The author declares no conflicts of interest.

Nomenclature

MPFU	Maternal-placental-fetal unit
HPG	Hypothalamus-pituitary-gonads axis
HPA	Hypothalamus-pituitary–adrenal gland axis
HPT	Hypothalamus-pituitary-thyroid axis
GnRH	Gonadotropin-releasing hormone
GnRHR-I and GnRHR-II	Gonadotropin-releasing hormone receptors I and II
FSH	Follicle-stimulating hormone
LH	Luteinizing hormone
β-hCG	β-Human chorionic gonadotropin
P4	Progesterone
MMP	Metalloproteinases
3β-HSD	3-β-hydroxysteroid-dehydrogenases
11β-HSD	11-β-hydroxysteroid-dehydrogenase
Th cells	Helper T cells
IL	Interleukins
APCs	Antigen-presenting cells
T	Testosterone
A4	Androstenedione
DHEA	Dehydroepiandrosterone
E1	Oestrone
E2	17β-Oestradiol
E3	Oestriol
E4	Oesterol
ESC	Endometrial-epithelial cells
IGF-1	Insulin growth factor type 1
PRL	Prolactin
DA	Dopamine
LepR	Leptin receptors
hPL	Human placental lactogen hormone
TSH	Thyroid Stimulating Hormone
TGB	Thyroxine-binding globulin
VEGF	Vascular-endothelial growth factor
CRH	Corticotropin-releasing hormone
GC	Glucocorticoids
T4	Thyroxine
T3	Triiodothyronine
TRH	Thyrotropin-releasing hormone
SLC	Small luteal cells
GDM	Gestational diabetes mellitus
GHb	Glycosylated Hemoglobin
FBG	Fasting blood glucose

Author details

Luz Irene Pascual Mathey
Faculty of Biological Pharmaceutical Chemistry, Veracruzana University, Gonzalo Aguirre Beltrán s/n, Zona Universitaria, Xalapa, Veracruz, Mexico

*Address all correspondence to: lupascual@uv.mx

References

[1] Voltolini C, Petraglia F. Neuroendocrinology of pregnancy and parturition. Handb Clin Neurol. 2014;124:17-36. doi: 10.1016/B978-0-444-59602-4.00002-2. PMID: 25248577.

[2] Lahita RG. The effects of sex hormones on the immune system in pregnancy. Am J Reprod Immunol. 1992 Oct-Dec;28(3-4):136-7. doi: 10.1111/j.1600-0897.1992.tb00775.x. PMID: 1285863.

[3] Costa MA. The endocrine function of human placenta: an overview. Reprod Biomed Online. 2016 Jan;32(1):14-43. doi: 10.1016/j.rbmo.2015.10.005. Epub 2015 Oct 27. PMID: 26615903.

[4] Behura SK, Dhakal P, Kelleher AM, Balboula A, Patterson A, Spencer TE. The brain-placental axis: Therapeutic and pharmacological relevancy to pregnancy. Pharmacol Res. 2019 Nov;149:104468. doi: 10.1016/j.phrs.2019.104468. Epub 2019 Oct 7. PMID: 31600597; PMCID: PMC6944055.

[5] Sasaki K, Norwitz ER. Gonadotropin-releasing hormone/gonadotropin-releasing hormone receptor signaling in the placenta. Curr Opin Endocrinol Diabetes Obes. 2011 Dec;18(6):401-8. doi: 10.1097/MED.0b013e32834cd3b0. PMID: 22024993.

[6] Hirano M, Igarashi A, Suzuki M. Dynamic changes of serum LH and FSH during pregnancy and puerperium. Tohoku J Exp Med. 1976 Mar;118(3):275-82. doi: 10.1620/tjem.118.275. PMID: 772883.

[7] Zen M, Ghirardello A, Iaccarino L, Tonon M, Campana C, Arienti S, Rampudda M, Canova M, Doria A. Hormones, immune response, and pregnancy in healthy women and SLE patients. Swiss Med Wkly. 2010 Apr 3;140(13-14):187-201. PMID: 20175004.

[8] Arck P, Hansen PJ, Mulac Jericevic B, Piccinni MP, Szekeres-Bartho J. Progesterone during pregnancy: endocrine-immune cross talk in mammalian species and the role of stress. Am J Reprod Immunol. 2007 Sep;58(3):268-79. doi: 10.1111/j.1600-0897.2007.00512.x. PMID: 17681043.

[9] Yang R, You X, Tang X, Gao L, Ni X. Corticotropin-releasing hormone inhibits progesterone production in cultured human placental trophoblasts. J Mol Endocrinol. 2006 Dec;37(3):533-40. doi: 10.1677/jme.1.02119. PMID: 17170093.

[10] Tuckey RC. Progesterone synthesis by the human placenta. Placenta. 2005 Apr;26(4):273-81. doi: 10.1016/j.placenta.2004.06.012. PMID: 15823613.

[11] Hızlı D, Köşüş N, Köşüş A, Kasap B, Kafali H, Turhan NÖ. First-trimester reference ranges for decidual thickness and its relation to progesterone levels. J Perinat Med. 2012 Sep;40(5):521-5. doi: 10.1515/jpm-2012-0035. PMID: 23104794.

[12] Leitao B, Jones MC, Fusi L, Higham J, Lee Y, Takano M, Goto T, Christian M, Lam EW, Brosens JJ. Silencing of the JNK pathway maintains progesterone receptor activity in decidualizing human endometrial stromal cells exposed to oxidative stress signals. FASEB J. 2010 May;24(5):1541-51. doi: 10.1096/fj.09-149153. Epub 2009 Dec 21. PMID: 20026682; PMCID: PMC2857868.

[13] Jeschke U, Mylonas I, Richter DU, Höcker I, Briese V, Makrigiannakis A, Friese K. Regulation of progesterone production in human term trophoblasts in vitro by CRH, ACTH and cortisol (prednisolone). Arch Gynecol Obstet. 2005 Jun;272(1):7-12. doi: 10.1007/s00404-005-0728-0. Epub 2005 Apr 16. PMID: 15834733.

[14] Makieva S, Saunders PT, Norman JE. Androgens in pregnancy: roles in parturition. Hum Reprod Update. 2014 Jul-Aug;20(4):542-59. doi: 10.1093/humupd/dmu008. Epub 2014 Mar 18. PMID: 24643344; PMCID: PMC4063701.

[15] Satué K, Marcilla M, Medica P, Ferlazzo A, Fazio E. Testosterone, androstenedione and dehydroepiandrosterone concentrations in pregnant Spanish Purebred mare. Theriogenology. 2019 Jan 1;123:62-67. doi: 10.1016/j.theriogenology.2018.09.025. Epub 2018 Sep 26. PMID: 30292857.

[16] Corcoran JJ, Nicholson C, Sweeney M, Charnock JC, Robson SC, Westwood M, Taggart MJ. Human uterine and placental arteries exhibit tissue-specific acute responses to 17β-estradiol and estrogen-receptor-specific agonists. Mol Hum Reprod. 2014 May;20(5):433-41. doi: 10.1093/molehr/gat095. Epub 2013 Dec 19. PMID: 24356876; PMCID: PMC4004081.

[17] Chang K, Lubo Zhang. Review article: steroid hormones and uterine vascular adaptation to pregnancy. Reprod Sci. 2008 Apr;15(4):336-48. doi: 10.1177/1933719108317975. PMID: 18497342; PMCID: PMC2408771.

[18] Gambino YP, Maymó JL, Pérez-Pérez A, Dueñas JL, Sánchez-Margalet V, Calvo JC, Varone CL. 17Beta-estradiol enhances leptin expression in human placental cells through genomic and nongenomic actions. Biol Reprod. 2010 Jul;83(1):42-51. doi: 10.1095/biolreprod.110.083535. Epub 2010 Mar 17. PMID: 20237333.

[19] Brunton PJ, Russell JA. The expectant brain: adapting for motherhood. Nat Rev Neurosci. 2008 Jan;9(1):11-25. doi: 10.1038/nrn2280. PMID: 18073776.

[20] King AE, Collins F, Klonisch T, Sallenave JM, Critchley HO, Saunders PT. An additive interaction between the NFkappaB and estrogen receptor signalling pathways in human endometrial epithelial cells. Hum Reprod. 2010 Feb;25(2):510-8. doi: 10.1093/humrep/dep421. Epub 2009 Dec 2. PMID: 19955102; PMCID: PMC2806182.

[21] Bai J, Qi QR, Li Y, Day R, Makhoul J, Magness RR, Chen DB. Estrogen Receptors and Estrogen-Induced Uterine Vasodilation in Pregnancy. Int J Mol Sci. 2020 Jun 18;21(12):4349. doi: 10.3390/ijms21124349. PMID: 32570961; PMCID: PMC7352873.

[22] Shao R. Understanding the mechanisms of human tubal ectopic pregnancies: new evidence from knockout mouse models. Hum Reprod. 2010 Mar;25(3):584-7. doi: 10.1093/humrep/dep438. Epub 2009 Dec 19. PMID: 20023297; PMCID: PMC2817566.

[23] Grattan DR. 60 YEARS OF NEUROENDOCRINOLOGY: The hypothalamo-prolactin axis. J Endocrinol. 2015 Aug;226(2):T101-22. doi: 10.1530/JOE-15-0213. Epub 2015 Jun 22. PMID: 26101377; PMCID: PMC4515538.

[24] Honjo H, Kitawaki J, Itoh M, Yasuda J, Yamamoto T, Yamamoto T, Okada H, Ohkubo T, Nambara T. Serum and urinary oestrone sulphate in pregnancy and delivery measured by a direct radioimmunoassay. Acta Endocrinol (Copenh). 1986 Jul;112(3):423-30. doi: 10.1530/acta.0.1120423. PMID: 3751457.

[25] Holinka CF, Diczfalusy E, Coelingh Bennink HJ. Estetrol: a unique steroid in human pregnancy. J Steroid Biochem Mol Biol. 2008 May;110(1-2):138-43. doi: 10.1016/j.jsbmb.2008.03.027. Epub 2008 Mar 29. PMID: 18462934.

[26] Yin P, Arita J. Differential regulation of prolactin release and lactotrope proliferation during

pregnancy, lactation and the estrous cycle. Neuroendocrinology. 2000 Aug;72(2):72-9. doi: 10.1159/000054574. PMID: 10971142.

[27] Soares MJ. The prolactin and growth hormone families: pregnancy-specific hormones/cytokines at the maternal-fetal interface. Reprod Biol Endocrinol. 2004 Jul 5;2:51. doi: 10.1186/1477-7827-2-51. PMID: 15236651; PMCID: PMC471570.

[28] Matalka KZ, Ali DA. Stress-induced versus preovulatory and pregnancy hormonal levels in modulating cytokine production following whole blood stimulation. Neuroimmunomodulation. 2005;12(6):366-74. doi: 10.1159/000091130. PMID: 16557037.

[29] Bachelot A, Binart N. Reproductive role of prolactin. Reproduction. 2007 Feb;133(2):361-9. doi: 10.1530/REP-06-0299. PMID: 17307904.

[30] Tessier C, Prigent-Tessier A, Ferguson-Gottschall S, Gu Y, Gibori G. PRL antiapoptotic effect in the rat decidua involves the PI3K/protein kinase B-mediated inhibition of caspase-3 activity. Endocrinology. 2001 Sep;142(9):4086-94. doi: 10.1210/endo.142.9.8381. PMID: 11517188.

[31] Nagaishi VS, Cardinali LI, Zampieri TT, Furigo IC, Metzger M, Donato J Jr. Possible crosstalk between leptin and prolactin during pregnancy. Neuroscience. 2014 Feb 14;259:71-83. doi: 10.1016/j.neuroscience.2013.11.050. Epub 2013 Dec 4. PMID: 24316468.

[32] Butte NF, Hopkinson JM, Nicolson MA. Leptin in human reproduction: serum leptin levels in pregnant and lactating women. J Clin Endocrinol Metab. 1997 Feb;82(2):585-9. doi: 10.1210/jcem.82.2.3731. PMID: 9024259.

[33] Ngala RA, Fondjo LA, Gmagna P, Ghartey FN, Awe MA. Placental peptides metabolism and maternal factors as predictors of risk of gestational diabetes in pregnant women. A case-control study. PLoS One. 2017 Jul 21;12(7):e0181613. doi: 10.1371/journal.pone.0181613. PMID: 28732072; PMCID: PMC5521813.

[34] Simpson S, Smith L, Bowe J. Placental peptides regulating islet adaptation to pregnancy: clinical potential in gestational diabetes mellitus. Curr Opin Pharmacol. 2018 Dec;43:59-65. doi: 10.1016/j.coph.2018.08.004. Epub 2018 Sep 7. PMID: 30199758.

[35] Licht P, Russu V, Wildt L. On the role of human chorionic gonadotropin (hCG) in the embryo-endometrial microenvironment: implications for differentiation and implantation. Semin Reprod Med. 2001;19(1):37-47. doi: 10.1055/s-2001-13909. PMID: 11394202.

[36] Field T, Diego M. Cortisol: the culprit prenatal stress variable. Int J Neurosci. 2008 Aug;118(8):1181. doi: 10.1080/00207450701820944. PMID: 18589921.

[37] Shams M, Kilby MD, Somerset DA, Howie AJ, Gupta A, Wood PJ, Afnan M, Stewart PM. 11Beta-hydroxysteroid dehydrogenase type 2 in human pregnancy and reduced expression in intrauterine growth restriction. Hum Reprod. 1998 Apr;13(4):799-804. doi: 10.1093/humrep/13.4.799. PMID: 9619527.

[38] Diego MA, Jones NA, Field T, Hernandez-Reif M, Schanberg S, Kuhn C, Gonzalez-Garcia A. Maternal psychological distress, prenatal cortisol, and fetal weight. Psychosom Med. 2006 Sep-Oct;68(5):747-53. doi: 10.1097/01.psy.0000238212.21598.7b. PMID: 17012528.

[39] Chan J, Rabbitt EH, Innes BA, Bulmer JN, Stewart PM, Kilby MD, Hewison M. Glucocorticoid-induced

apoptosis in human decidua: a novel role for 11beta-hydroxysteroid dehydrogenase in late gestation. J Endocrinol. 2007 Oct;195(1):7-15. doi: 10.1677/JOE-07-0289. PMID: 17911392.

[40] Myatt L. Placental adaptive responses and fetal programming. J Physiol. 2006 Apr 1;572(Pt 1):25-30. doi: 10.1113/jphysiol.2006.104968. Epub 2006 Feb 9. PMID: 16469781; PMCID: PMC1779654.

[41] Myatt L, Sun K. Role of fetal membranes in signaling of fetal maturation and parturition. Int J Dev Biol. 2010;54(2-3):545-53. doi: 10.1387/ijdb.082771lm. PMID: 19924634.

[42] Rosen T, Krikun G, Ma Y, Wang EY, Lockwood CJ, Guller S. Chronic antagonism of nuclear factor-kappaB activity in cytotrophoblasts by dexamethasone: a potential mechanism for antiinflammatory action of glucocorticoids in human placenta. J Clin Endocrinol Metab. 1998 Oct;83(10):3647-52. doi: 10.1210/jcem.83.10.5151. PMID: 9768679.

[43] Street ME, Smerieri A, Petraroli A, Cesari S, Viani I, Garrubba M, Rossi M, Bernasconi S. Placental cortisol and cord serum IGFBP-2 concentrations are important determinants of postnatal weight gain. J Biol Regul Homeost Agents. 2012 Oct-Dec;26(4):721-31. PMID: 23241122.

[44] Tian CF, Kang MH. Common stress and serum cortisol and IL-12 levels in missed abortion. J Obstet Gynaecol. 2014 Jan;34(1):33-5. doi: 10.3109/01443615.2013.830089. PMID: 24359046.

[45] Marsman R, Rosmalen JG, Oldehinkel AJ, Ormel J, Buitelaar JK. Does HPA-axis activity mediate the relationship between obstetric complications and externalizing behavior problems? The TRAILS study. Eur Child Adolesc Psychiatry. 2009 Sep;18(9):565-73. doi: 10.1007/s00787-009-0014-y. Epub 2009 Apr 8. PMID: 19353232; PMCID: PMC2721131.

[46] Springer D, Jiskra J, Limanova Z, Zima T, Potlukova E. Thyroid in pregnancy: From physiology to screening. Crit Rev Clin Lab Sci. 2017 Mar;54(2):102-116. doi: 10.1080/10408363.2016.1269309. Epub 2017 Jan 19. PMID: 28102101.

[47] Thorpe-Beeston JG, Nicolaides KH. Fetal thyroid function. Fetal Diagn Ther. 1993 Jan-Feb;8(1):60-72. doi: 10.1159/000263749. PMID: 8452651.

[48] Temboury Molina MC, Rivero Martín MJ, de Juan Ruiz J, Ares Segura S. Enfermedad tiroidea autoinmunitaria materna: repercusión en el recién nacido [Maternal autoimmune thyroid disease: relevance for the newborn]. Med Clin (Barc). 2015 Apr 8;144(7):297-303. Spanish. doi: 10.1016/j.medcli.2013.10.024. Epub 2014 Jan 30. PMID: 24486115.